More Praise for *To Know and Honor:* *Building a Culture of Person-Centered Decision-Making*

"Linda Briggs is a pioneer in the work to shift the culture of care so that person-centered decision-making is threaded through all aspects of care. This book is an invaluable resource to professionals who share this vision. It provides an excellent review of the elements essential to successfully implement comprehensive advance care planning in their health care organization. Her accumulated wisdom will benefit the next generation of leaders to continue to make the culture of person-centered decision-making a reality accessible to all."

> **—Susan Hickman, PhD**, Professor,
> Indiana University School of Nursing

"Anyone who is interested in honoring patients' wishes must read this book. Linda is a luminary in the field of advance care planning, and we are so fortunate that she has distilled her 20 plus years of experience into key, pragmatic solutions to create a patient-centered, decision-making healthcare culture. I agree with Linda that 'There is no other imperative in healthcare that is more important' and that we must 'make and keep promises to our patients.' Through engaging and illustrative stories and helpful thought exercises, Linda has created a step-by-step roadmap for systems change that includes content on "disruptive" leadership, systems redesign and needed clinical infrastructure, community engagement, sustainability, and quality improvement. This book is a gift that will challenge you to think outside of the box and will provide the much-needed clarity and concrete steps to honor our patients' wishes."

> **—Rebecca Sudore, MD**, Professor of Medicine,
> University of California, San Francisco, Creator of
> PREPAREforYourCare.org

"Respecting Choices has always aimed to transform health care into a person-centered care system…especially when facing crucial health care decisions. Linda Briggs's book is an outstanding guide to creating such a person-centered care system. Arguably, Linda was ideally positioned to write this in-depth, nuanced guide. Linda's writing is based on the rich and mature theory of Respecting Choices as well as a vast, practical experience of implementing Respecting Choices programs in numerous settings and institutions, big and small, domestic and international. In addition, it is grounded in the insights and wisdom of numerous research findings, many of which Linda was closely involved in. If you want to improve care by creating a person-centered culture, Linda's book is probably the only book that can successfully help you achieve that end."

—**Bernard "Bud" Hammes, PhD,** Executive Director
Emeritus of Respecting Choices, A Division of
C-TAC Innovations

"Linda Briggs' years of experience pour out onto the page in a way that makes you feel like you are joining her on her life journey and mission to transform the way healthcare organizations engage people in advance care planning. Each chapter is filled with Linda's valuable clinical and research knowledge on the topic, and it is shared in a way that highlights her love for teaching others to systematically implement and evaluate this important work. Our team feels blessed to have worked with Linda, and we blossomed under her training and commitment to helping us be change agents and leaders."

—**Kaiser Permanente Colorado Life Care Planning/
HealthPlan Team**

TO KNOW AND HONOR:

BUILDING A CULTURE OF PERSON-CENTERED DECISION-MAKING

LINDA BRIGGS, MSN, MA, RN,

IS THE CO-FOUNDER OF RESPECTING CHOICES®,
AN INTERNATIONALLY RECOGNIZED ADVANCE CARE PLANNING PROGRAM

ISBN: 978-1-66780-172-8 (print)
ISBN: 978-1-66780-173-5 (eBook)

About the author

With 25 years of nursing experience as a critical care staff nurse, nurse manager, clinical nurse specialist, and educator, Linda Briggs joined Respecting Choices in 1999 to provide leadership in the development and dissemination of the internationally recognized program.

Briggs has consulted with healthcare leaders, organizations, and communities around the world, providing education and support in implementing the principles of effective and sustainable person-centered decision-making programs. Her clinical and research interests have focused on the disease-specific planning needs of patients with advanced illness and their families.

Briggs has led the development of the Respecting Choices curriculum, co-authored several Respecting Choices manuals and programs, and published numerous articles on advance care planning and end-of-life care. In 2015, Briggs received recognition from the Tribeca Disruptive Innovation Awards for the impact of the Respecting Choices program. In 2019 Briggs transitioned to a consultant role. She resides in Madison, WI.

With Heartfelt Thanks...

...to the individuals, patients, families, worldwide implementation leaders and researchers, Respecting Choices faculty and staff, colleagues, family, and friends who have inspired me personally and professionally. I hope that the lessons I have learned from you — recorded in these pages — will motivate others to continue their journey to improve person-centered care.

...to my editor, Annie Beth Donahue.

...to my book advisory group members who were invaluable in giving feedback and improving the book's mission "to know and honor" individual's goals, values, preferences, and healthcare decisions:

Sanders Burstein, MD
Kathryn Detwiler, parent
Nancy Greenstreet, LCSW
Bernard "Bud" Hammes, PhD
Susan E. Hickman, PhD
Maureen E. Lyon, PhD
Carole Montgomery, MD, FHM, MHSA
Joyce Smerick, BS
Christine Swift RN, MSN, CHPN

Contents

Part One

3

Part Two

39

Part Three

115

Part Four
163

Part Five
227

Part Six

293

Part Seven

371

Foreword

Over the past three decades, a plethora of programs, guidelines, tools, and techniques have emerged to improve person-centered care: "Care that is respectful of and responsive to individual patient preferences, needs, and values, ensuring that patient values guide all clinical decisions,"[1] yet implementation remains largely an aspiration. Individual's goals and values are often unknown, which leads to uncertainty, over and under treatment, avoidable suffering, increased costs of care, and moral distress for healthcare providers.

Fulfilling the promise of person-centered care mandates the creation of a culture that seamlessly integrates person-centered decision-making programs to assist individuals in making *current* and *future* healthcare decisions *and* designs systems capable of knowing *and* honoring an individuals' goals and values. Creating a culture of person-centered decision-making is no easy task.

The co-creator of the nationally recognized Respecting Choices® program shares implementation experiences from twenty years creating a national curriculum and consulting with over thirty organizations around the U.S. and in five countries to disseminate the principles of two person-centered decision-making programs, Advance Care Planning (ACP) and Shared Decision-Making in Serious Illness (SDMSI). The perspectives and lessons learned are not intended as a panacea to resolve the daunting challenge in creating cultural transformation, but to promote conversation and consensus on the work yet to be done.

The Respecting Choices "Promises" framework is used to explore five elements in designing a culture of person-centered decision-making: leadership, systems redesign, education and competency, community engagement, and continuous quality improvement.

Book Part Outline:

Part One: Who Am I and Why Do I Have Something to Say?

Part Two: The Promise of Leadership in Building a Culture of Person-Centered Decision-Making

Part Three: The Promise of System Redesign in Supporting a Culture of Person-Centered Decision-Making

Part Four: The Promise of Education and Certification in Building a Culture of Person-Centered Decision-Making

Part Five: The Promise of Community Engagement and Education in Promoting a Culture of Person-Centered Decision-Making

Part Six: The Promise of Quality Improvement, Research and Evidence-Based Practice in Building a Culture of Person-Centered Decision-Making

Part Seven: The Promise of Pediatric Advance Care Planning

Part One

Introduction:
Who Am I and Why Do I Have Something to Say?

But the Surgery Went Well

James was a patient in his mid-twenties who experienced intraoperative complications during high-risk cardiac surgery. He suffered significant intracranial bleeding that resulted in permanent brain damage. "But the surgery was successful," the surgeon told the family. "His heart is working well."

After many days, however, his heart was the least of his problems. James never awoke and could not be weaned from the ventilator. While caring for him one evening, his family approached me with a request to remove the ventilator keeping his lifeless body functioning. The family had labored over his situation and had come to the consensus that James would not choose to continue to fight to stay alive, given the consequences of his damaged brain. He had enjoyed an active life and was intelligent with a promising career. As they observed James display physical signs of distress, such as grimacing and bucking the ventilator, they wondered if he was suffering.

I called the surgeon with these observations and the family's request to withdraw the ventilator. After shouting at me and telling me he could not "kill his patient" [if he approved the ventilator withdrawal], he ordered more sedation so that "the nurses and family" could not observe the patient's symptoms. As he slammed down the phone, he instructed me not to call him back. The nursing supervisor offered no alternative but to follow the surgeon's orders.

Distraught, I gathered my composure and informed the family of my conversation with the surgeon and the mandate to continue the ventilator. Upon hearing this decision, two family members got down on their knees (literally) and begged me to remove the ventilator. "We won't tell anyone. It will be our secret."

That evening lasted a lifetime. I was a nurse who believed she was inflicting more harm than good for this patient and his family. I felt helpless. Over the ensuing four weeks, I witnessed the ripple effects of suffering. Nurses requested not to take care of James. Some family members never returned to the hospital. The surgeon did not talk to me for days. Eventually, James developed an overwhelming infection. And after an attempt at cardiopulmonary resuscitation (CPR), he died in the intensive care unit (ICU) with few family members at his side.

James is a personal story of regret. Many clinicians have similar stories. Why do such stories linger within us and, if we choose, propel us to action?

An Investment in Person-Centered Decision-Making

The first twenty-five years of my career were devoted to cultivating my expertise as a clinical nurse specialist (CNS) in the critical care arena. These edifying years unearthed the wonders of medical science. I became a technology geek and marveled at how we could use scientific advances to help patients recover successfully from illness or injury.

Over time, however, I became confused and overwhelmed by a plethora of questions about the limits of this technology and the potential loss or mitigation of the patient's voice in the decision-making process. There were few morally satisfying answers — until I discovered Respecting Choices in 1999.

I was recruited to provide leadership in building a national platform for the dissemination of this evidence-based program that originally gained notoriety for its advance care planning (ACP) strategies and outcomes. As the mission of Respecting Choices evolved, it became more accurately described as a "person-centered decision-making" system that encompasses ACP and Shared Decision-making in Serious Illness (SDMSI) programs — programs that have the power to transform the healthcare culture.[1]

But what is "person-centered decision-making," and why did I dedicate 20 years of my professional career to this mission? Person-centered decision-making is the core attribute of person-centered care, "Care that is respectful of and responsive to individual patient preferences, needs, and values, ensuring that patient values guide all clinical decisions."[2]

Who would debate the worth of preserving the "person" in person-centered decision-making as a moral imperative? But I learned that delivering personalized care is easier said than done. This book describes strategies to operationalize the commitment "to know and honor" individuals' goals, values, preferences, and decisions — a commitment that will require cultural change at the individual, professional, organizational, and community levels.

For the first seven years in the development of a national platform for the dissemination of Respecting Choices (RC), I was part of a two-person team forging new territory. We were accountable for: identifying the core content for program dissemination, creating, delivering, and revising curriculum, consulting with national and international implementation teams, conducting quality improvement projects, planning for and presenting at educational conferences, participating as co-investigators on relevant research studies, designing marketing strategies, maintaining financial viability, and publishing. The program evolved and improved with the expansion of its staff, leadership, products, and talent.

But this book is not intended to be about me or one program. This book is intended to share lessons learned from over twenty years of consulting with over thirty organizations around the U.S. and five other countries. It is intended to disseminate the principles of person-centered decision-making.

In part, this book will reflect a rich history of implementation anecdotes and experiences. But it will also be useful for healthcare leaders currently struggling to operationalize the delivery of person-centered care.

How This Book is Organized- To Know and Honor:
Building a Culture of Person-Centered Decision-Making (PCDM)

Implementation of comprehensive and sustainable person-centered decision-making programs is complex. To digest and understand this complexity, RC crafted a "promises" framework to communicate the principles in building a culture of person-centered decision-making — promises devoted to the design of five essential elements for successful outcomes: leadership, systems redesign, education and competency, community engagement, and continuous quality improvement.

The chapters that follow will illustrate each of these promises, integrating national recommendations and personal experiences. Along with this Introduction, Part One includes three chapters that delve into my personal journey and interest in person-centered decision-making, providing context for the stories and experiences throughout this book.

Part Two illustrates the indispensable role of leadership in building a person-centered decision-making culture by exploring three questions: 1) Why should leaders invest in cultural transformation? 2) What are the initial leadership strategies in implementing a PCDM program, and 3) What actions can leaders take to promote program dissemination and sustainability? Included in Part Two is a brief history of the RC program.

Part Three highlights the inextricable link between systems design (and redesign) and the ability to successfully disseminate and sustain person-centered decision-making programs. Four specific microsystems are explored that form the foundation for successful outcomes: leadership, planning documents, medical record storage and retrieval, and the interdisciplinary team approach to person-centered decision-making.

Part Four explores the barriers to and imperative for developing national certification standards for competency in person-centered decision-making communication. The design and evolution of the RC communication programs are described: programs that are grounded in a competency-based approach to education, adaptable delivery modalities (such as blended learning and virtual platforms), instructor certification, and organizational commitment to interdisciplinary team dissemination. Real-life conversations are depicted that exemplify the power of person-centered decision-making communication skills and the harmful impact when these skills are absent.

Part Five explores the promise in building community engagement and education campaigns to promote person-centered decision-making behaviors. Community partnerships are identified that recognize the intrapersonal, interpersonal, organizational, community, and public policy influences that shape behavior change. Examples of community engagement activities are depicted that represent diverse cultures, ethnic and religious communities across the U.S and in other countries, including Australia, Canada, Germany, Singapore, and Spain.

Part Six illuminates the RC commitment to quality improvement, research, and evidence-based practice, including the Five Promises framework and relevant quality improvement and research studies. Program adaptations from the U.S and other countries are presented — adaptations consistent with the RC "freedom within a framework" philosophy. In addition, Part Five hosts a discussion of the measurement conundrums within ACP research, the evolving creation of an ACP Outcomes framework and future research agenda, and summarizes the author's reflections on the lessons learned through multiple research partnerships. In addition, Part Seven provides background, clinical experiences, parent perspectives, and research partnerships to promote the dissemination of pediatric ACP.

Each Part begins with a real-life story that illustrates key messages and content described throughout the Part, ending with a summary for future direction and a personal reflection exercise. Although Parts can be read in any order, no one promise can stand alone. Each promise works synergistically to provide an environment where person-centered decision-making becomes the cultural norm.

To Know and Honor: Thoughts on How to Read This Book

"What do you hope for with your current medical plan of care?" This formidable question is among the most noteworthy in a person-centered decision-making conversation guide for individuals with serious illness that I helped create in 2002, near the beginning of the journey described in this book.

The answers to this question have moved me. More importantly, the question has inspired patients to think critically about what is most important in their lives, opening doors to enhanced communication and understanding among patients' families and their healthcare team. But make no mistake, this is more than a simple question intended to be casually asked and answered. It is an exploration.

Chris Feudtner, physician and author, offers the following hypothesis about the power of hope exploration:

> The explicit and skillful management of hope in the process of medical decision making can facilitate a transformation in how individuals think and feel about their situation, which consequently has a direct impact on the decisions that they make and their subsequent experiences, including the experience of healing at the end of life.[3]

Hope exploration is tough. Asking individuals to talk about their hopes in the face of serious illness may appear, at first glance, to risk "taking away hope." However, an adept interviewer, allowing time for responses to percolate and accepting the accompanying emotion, will experience the therapeutic power of hope exploration. Patients self-discover that their hopes vary from the miraculous to the mundane. Clinicians discover previously unidentified hopes that they can help individuals attain.

Hope among patients with serious illness is multi-dimensional. A thoughtful and thorough examination of hope exposes its multiple layers. The first layer is often one that clinicians tend to label as "unrealistic," for example, "I hope they find a cure for my cancer," or "I hope for a miracle." While most patients possess the self-awareness that miracle hopes may not be achieved, expressing them in the presence of a non-judgmental listener serves to communicate the losses they are grappling with.

Hollie Coleman, a patient with gallbladder cancer and newly diagnosed lung cancer, expressed this first layer of hope in a conversation I facilitated with him and his daughter Pam, his designated healthcare agent:

I hope that the doctors are wrong, that they tell me,
Hollie, you do not have cancer.

But this was not Hollie's only hope. When prompted with, "Anything else you hope for?" a series of qualitatively different responses emerged:

I hope for healing.

I hope I can get back to doing the things I used to do.

I want to walk and go do things.

Hollie had bought a red sports car after his initial cancer diagnosis. He was often seen cruising the La Crosse landscape to fulfill his hope of "getting out and doing things."

The final enduring question in the hope exploration is harder to ask and harder to answer: "If these hopes don't come true [to have the cancer be gone, to control your pain], then what would you hope for?" This question probes

11

the essence of this crucial exploration for patients with serious illnesses. It acknowledges an individual's hopes for the best possible outcomes yet identifies the outcomes that, for each individual, are worse than death.

Hollie took a deep breath, sat back in his chair, and resolutely responded. "I hope I just die. I don't want to die, but you have to have this kind of pain to understand."

With this response, fresh insights into what mattered most to Hollie were exposed, including the role his daughter Pam would play in honoring his decisions and his life. They discussed the meaning of "die with dignity" and celebrated their daughter/father relationship. Pam's tears reflected her immense respect for her dad, who had served in two world wars, and a bit of anticipatory grief for the day he would no longer be with her.

This mode of hope exploration has guided patients with serious illness, their loved ones, and me through tough conversations. Individuals are allowed the hospitality to dream about possibilities, to lament their losses, to express affection for those they love, and to outline the boundaries of what they are willing to endure and what they are not willing to endure. It is a gift that patients give and one that families receive. It is a privilege to witness hope's therapeutic power.

I invite you to explore the hopes you have as you read this book. Why are you reading this book? Where are you in your personal journey in caring for individuals with serious illness? What experiences have shaped your perspectives? What promises have you made to provide person-centered care? What promises have been broken? As you think about this question, I will confess *my* hopes as you read this book.

I hope you recognize the themes that transcend the personal stories and experiences — themes that resonate with the work that you are currently doing to provide person-centered care. I hope you take the time to reflect on your experiences and acknowledge what you have already learned and what you still yearn to discover. If you have struggled with moral distress in the care of individuals with serious illness, I hope you can resolve the angst that you may carry with you and begin to heal the wounds that have festered for years — wounds that may have tainted your vision of what is possible. May you learn from my mistakes and mis-steps and envision the return on investment that a commitment to person-centered decision-making promises can give. May you realize the immense responsibility you have in creating an ethical environment for your patients, families, and the healthcare team.

I hope you see the power of mentorship and collaboration — learning from each other, easing each other's struggles, encouraging others to succeed. Perhaps these reflections will make you smile, laugh, or cry. I hope that you identify with the courage required to honor the goals and values of the people you are privileged to serve and realize how this courage can free you to become the healer you set out to be.

However, if these hopes do not come true, then I unassumingly hope that my family and friends will know me a bit more. I hope they will know how I have treasured the career path that I followed, that my professional work has made me a better person, mother, wife, and friend, sustaining me through personal challenges. I hope my family will understand why I missed some of their life events, why I was distracted at the dinner table, or why I lost my temper for no apparent reason. Lastly, I hope my grandchildren find a future pathway full of passion and reward.

Chapter 1: Preparation for an Undefined Future

Why Nursing?

When my granddaughter was four years old, she announced, "Gamma, when I grow up, I want to be a nurse (or maybe a doctor), a schoolteacher, a piano and gymnastics teacher, and a firefighter." I smiled, proud of her diverse aspirations, and responded with the feminist platitude, "Camryn, you can be anything you want to be."

This was not the message that I received as a high school senior contemplating my future after graduation from a Catholic high school in a small Iowa town. I loved the sciences, especially biology, and was encouraged by the school counselor to be a nurse, or the only other alternative, a teacher. Although my career path exploration was not remotely close to Camryn's world of possibilities, nursing seemed a good fit. Nursing offered a path to fulfill my altruistic nature, but I will avow that in 1970, my motivations were more egocentric. I wanted to move as far away as possible from the small Iowa town in which I grew up.

Needing tuition assistance, I enrolled in the only college that gave me a scholarship. I was the first sibling in the family who aspired to a four-year education, despite my father's directive that I become a licensed practical nurse (LPN), because "a nurse is a nurse." His insistence on my becoming an LPN was one more incentive for me to do the opposite, despite the ten years I would spend repaying four years of student loans. Subliminal at the time, or just the luck of the draw, the decision to pursue a Bachelor of Science degree in nursing was the perfect pathway. I had no idea *how* perfect.

14

I entered nursing education in the 1970s, a time when nurses still wore uniforms. During clinical rotations in the hospital, the female nurses wore white hats (with cool blue stripes), navy blue uniforms with huge white aprons (not so cool), white nylons, and spotless white shoes. Four years later, while leaving behind these nursing symbols at the graduation ceremony, I never left behind the pride and promise of being a nurse. This pride was energized by several remarkable mentors I encountered in my professional life that you will meet throughout this book.

The first was a unique female nun in the Catholic college I attended. Contrary to the stilted education I thought I would receive in this religious institution, I was "blessed" to encounter the smartest woman I had ever met. She guided my classmates and me to comprehend that being a caring nurse (although a quintessential quality) was insufficient to fulfill the ethos of nursing — the protection, promotion and optimization of health, prevention of illness, and alleviation of suffering through the diagnosis and treatment of human responses and advocacy in the care of individuals, families, communities, and populations (ANA definition).

She insisted that we understand what we were doing and embrace the science behind our nursing actions. She taught human anatomy, biology, and my personal favorite, physiology. She fueled my desire to grasp how the body worked: how an antibiotic could fight an infection, the gate control theory of pain, the precise muscle in the buttocks in which I would give my first intramuscular injection, the function of the mitochondria as the power-house of the cells, and how heart failure complications could lead to kidney disease. I was intrigued with how this knowledge could abet my promise to be a patient advocate, allow me to be an effective liaison between the patient, family, and healthcare team, and help me prevent complications and avoid suffering.

I begged to be one of the student nurses assigned to one of the limited intensive care unit clinical rotations that were available. The four days that I spent in the ICU sealed my career pathway for the next 25 years. Upon graduation, I was fortunate to be offered a position in a medical-surgical critical care unit. The environment was energizing. Exposure to state-of-the-art technology and science. Fast-paced. Intelligence required. New graduates were scheduled on the night shift, and while initially, I thought this was a penalty, it was an unforeseen advantage to be paired with a seasoned nurse.

Night after night, she challenged me to be a critical thinker, to anticipate problems, and to react quickly and competently to impending disaster. While sitting in front of the cardiac monitors one evening, I spotted ventricular tachycardia from one of my patients. Proud that I had recognized this lethal arrhythmia, I sat motionless. Recognizing the fear on my face, my mentor calmly said, "You know what to do. I will be right behind you."

I will never forget the impact of that first defibrillation and my patient's heart returning to sinus rhythm. He opened his fear-filled eyes, asking, "What happened to me?" He was totally unaware that my hands were still shaking, that I was amazed the defibrillation worked, and that I was more frightened than he was.

I was hooked. I immediately wanted to learn more and enrolled in a graduate-level histology course, a preclinical requirement for medical students. The plan was to begin post-graduate education while gaining clinical experience in critical care. It was a two-hour early morning course following the night shift, and the activity of looking under a microscope and identifying cells, tissues, and organs kept me wide awake.

I was intrigued with how the structure of epithelial cells, cilia, neutrophils, and plasma cells influenced their biologic function and clinical presentation. I now understood how the cilia (those tiny hairs that line the inside of bronchial tubes) of patients with chronic bronchitis had been destroyed and were unable to function normally to move mucous upward and out of the bronchi. It now made sense to me why we needed to treat the infection that caused the cilia inflammation, why we needed to ensure adequate hydration to liquefy the mucus, and why we had to assist with the removal of the copious amounts of mucous that were interfering with oxygen transport.

This interest sounds nerdy to me now, but my clinical experience enhanced my ability to immediately integrate this information in practical ways. I was surrounded by first-year medical students who, with little clinical experience, often probed me on my latest ICU adventures. During this semester-long course, I encountered a recurring question I would hear over the years, "Linda, you are so smart, why don't you become a doctor?" I have known many nurse colleagues who have, like me, bristled at the mere implication that nurses do not need to be smart. But this unwitting question is likely what sparked my cravings to advance my knowledge and contribute to the credibility of the nursing profession. And I was fortunate to receive a federal grant to pursue a master's degree in nursing.

The Power of Research

Over the next two years in graduate school, I constructed a variety of experiences that would assimilate my thirst for critical care expertise with organizational culture, research, and leadership. As is the case for many women, I confronted the challenge of integrating professional aspirations with the joys of motherhood. I always knew I wanted to be a mother but did not envisage becoming pregnant during my first year in graduate school. Joshua was not due to be born until the end of my first year, allowing me to orchestrate my class schedule so that I would complete the required exams and clinicals before he was born.

However, my son had different plans, deciding to make his entrance into the world one month premature — and one week prior to a midterm exam. Hoping that labor would be stalled, I brought study materials with me to the hospital. (They remained unopened in a pile on the bedside stand.) Despite my notice to the nursing instructor of my situation, she was not sympathetic and informed me that I would need to accept an incomplete if I could not be present for the exam. My stubborn attitude forced me to forge ahead, showing up at the exam just four days after Joshua was born and begrudgingly accepting the first "B" of my graduate education. This would not be the last time that my children would teach me the value of setting priorities.

During this graduate education, I was exposed to research, and the requirement to choose a topic for my master's level thesis. There was a plethora of critical care topics I could have chosen, but I was intrigued with the nebulous issues surrounding informed consent. While my nursing career began in an age of paternalism, a person's right to self-determination through the process of informed consent was being scrutinized in the courts.

The case of Canterbury v. Spence was one landmark case that changed the informed consent standards.[1] Canterbury suffered permanent paralysis after a laminectomy performed by Dr. William Spence. Canterbury sued for malpractice based on negligence, claiming he had never been informed of the risk of paralysis. During his trial, the defense team could not provide an expert witness, likely the result of a "conspiracy of silence" that thwarted physicians from testifying against other physicians. Moreover, Dr. Spence admitted that he had only informed Canterbury of the risk of weakness (not paralysis) for fear he would not consent to the surgery. Although the jury ruled against Canterbury, the ramifications of this case left their mark on the clinical and legal landscape.

The disclosure standard for informed consent formally shifted from a "professional practice" standard (revealing information that a reasonable physician would provide) to disclosing information that a reasonable person would need to decide about the risks of an impending procedure or surgery. The case also undermined the common practice of physicians not testifying against each other and essentially opened the door to malpractice litigation. The clinical impact of this case left many unanswered questions about the informed consent process. What specific information would a reasonable person find critical in making a decision? What type of consent form should be crafted to convey this disclosure? Who should provide this information and witness a person's signature? Most importantly, how would a person's understanding of the information be adequately assessed?

I had felt the tension of inconsistencies in the informed consent process in the clinical arena. I had witnessed patient signatures, reviewed insipid consent forms, and listened to information being provided to patients about their impending surgery or procedure. The process left me with the uncomfortable realization that some patients lacked a full understanding of what would be happening to their bodies.

One evening, while caring for an ICU patient scheduled for a mitral valve replacement surgery the next morning, I fielded a series of questions. How long would the surgery take? How long would he be in the ICU? And "How many bypasses will they put in me?"

I corrected his misunderstanding of the type of surgery he would be having; it was a valve replacement and not bypass surgery. I reviewed the medical chart for more explanation of the informed consent discussion but found scant details of what was discussed, such as "the risks and alternatives of the surgery were discussed." The patient did not remember having any conversation with the surgeon. He recalled that his wife had told him he would be having bypass surgery. I felt uneasy and suggested that I call the surgeon who could come again and talk to him. The patient refused, saying, "He knows what he is doing, and you don't need to disturb him." The tension with the informed consent process lingered.

As I deliberated my interest in exploring an informed consent topic with my research committee, I was given a unique opportunity to be mentored by Dr. Norman Fost, an ethicist I had long admired. Dr. Fost directed the Department of Pediatrics residency program at the University of Wisconsin in Madison for 20 years, founded the organizations' bioethics program, and chaired the Institutional Review Board and clinical ethics committee for 30 years. He was a member of many national committees and a frequent media guest in ethics, and an accomplished author.

I attended many of his lively and provocative presentations. He agreed to be a member of my research committee and suggested I merge my interest in informed consent with a current controversy surrounding the medical necessity of male circumcision immediately after birth.

Male circumcision? This was not my clinical area of expertise. But a local healthcare organization was enthusiastic and supportive of this investigation — at least initially. I learned about research design, collection of data, informed consent, and the controversy over the medical necessity of newborn circumcision. After months of development and meetings with the clinical team, the study was ready to be implemented. This investigation included interviewing parents of male newborns to assess their understanding of the circumcision procedure *after* they had signed the requisite consent form.

A few days before the study was to begin, I was informed that I could not proceed. I was never given an official rationale. However, I learned that in the process of designing the study, procedural concerns with obtaining informed consent from parents for circumcision were uncovered. These concerns had legal and public exposure consequences.

Although I lost the experience of conducting a study, my thesis committee believed that I had accomplished the necessary intent of the research activity. Moreover, the simple act of designing the study changed practice by exposing the inadequacies of the existing informed consent process. This was likely my first exposure to quality improvement and evidence-based practice. In lieu of conducting the study — and to fulfill my research credits for graduation — I was directed to publish an article to demonstrate my learning about circumcision and informed consent.[2] Although it would be years before I would publish again, the experience piqued my interest in research and the ethics of informed consent.

The Changing Culture of Decision-Making:
From Paternalism to Self-Determination

My true passion during graduate school was to improve my critical care experience and expertise. I elected as many clinical field studies as possible, including my first exposure to a neurosurgical ICU where I cared for patients with traumatic brain and spinal cord injury and witnessed the aftermath of living with mental and physical disability.

Inspired by two all-star clinical nurse specialists, I was destined to follow in their footsteps. I admired how these amazing women combined their clinical expertise with leadership strategies to champion and enhance patient care. I landed a position as a CNS in a medical-surgical ICU from 1978-1989 in an organizational culture infused with exceptional healthcare professionals, administrators, and mentors who nurtured me and helped me hone my leadership skills.

The CNS, an emerging healthcare role, was an advanced practice nurse with expertise in a selected area of patient care, such as cardiology or gerontology. The CNS is responsible for direct patient care, consultation, education, research, and administrative management. This role energized my feminist inclinations to lead, become an equal member of the healthcare team, and influence the nursing profession's stature and credibility.

I was particularly focused on my responsibility of managing the nursing staff's clinical expertise by providing education, preceptorship, and mentoring to an amazing group of nurses who cared deeply about what they were doing. The critical care course I designed was jam-packed with information, problem-solving scenarios, and technical skill development. The goal of this education was to elevate the competency of the nursing staff to critically use data and science to provide exceptional patient care. I role modeled these expectations by becoming certified as a critical care registered nurse (CCRN) and Advanced Cardiac Life Support (ACLS) Instructor.

The culture and role of the critical care nurse was evolving. The younger nurses were energized and eager to learn. Still, the older nurses who had years of clinical experience were a bit intimidated because they had grown up in a different environment. They were accustomed to following doctor's orders and received on-the-job critical care education.

For some, the cultural shift was palpable. One nurse, well respected for her technical ability and caring attitude toward patients, relayed the story of how she learned to interpret dysrhythmias when cardiac monitoring was initially implemented in the ICU as a standard of care. A doctor scribbled an image of what we now know as ventricular tachycardia on a piece of paper saying, "If you see this image on the cardiac monitor, call me immediately." This was a far cry from the new expectations to recognize, interpret, and communicate potentially lethal arrhythmias.

Nurses were taught to interpret a 12 lead electrocardiogram (ECG) — not to merely know how to hook up the leads to the machine. They learned to recognize bundle branch blocks, and the implication of ST segment elevation for a cardiac patient. Strategies for how to use this new information and the impact on patient care were outlined. Armed with knowledge, the nurses began communicating with physicians in a novel way, offering their analysis of a patient's symptoms, anticipating problems, and consequently, preventing complications.

The outcome of this cultural transformation did not go unnoticed by physicians, other staff, and administrative leaders. Over time, the physicians came to respect and rely upon the expertise of this critical thinker at the bedside. Patient care improved, safety was maintained, and adjustments to the treatment plan expedited and enhanced. This critical thinking atmosphere, however, had another unforeseen consequence.

Medical decision-making in the seventies and early eighties was straightforward. Paternalism was the norm, and the Patient Self Determination Act was a decade in the future. Doctors made recommendations and decisions which, with little discourse, were accepted by the patient and family. As a neophyte CNS, there were times I was uncomfortable with this decision-making process, creating a nagging feeling in the pit of my stomach. This feeling would recur many times throughout my clinical experience.

The nursing staff began to ask questions about the life-sustaining treatment that was being delivered to some patients. Are we doing the "right" thing? How long would we wait to see if these interventions would work? Were we inflicting more harm than good? These were prickly questions. We were uncomfortable and had no mechanism to understand what we were observing and feeling. There was no clear direction on how a patients' voice could be integrated into the process of medical decision-making.

I encouraged open communication about these questions with the medical team. This initial questioning was not well received by all the ICU physicians. One cardiologist, admired for his clinical expertise and patient care, was harsh in his reactions to any questions that surfaced from me or the nursing staff regarding the goals of continuing life support for patients who seemed to be on the edge of death. He labeled us as the "rush to flush" nursing staff, a phrase that cut us to the core. It was far from the reason why we were questioning the medical plan of care. It denigrated the role of patient advocate that we were attempting to fulfill. The aftermath of these unskilled dialogues with each other and our physician colleagues were further exemplified in ethical dilemmas that emerged on the national scene.

The Influence of National Right to Die Cases

Karen Quinlan, the first right-to-die case in the United States, introduced me to the field of clinical bioethics.[3] Ms. Quinlan was a young woman who suffered brain damage after a car accident where she lost consciousness for a prolonged period. Her life was sustained with a ventilator and tube feedings. Physicians refused to honor the request of her parents to remove the ventilator. Quinlan's parents fought the judgment through several court battles. Eventually, the courts agreed to allow the ventilator to be removed, based on an individual's right to privacy. Her tube feedings, at the time considered ordinary treatment, were continued. Able to breathe on her own, she survived another ten years in a persistent vegetative state.

As this case unfolded on the national scene, I experienced an eerily similar situation in the ICU that was markedly different from the Quinlan saga. The young woman I cared for had suffered a cerebral aneurysm and was not expected to recover her cognitive abilities. Through several conversations, the medical team and family made the decision to remove her from life support, allowing her to die. There were no court battles, no media sensation, no obvious uncertainty. There was emotion and intense grief. The family came to say goodbye, tears flowed, she was removed from the ventilator, and she died in the ICU. What made this case different from what Karen Quinlan's family experienced?

Another influential case in my early exposure to the emerging field of bioethics was the story of Nancy Cruzan, a 25-year-old woman who was in a car accident in Missouri in 1983. She was found unconscious, face down beside her overturned car. Initially presumed dead, CPR was attempted that resulted in a "successful" resuscitation. The meaning and consequence of "success" would be debated for years. She never regained consciousness, and after five years on life support, Cruzan's parent's request to have her artificial feeding tube removed was denied by the medical team and hospital.

It was years later and after several court battles before Nancy's tube feeding could be discontinued. Her parents fought for seven years to do what they believed Nancy would want them to do. The U.S. Supreme Court, in addition to granting Cruzan's parent's request, additionally established the important precedent that the court does not distinguish between the withdrawal of a tube feeding and other life-sustaining treatment. This case laid the foundation for the Patient Self-Determination Act (PSDA) of 1990. It also laid the foundation for my ongoing distress of observing the agony and burden of family decision-making in the midst of uncertainty and differing opinions.

One aspect of this agony was relayed in a book by the Cruzan family attorney, William Colby, entitled "The Long Goodbye: The Deaths of Nancy Cruzan."[4] Amid dealing with the heart-wrenching process of losing their daughter, Joe and Joyce Cruzan faced opposition to their request to remove life support from the Missouri attorney general and the U.S Conference of Catholic Bishops.

Despite eventual court approval of the withdrawal of the feeding tube, protesters from around the country converged on the facility where Nancy received care, attempting to force the reinsertion of her feeding tube. Nancy's parents were outraged at the protester's actions at a time when they simply longed to have the opportunity to say goodbye to their daughter. On one occasion, protesters stormed the hallway outside of Nancy's room and — refusing to leave — were removed one-by-one by armed officers. One of the protesters confronted an officer with a glass of water intended for Nancy. Thwarted, the protester yelled at the officer, "You're a party to murder. Why not just take a pillow and smother her?"[5]

I was outraged as I learned about these actions. How could complete strangers feel they had the right to trespass on a family's private tragedy? Nancy's father wrote the following tribute upon her death:

> Today, as the protester's sign says, we give Nancy the gift of death. An unconditional gift of love that sets her free from the twisted body that no longer serves her. A gift I know she will treasure above all others, the gift of freedom. So, run free, Nan, we will catch up later.[6]

These observations on the ethics of clinical decision-making left an indelible mark on my perceived responsibility as a patient advocate and nursing leader. In 1980, just two years after I started my career as a critical care CNS, I volunteered to be on the organization's first ethics committee, formed in response to The Joint Commission's mandate that every organization have a mechanism to resolve ethical dilemmas.[7]

As new ethics committee members, most of us had no experience, preparation, or background in our newfound role. But we were eager to learn. We inhaled the emerging bioethics literature, debated national cases, encouraged conflicting views, and gradually prepared our healthcare teams to integrate the principles of bioethics.

I now had a new avenue to explore the promises that I had made as a nurse. The exploration into bioethics filled a deep hole in my yearning to understand the tension that existed between technology and an individual's right to navigate their healthcare decisions, even when decision-making capacity is lost.

For years, my involvement in this ethics committee and case consultations sustained me. Although I did not appreciate the importance of organizational culture and climate at that time, I was privileged to learn in an environment that took to heart the mission of supporting an environment of ethical inquiry. Differing points of view were supported, ethics consultations enhanced, interdisciplinary respect expanded, and patients' goals and values acknowledged. Soon, I would learn that not all organizations share this mission.

Chapter 2: A Clinician's Moral Distress

In 1989, I made a career move to a large university medical center, accepting a position as a critical care CNS with a focus on the cardiothoracic surgical and medical ICUs. State-of-the-art heart surgeries and procedures — cardiac bypass, heart, and lung transplantations, left ventricular assist devices — were performed with renowned cardiac surgeons. It was technology heaven. I was excited to continue to expand my clinical expertise in an environment devoted to the power of evolving science and life-sustaining interventions. I wanted to share my expertise as an educator, consultant, patient advocate, and nursing leader.

I would next make a career decision that would shock my inner core. It would be a decision that I initially would regret for years to come. I accepted the request by the nursing administration to take on an additional role as nurse manager of the cardiothoracic surgical ICU. The request tugged at my heartstrings. The culture of nursing care in this ICU was in shambles. Recruiting (and keeping) qualified nurses had become impossible.

At the time, eight full-time positions were being filled by traveling nurses committed to three-month rotations. Nurse managers rarely stayed for more than one year. Disturbing nursing behavior had become routine among key senior staff, including cursing at patients recovering from surgery, engaging in personal and inappropriate bedside conversations, and refusing to support the novice practitioners during orientation.

I yearned to make an impact on this environment and, ultimately, on the nursing profession. I became engrossed in establishing and enforcing rules of behavior that had never existed and were unpopular. I became unpopular.

This was a lonely time in my nursing career even though my actions were lauded by administrators (and secretly by a few nurses). I missed the nursing culture from my previous organization. Where were the critical thinkers, the mentors, the visionary leaders? I felt a disconnect from my professional objectives that worsened as I encountered disturbing ethical controversies.

The high-tech environment of the cardiothoracic ICU was picture-perfect fodder for legal, moral, and ethical dilemmas. One highly influential cardiac surgeon was often at the center of these dilemmas. This surgeon initially appreciated my clinical expertise and competence. I was upgrading the skills of the nursing staff and setting new expectations for performance and behavior. His enthusiasm for my expertise soon waned as I tackled ethical dilemmas involving his patients. This surgeon was the antagonist in the opening story about James — a story forever etched in my memory.

As I recant the experience on these pages, it is as if it happened yesterday. It took me years before I told this story to anyone. I was embarrassed that I did not relieve the suffering for this patient and family. I had broken my promise as a patient advocate and a clinical role model. I felt unsupported by others in the organization. I wondered why others did not react to this situation. Did they recognize the suffering? Or were they simply conditioned to accept the cultural norms that had been established? The remnants of this specific case lingered and festered within me. I lost sleep, and for the *only* time in my nursing career, loathed going to work. This was my first experience with what I eventually came to understand as moral distress, a phenomenon first described as "knowing what to do in an ethical situation, but not being allowed to do it."[1]

There are many causes of moral distress, including the continuation of life-sustaining treatment under conditions of uncertainty, poor communication among healthcare providers, patients, and family, and false hope given to patients. Moral distress is accompanied by a sense of powerlessness, anxiety, and self-doubt. In retrospect, this is exactly what had happened to me, though I had no understanding or path to its resolution.

This distress undoubtedly influenced how I reacted to the next ethical dilemma in this clinical setting.

The Case That Would Permanently Change My Future

Another cardiac surgery had been completed "successfully" that unfortunately resulted in postoperative complications. After an aggressive plan to attempt to reverse the patient's complications, one by one, his organs failed. Recognizing the futility of the situation after several weeks, the family requested life support be discontinued. Although there was no advance directive, the family was in consensus. As in the opening story, the cardiac surgeon refused to comply with the family's request — refused to talk to them. Believing the family had a right to have their voices heard, I confronted the surgeon with a request to sit down with the family and have a conversation.

This was mistake number one. With the aftermath of the opening story fresh in his mind, I was exposed to his verbal abuse in the middle of the ICU. He accused me of insubordination (as if I worked for him). Although humiliated, a fire within me had ignited. What type of patient advocate was I willing to be? The family came to me to express their suffering and frustration. I considered recommending that they request a transfer of care to a different physician who might be more open to their request. That might have been mistake number two. Instead, I offered the family an opportunity for an ethics consultation. The existing organizational policy allowed *any* staff member to make a referral. The family welcomed the opportunity. Would this be mistake number three?

The head of the ethics committee assured me of the appropriateness of the consultation and began the investigation that included meetings with the family, the medical team, the surgeon, and nursing staff, among others. After deliberation, the ethics committee recommended that the surgeon comply with the family's request, based on family consensus, evidence of the patient's values, and the medical team's conclusion that the patient was likely to die regardless of any further efforts. These recommendations were consistent with ethical principles, but clearly had not been disseminated into clinical practice, understanding, or acceptance. The cardiac surgeon refused to comply, and when the ethics committee recommended he transfer care to another surgeon, he agreed. Eventually, the family's request was honored.

At the final ethics committee meeting, the vice president of nursing, who participated in the entire investigation, pulled me aside as we exited the room. With arms crossed and an icy cold stare, she said emphatically, "Linda, I see that you have won this battle, but you have clearly lost the war. You will no longer be effective as the nurse manager if you can't get along with this cardiac surgeon." The nagging feeling in the pit of my stomach returned.

I had encountered a new type of ethical dilemma — one created by bureaucracy. The tone of an ethical environment comes from organizational leaders and the culture they create. To understand what I had experienced, I delved into the literature on the emergence of organizational ethics. "If an institution is not clear about what it values, then its employees will have only their individual values to guide their actions…this will contribute to confusion about what constitutes appropriate behavior."[2]

I was disillusioned, frustrated, and marginalized. My actions as a patient advocate ran contrary to the deference given to the more powerful surgeon. The imbalance in power was reinforced by the messages delivered to me by nursing administration, by the very profession that I had thought would provide moral and ethical support. I learned that patient advocacy had its price. A few months later, I left hospital nursing and never returned.

It took me years to understand what had happened with this experience. I failed to succeed in this new role as a nurse manager in this new organization. I was unable to fulfill my perceived obligations as a patient advocate due to value conflicts, lack of managerial skills, organizational oversight, and ineffective communication. I felt abandoned by nursing colleagues. My moral compass was in disarray. How would I find a path forward? Over time, I would come to appreciate and value the lessons I had learned.

Nursing management is challenging. I gained an appreciation for the responsibilities and skills necessary for success. My experience as a clinical expert and consultant did not prepare me for the skills needed to be an effective manager. I missed my role as a CNS consultant and educator. I was intrigued by the impact of leadership and organizational culture on professional behavior. I became invested in the emerging field of clinical bioethics. I felt the effect of personal values and their inadvertent yet potentially harmful impact on patient outcomes.

Although it took me much longer, I eventually came to understand (well, kind of) the cardiac surgeon's actions. He received his medical education within an ethos that taught him to sustain human life at all costs; paternalism was still the norm; the PSDA had no real impact mainly because there were so few advance directives completed. Family decision-making was not the norm.

Withdrawing life support was viewed differently than withholding life support. Surgical survival rates were important to maintain. Moreover, the impact of personal values on medical decision-making was not openly examined nor acknowledged. I admit that I never would come to understand the behavior of the vice president of nursing, who, rather than celebrate my actions of patient advocacy, abandoned me.

While it appeared that nothing good came out of this three-year experience, I was wrong. I discovered what was important to me as a nurse leader, what skills were natural for me, and what I wanted for my future. I answered a job posting for a nurse consultant role for the Rural Wisconsin Healthcare Cooperative. This role would enhance my leadership skills, give me new opportunities to learn about collaboration, and continue my quest to impact nursing competency and roles as patient advocates. It would also expose me to new mentors.

The Ethics Connection

The Rural Wisconsin Healthcare Cooperative (RWHC) is a shared services organization committed to providing affordable programs to its rural healthcare partners.[3] My role was focused on critical care education, competency-based program development, nursing leadership, and consultation. I facilitated several RWHC's professional roundtables, which are quarterly meetings that provide an opportunity to network with peers, discuss common issues, exchange ideas, and participate in selected projects. I led several existing nursing roundtables, such as medical-surgical, critical care and leadership, but established novel opportunities for networking, including the development of competency-based education (CBE) and ethics committee roundtables.

The CBE roundtables provided structure on how to orient and maintain the skills and expertise of the nursing staff. Influenced by my previous experiences and interest, I formed the first RWHC Ethics Committee in 1991. This Committee serves the needs of smaller organizations that do not have ethics resources by providing ethics education, policy and procedure development, and a forum for ethics case consultation reviews.

As a core component of my role with RWHC, I traveled to several communities in rural Wisconsin, providing monthly consultation in areas of critical care nursing, ethics committee facilitation and consultation, policy and procedure development, leadership mentorship, and other projects determined by the contracted organization. For the next six years, I expanded my personal leadership skills in facilitation, relationship building, collaboration, conflict resolution, negotiation, and quality improvement strategies.

Because I loved to teach and had conducted many critical care seminars, I ventured into the entrepreneurial world. I created a business as an independent consultant, providing critical care education in 12 lead ECG interpretations, advanced arrhythmias, and cardiac assessment and critical thinking. This business included contracting with a few law firms to serve as a nurse expert witness.

My obsession with the process of ethical decision-making continued. The RWHC financially supported my desire to pursue a master's degree in bioethics. It was an arduous four-year journey that required a weekly 130-mile commute to attend the classroom curriculum. I was not confident that I would complete the entire curriculum, but it was inspiring to learn from and interact with renowned ethicists and people from all walks of life who were interested in the field of ethics.

These interactions were motivational and fueled my desire to become a clinical ethicist. This new aspiration offered an avenue to fill the gaps I had experienced in medical decision-making and patient self-determination. Perhaps this would be a solution to the promises I hoped to achieve as a patient advocate? My experience as an ethics committee member and in developing competency-based education helped me select my master's thesis: the development of a Competency-Based Curriculum for Ethics Committee members. This manual was eventually published and distributed by Gundersen Medical Foundation.

The ethics committee educational manual I created was spurred in graduate school through an ethics consultation clinical that would provide mentorship and experiences in the requisite skills for ethics consultations. I observed ethics committee meetings and participated in consultations at several healthcare organizations. My bioethics student colleagues shared their collective experiences, discussed consultations, and debated recommendations that emerged.

We discussed Daniel, a 32-year-old man who had permanently fractured his spine in a diving accident. He would never be able to move his arms, move his legs, or breathe on his own for the rest of his life. An ethics consultation was called to review his request to be removed from the ventilator. He was competent, made repeated requests, but no one on the medical team felt comfortable honoring his request. The ethics team, in concert with the medical team, spent many hours deliberating. Would he eventually change his mind? There is evidence that spinal cord patients, over time and a period of adjustment, change their minds about their capacity to live with disabilities. Was he depressed? Would this be considered suicide? Would the family take legal action against the hospital? The dilemmas were overwhelming.

The decision was made to require Daniel to participate in counseling and to comply with a course of antidepressant therapy. After three months of compliance, Daniel's request to be removed from the ventilator persisted. "I have done everything you have asked me to do," he said. His request was honored. Daniel's case was among the many that illustrated the skill and expertise to conduct ethics case consultations: applying the principles of bioethics (autonomy, nonmaleficence, beneficence, justice) with an ethics of care (relationship-based).

I hoped to use this newfound knowledge and experience but was unsure how to craft a path forward. Four and one-half years later, I realized that I would have a bioethics degree but few prospects of a clinical ethics position. As I approached graduation, another mentor was there to offer advice, support, and opportunity.

Dr. Bernard ("Bud") Hammes, was a clinical ethicist at Gundersen Medical Foundation in La Crosse, Wisconsin, and founder of the local Respecting Choices program. I had formed a professional relationship with him on several levels. As a faculty member in the bioethics program, I elected a clinical ethics consultation field study with Bud to observe his organizational ethics role and receive ongoing mentorship in ethics case consultations. Bud was also one of my thesis advisors on the development of a competency-based curriculum for Ethics Committee members.

Most importantly, he exposed me to the Respecting Choices program in a memorable presentation he delivered after the publication of the La Crosse Advance Directive Study (LADS).[4] The outcomes achieved after two years of implementation were impressive. In a review of 540 deaths in the La Crosse community, 85% had completed a written plan, 95% of these were in the medical chart at the location of the death, and 98% of the time there was evidence that the plan had been followed; the care was consistent with the patient's previously expressed preferences and decisions.

But more impressive to me than these results was the vision he described about the power of advance care planning. This vision was not merely focused on the completion of documents, or patient autonomy, or compliance with the PSDA. Rather, advance care planning was a pathway to provide person-centered care for those we love. It was a program developed to help individuals reflect on their situation, goals, and values, and prepare their loved ones for making substitute decisions if needed. The program was designed to create systems that would help busy professionals do the right thing and facilitate skilled conversations. Creating effective systems involved much more than a simple question on admission, "Do you have an advance directive?" These were new messages. I was intrigued.

The publication of LADS stimulated interest by other communities across the country. How were the unprecedented outcomes achieved? What strategies could be shared? What replication was possible? To support this national interest, Gundersen Medical Foundation agreed to support the development of a national curriculum for program dissemination. I was recruited to fill the one position allocated to this program development. The position would include a role as a clinical ethicist. The stars aligned. Finally, I understood that everything I had accomplished, the experiences that I had encountered, the patients I had cared for, and the mistakes I had made, were there to prepare me for this new role. It prepared me for my next twenty years as an advocate for the person-centered decision-making approach that is detailed in the remainder of this book.

Chapter 3: But the Surgery Went Well Revisited

Remember James? My evolving role with Respecting Choices provided an opportunity to prevent similar stories. In a culture of person-centered decision-making, James' story would look different:

James was a patient in his mid-twenties scheduled for high-risk cardiac surgery. During a shared decision-making conversation with his surgeon and parents, the risks of surgery and alternatives to treating his advanced heart failure were explored. Surgery offered him the best option to help meet his goals of returning to an active physical and mentally fulfilling life. He understood the risks involved.

As a component of his preoperative preparations, he and his parents met with a social worker to further discuss advance care planning, designating his father to be his healthcare agent if he were to become unable to make his own decisions. They discussed his hopes for the surgery and his perspective on unacceptable outcomes. He was willing to fight through the high-risk surgery, potential complications, and long hospitalization. There were two outcomes he would not be willing to endure: the loss of his mental capacity and not being able to communicate. His plans were documented in the medical chart and shared with the rest of his family.

Unfortunately, James suffered significant intracranial bleeding that resulted in permanent brain damage. After many days, James never awoke and could not be weaned from the ventilator. A family conference was called to discuss the situation with the care team. The surgeon provided information on the clinical situation and answered the family's questions. He assured the family that multiple tests and expert opinion had confirmed that James would not regain his mental capacity due to the extensive brain damage. He would never be able to care for himself, and his ability to communicate in meaningful ways was doubtful.

The surgeon reviewed James' documented goals for the surgery with his family, and the written plan that had been created with his father, his designated healthcare agent. "Based on this information, what do you think James would want us to do?" the surgeon asked, "How can we best honor James at this point in time?"

There was no family disagreement, no surgeon's angst over decisions that would result in "killing my patient," no late-night calls from a frantic nurse, no lasting moral distress from the staff, no physician/nurse conflict, and no uncertainty about what James would want if he could speak.

Summary

Are the promises described in this book the essential elements in creating a person-centered decision-making culture? There is no imperative in healthcare that is more important than answering this question. If healthcare can agree on a core set of promises, there is no better return on investment. Making and keeping promises allows us to deliver the best care medical science has to offer — care that is aligned with an individual's goals and values.

Promises hold healthcare leaders accountable to create systems to honor patient goals and values and, in the process, improve safety and fidelity to the caring relationship. Keeping promises allows patients and families to trust healthcare providers and experience satisfaction with care. When promises are made and kept, the costs of unwanted care decrease and avoidable suffering is averted. Lastly, the return on the investment to make and keep promises to our patients leaves its mark on those who provide care. Moral distress among providers decreases, thereby improving professional satisfaction.

As Part One of this book has revealed, personal experiences inform our perspectives in both positive and negative ways. These perspectives influence the choices we make for our future endeavors. I invite you to review the following questions. Reflect on your own journey and allow this exploration to guide and fuel your passion for person-centered decision-making.

Personal Exercise

1) What is your story? How did it bring you to this book?

2) What experiences have you had with moral distress? Are there wounds that continue to fester?

3) What is your current role in creating a culture of person-centered care?

4) Identify mentors that may help you continue to find the courage to forge new pathways toward person-centered decision-making.

Part Two

Chapter 4:
The Promise of Leadership in Building a Culture
of Person-Centered Decision-Making

No Turning Back

Throughout the early months of implementation of the Respecting Choices (RC) First Steps®, Next Steps, and Advanced Steps advance care planning programs at a large healthcare system, the executive sponsor repeatedly delivered the following messages to multiple audiences:

> This decision-making program will transform how we will deliver healthcare in our organization. This is not a project. There is no turning back. You are the early adopters, but others will follow your lead. Thank you for your courage in being the first to learn about the changes that will be required, to test them, and to make them better for our patients and families.

Overview

The actions — or inactions — of a relatively small group of leaders in an organization can have a vast impact on how, and if, an innovation gets adopted, disseminated, and sustained. This realization has been an evolution for me personally and programmatically. I often wondered why the changes we attempted to implement were not sustained; why momentum waned. As a consultant, it was disheartening when an organization or community abandoned its efforts to fully support and implement the person-centered decision-making (PCDM) program that they were originally excited about

— one that was fully endorsed and financially funded. I wondered if I missed opportunities to connect the innovation more intimately to the existing characteristics of the culture. I ruminated over this reality and yearned for more expertise in organizational culture change and design.

Building a culture of person-centered decision-making is really, really hard work. Despite the programmatic failures and personal disappointments, organizations and communities changed their cultures for the better; decision-making practices moved in the right direction. I am ever convinced of the power of PCDM as an indispensable innovation in the quest to keep promises to our patients, families, and ourselves. I am ever convinced of the power of leadership to tackle the challenge of building a person-centered culture. Leaders who take on the toughest challenges are the ones who leave legacies that last.

This Part will explore three main questions:

- Why should leaders invest in building a culture of person-centered decision-making and how does the Respecting Choices program assist with this investment? (Chapter 4)

- What are the initial leadership strategies in implementing a person-centered decision-making program? (Chapter 5)

- What actions can leaders take to promote program dissemination and sustainability? (Chapters 6 and 7)

In the chapters that follow, seven recommendations for leaders are described.

Leaders:

---

1) Understand and lead the cultural change

2) Create engagement activities

3) Create a plan for sustainability from the beginning of the innovation

4) Embrace the innovation and conduct a cultural assessment

5) Create and communicate the vision and align the vision with strategic priorities

6) Lead by example

7) Expect setbacks and remove barriers

These leadership recommendations are based on personal experiences observing, mentoring, admiring, learning from, and evaluating courageous individuals and teams who aspired to construct a person-centered decision-making environment for all patients, families, and healthcare providers. I became an inquisitive student who learned every day. I evolved — am still evolving — in my thinking, competence, and beliefs about leadership.

The history and evolution of the RC program can be found in Chapter 8 — content that reflects my personal leadership perspectives and program development experiences, experiences that provide background on the recommendations in the remainder of this Part.

My observations, success stories, disappointments, and failures influenced my transformation as a consultant providing guidance and mentorship for implementation teams and as a program director responsible for creating materials and strategies for replication. Some of my discoveries occurred too late to make a difference; some I am discovering as I write this book. If

I were to start over in these roles, I would do some things differently. If you are currently in a leadership role, I hope you find guidance.

Why Should Leaders Adopt a Person-Centered Decision-Making Innovation?

First and foremost, building a culture of person-centered decision-making is the core attribute in delivering person-centered care: "Care that is respectful of and responsive to individual patient preferences, needs, and values, ensuring that patient values guide all clinical decisions."[1]

Who would negate the magnitude of preserving the "person" in the delivery of person-centered care? This intent has clearly been at the forefront of a plethora of programs, guidelines, tools, techniques, and measurement concepts over the past three decades. Yet, the promise of person-centered care remains largely an aspiration, but not a new phenomenon.

Person-Centered Decision-Making is the Core Attribute in Providing Person-Centered Care (PCC)

The appeal for person-centered care is not a new phenomenon. Even a superficial glance at the history of PCC reveals a slow, painful, and arduous pathway. "In fact, thirty years ago, when the idea [of patient-centered care] first emerged as a return to the holistic roots of health care, it was swiftly dismissed by all but the most philosophically progressive providers as trivial, superficial, or unrealistic. Its defining characteristics of partnering with patients and families, of welcoming—even encouraging—their involvement, and of personalizing care to preserve patients' normal routines as much as possible, were widely seen as a threat to the conventions of health care where providers are the experts, family are visitors, and patients are body parts to be fixed. Indeed, for decades, the provision of consumer-focused health care information, opportunities for loved ones' involvement in patient care, a healing physical environment, food, spirituality, and so forth have largely been considered expendable when compared to the critical and far more pressing demands of quality and patient safety—not to mention maintaining a healthy operating margin."[2]

While the remnants of this history exist, over the last two decades, healthcare has embraced the transition from a culture of treating diseases to a culture that cares for individuals — a transition enriched by leaders, national organizations, and researchers.

For example, the Planetree organization, dedicated to making patients partners in care with their providers, was envisioned by Angela Thieriot, who, after experiencing several challenging healthcare events as a patient, was intent on changing the healthcare culture. Hospitalized with a "mystery virus," Ms. Thieriot found herself in an environment where no one seemed to care: "…there was little human warmth or healing energy…people talked about me as if I weren't there." She was convinced she was going to die. After a few days of hospitalization, she credits two nurses who "saved my life." Why? Because they talked to her in a way that communicated caring. After she recovered, she vowed to make a difference, and in 1978, she started the Planetree organization.[3]

Today, Planetree is a nonprofit organization whose vision is to promote "the development and implementation of innovative models of healthcare that focus on healing and nurturing body, mind, and spirit."[4] Planetree describes three "simple" pillars for the delivery of patient centered care: purpose (communicate a shared mission and promote consistency and continuity for all patients and their families), process (create a systematic approach that is replicated for all patients, systems, and a formal approach to engaging patients), and practice (turn patient goals into actions, establish, monitor, and improve the system). Nearly 40 years after its development, Planetree's mission remains as essential as ever, but there is nothing "simple" about what is required to create this healthcare culture.

The origin of the term "person-centered care" has been credited to The Picker Institute, formed in 1986 by Jean and Harvey Picker, as the aftermath of

Jean's treatment for terminal cancer. The Picker Institute is a nonprofit organization dedicated to improving the healthcare experience for patients and families.[5] The Institute has published resources and tools, including its eight principles of person-centered care, and partnered with researchers, universities, hospitals, and charities to investigate, document, and communicate patients' healthcare experiences. The work of the Institute has been used by governments and regulators to influence health and social care policy.

In 2008, and with funding from the Picker Institute and Planetree, a panel of national experts published a "Patient Centered Care Improvement Guide" declaring that patient-centered care is "an idea whose time has come."[6] The guide provides a rich description of best practices and specific tools to promote person-centered care, contributed by United States hospitals committed to sharing their successful strategies. In a tribute to the founder of the Picker Institute, the foreword of the report states: "Harvey Picker's vision for a health care system organized around the patient perspective was—and continues to be—the driving force of the Picker Institute. Days before Mr. Picker died, his request to all champions of patient-centered care was to "Carry on." These words of encouragement are needed as much today as then.

To address the slow indoctrination of person-centered care, the National Academy of Medicine's Leadership Consortium convened a Scientific Advisory Panel (SAP) to address the uncertainty about how and if this person-centered approach will lead to improved patient outcomes and to support its integration into the healthcare culture. In 2017, the SAP published a guiding framework for "patient and family engaged care" that offers an updated definition of person-centered care and identifies the characteristic of leadership as instrumental in creating cultural transformation:

> Patient and family engaged care (PFEC) is care planned, delivered, managed, and continuously improved in active partnership with patients and their families (or care partners as defined by the patient) to ensure integration of their health and health care

goals, preferences, and values. It includes explicit and partnered determination of goals and care options, and it requires ongoing assessment of the care match with patient goals.[7]

The SAP framework describes four foundational elements for achieving PFEC:

- organizational leadership and levers for change

- strategic inputs that include structures, practices, skill-building, and connections

- practice outputs

- engagement strategies; elements connected to the achievement of the Aim outcomes

The SAPs framework — analogous to the RC five promises for systematic program improvement outlined in this book — requires an intentional approach to weave the variables of a chosen innovation into the fabric of the organization, into the behaviors of *all* providers and staff and available to *all* patients and their families. Absent a guiding framework, "…PFEC continues to be a 'nice to have' rather than a 'must have' to achieve high-quality, safe, and efficient care."

Person-Centered Decision-Making Assists in Achieving the Quadruple Aim

Don Berwick, past president of the Institute for Healthcare Improvement (IHI) and an unflinching champion for healthcare improvement, reflected on his personal meaning of patient-centered care at an International Forum in Berlin in 2009. Dr.Berwick asserted: "What I fear is the loss of dignity. It is the doctor saying, 'we think' rather than. 'I think'… It scares me to remain ignorant when I want to know. To be told, when I wish to be asked…

[patient-centered care]... is that property of care that welcomes me to assert my humanity and my individuality and my uniqueness and if we be healers then I suggest to you that that is not a route to the point, it is the point."[8]

Intuitively, the investment in innovations in person-centered care yields a potential promise on a host of healthcare outcomes. The creation of a person-centered care culture is the vehicle to achieve the IHI Triple Aim: better care, better health, and lower per capita cost of healthcare.[9]

Central to the achievement of the Triple Aim is the simultaneous attention to each aim. How one measures progress on the attainment of these aims remains an evolving debate. Don Berwick and contributing authors reflect on how an organization might measure its achievement toward the Triple Aim. "First, hospitals involved in the Triple Aim would be emptier, not fuller. They would celebrate success that the hospital is less and less often needed by the population. Second..., they would observe that the dynamics of supply-driven care are no longer strong and that patients pull resources, rather than vice versa. And third, patients would say of those who try to maintain and restore their health: 'They remember me.'" [10]

The Triple Aim's addition of a fourth aim — the Quadruple Aim — to improve the experience of those that provide healthcare, is also supported by IHI.[11] The prevalence of burnout and disengagement of healthcare providers must be addressed for person-centered care to become a reality. The delivery of person-centered care cannot be divorced from those that are delivering it. The IHI warns, however, that the focus of the Triple Aim is on patients and should remain healthcare's priority.

The IHI has continued to marshal strategies and innovations to achieve the Triple Aim, for example, by establishing a Research and Development team that created a process to spark new thinking about the delivery of patient care. In 2017, the team studied leaders from industry, manufacturing, and energy, adapted their techniques, and published "10 IHI Innovations to Improve Health and Healthcare" — a report whereby leaders of these innovations share their implementation experiences and challenges to integrate systematic approaches that improve health and healthcare.[12]

In summary, leaders who commit to the development, dissemination, and sustainability of person-centered decision-making programs have improved opportunities to deliver person-centered care and produce better care (individuals receive care that aligns with their goals and values), better health (increased satisfaction with the plan of care and prevention of avoidable suffering), lower costs (preventing unwanted care), and provider satisfaction (decrease in moral distress associated with uncertainty in medical decision-making).

This is the mission of the Respecting Choices PCDM programs.

The Respecting Choices Person-Centered Care Innovation: Building a Culture of Person-Centered Decision-Making

Building a system of person-centered decision-making is the innovation described in this book to assist organizations and communities in delivering on the promise of person-centered care. Naturally, it is not the only innovation, nor is it perfect. My experiences developing, disseminating, and improving the RC person-centered decision-making programs have revealed the power of this innovation to change behaviors, to impact the lives of patients, families, and healthcare professionals, and to achieve the Quadruple Aim. My aspiration is that the description of these experiences will inform other innovation efforts and requisite leadership responsibilities.

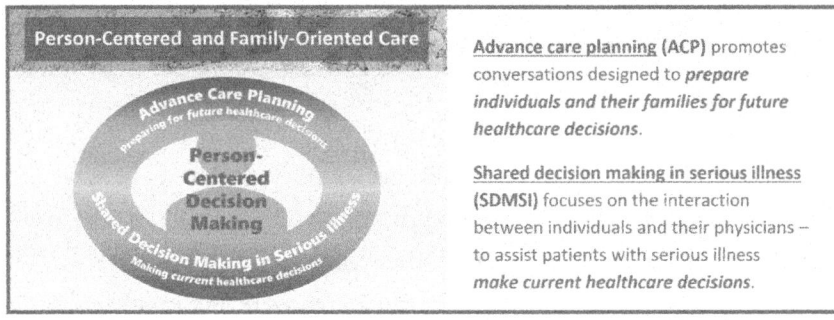

Person-Centered and Family-Oriented Care

Advance care planning (ACP) promotes conversations designed to *prepare individuals and their families for future healthcare decisions*.

Shared decision making in serious illness (SDMSI) focuses on the interaction between individuals and their physicians — to assist patients with serious illness *make current healthcare decisions*.

Respecting Choices has two person-centered decision-making programs: Advance Care Planning (ACP) and Shared Decision Making in Serious Illness (SDMSI), which work synergistically to build a culture of person-centered and family-oriented care.[13]

The initial person-centered decision-making program developed and disseminated for over two decades is branded as advance care planning, designed to prepare individuals and their families for future healthcare decisions. However, advance care planning is not a "one size fits all" intervention. The type of future healthcare decisions people must be prepared to contemplate varies with the individual's stage of illness; decisions become more specific regarding advancing illness, age, and risk of complications. To address this reality, there are three stages of advance care planning: First Steps, Next Steps, and Advanced Steps.

First Steps planning is designed to motivate any adult to participate in the planning process, assist in the selection of a healthcare agent, provide instructions for goals of care for an event that results in permanent brain damage and a poor cognitive outcome, and completing a written plan.

Next Steps planning is intended for those living with a serious illness, actively engaged in treatment, but experiencing complications. These individuals face future healthcare decisions that are context, or disease, specific and can be anticipated as serious illness progresses.

Advanced Steps planning is for individuals at risk of a life-threatening complication due to serious illness, advanced age, or frailty. It integrates the national POLST program and its system for converting decisions into medical orders.

The Next Steps and Advanced Steps populations comprise millions of individuals living with serious illness who are at risk for complications, and — beyond the need to think about future healthcare decisions — face current complex preference-sensitive treatment decisions every day. These complex treatment decisions, typically facilitated by physicians and advanced practitioners, require a person-centered approach. The person-centered decision-making skills, strategies and systems created for the ACP programs were applied in creating a complimentary program: "Shared Decision Making in Serious Illness." This program was specifically designed for physicians and advanced practitioners to assist patients and their families with serious illness make current treatment decisions aligned with their goals and values.

Together, these two programs — ACP and SDMSI — create an interprofessional person-centered approach to engaging and supporting individuals on their journey through their decision-making process.

Respecting Choices, and this book, use the term "person-centered decision making" interchangeably with shared decision-making — to reflect the principles of active partnership and engagement with individuals and their families, with the goal of reaching decisions that incorporate the best evidence science has to offer with personal values and "what matters most" in arriving at healthcare decisions.

Shared decision-making is often referenced as the "gold standard for the cooperation of doctor and patient," although there is a lack of consensus on the implementation principles of shared decision-making. In a systematic review of outcome-relevant effects of shared decision-making, an analysis of 22 randomized controlled trials of shared decision-making acknowledged a wide variation in the methods used and the extent of their full implementation.[14] "It needs to be borne in mind that the approach of patient participation is continually evolving. Depending on the respective perceptions of shared decision-making and the context, the implementation may differ. Irrespective of this, SDM is a gold standard for the cooperation between doctor and patient. Studies have shown, however, that SDM has not yet comprehensively been adopted in clinical practice. Decisions about treatment are often still unilaterally made by doctors although patients have a fundamental need to be involved in such decisions."[15]

In contrast to the wide variation and implementation of shared decision-making concepts and strategies, the RC person-centered decision-making programs have a rich history of development and experiential and research-based evidence. The structure, goals, and strategies have been tested, improved, and implemented in a variety of settings, providing a strong foundation for replication. To achieve the goal "to know and honor individual preferences and decisions," person-centered decision-making skills set the environment for robust conversations between patients, their families, providers, and others to reveal "what matters most to individuals."

These conversations are standardized and focused on understanding the patient's illness representation, providing information, eliciting the patient's values and beliefs, building trusting relationships, displaying compassion and empathy, and identifying needs and services to assist patients in living well. In contrast to shared decision-making concepts as "the gold standard for the cooperation of doctor and patient," the RC person-centered decision-making skills are not limited to the role of the physician or other provider. To the contrary, the premise for implementation is that all staff develop a core set of skills that allow them to work as a team in helping individuals make both future and current healthcare decisions aligned with their goals and values. Patients and families reap the benefits of consistent communication approaches delivered by the entire healthcare team.

However, ACP or SDMSI conversations are inadequate to meet the promise of person-centered care. *Conversations* alone do not constitute a PCDM *program,* nor will they result in the ability "to know and honor" individuals' goals, values, preferences, and decisions. The RC framework for building a system of person-centered decision-making includes five key elements for program sustainability: leadership systems redesign, education and competency, community engagement, and continuous quality improvement. Each of these key design elements are described in other chapters of this book.

The RC framework parallels, precedes, and is consistent with the guiding framework offered by the National Academy of Medicine. Systems are needed to allow transparency between the conversations and episodic hospitalizations and doctors and Emergency Department visits, making individualized plans available to those providing care so they can guide that care effectively. The system includes the education of others on their roles in supporting person-centered decision-making and strategies to honor these plans and respect an individual's goals, values, and preferences. Ultimately, a system must monitor whether patients received concordant care.

Chapter 5 describes two initial leadership recommendations to begin implementation of a PCDM program.

Chapter 5: Initial Leadership Recommendations in Building a Culture of Person-Centered Decision-Making

In preparation for the implementation of a PCDM program, such as ACP or SDMSI, leaders must first: 1) understand the goal and challenges of cultural transformation and 2) create engagement strategies that enlist participation of the entire organizational or community leadership team. A few committed champions are not capable of changing a culture. It takes a village.

Leadership Recommendation #1: Understand and Lead Cultural Transformation: The Rigor of the Work Makes it Real

Hospital mission statements that include "person-centered care" phrases are ubiquitous in modern healthcare. Moving to a culture of person-centered care, however, is not. This culture will not occur with a training program, a logo, or a mantra repeated oft enough that it will magically happen. It will require disruption at the organization, team, and individual levels. It will require leaders who understand cultural transformation.

The path to successfully integrate an innovation into the culture of an organization or community is thorny. The interconnection between leadership and culture in fostering innovations is reported in a manuscript that analyzed 12 years of research on leadership and organizational culture in the top eight management journals. "Organizations that want to achieve their goals with high performance should enhance the conjunction of leadership and organizational culture."[1] Organization culture and leadership is intimately intertwined, and both are needed in order to successfully innovate.

What is Culture and Cultural Transformation?

Culture is often thought of as something big and massive, something that we are the victims of, something that happens to us rather than something we have the power to create. Culture is how things "are done" in an organization and defines the range of acceptable behaviors — behaviors articulated, recognized, reinforced, and measured by its leaders. Few organizations think about designing their culture; rather, they hope that enough strategies and planning will create change and deliver results. Peter Drucker's often quoted "Culture eats strategy for lunch" reflects the importance of paying attention to transformation strategies.[2]

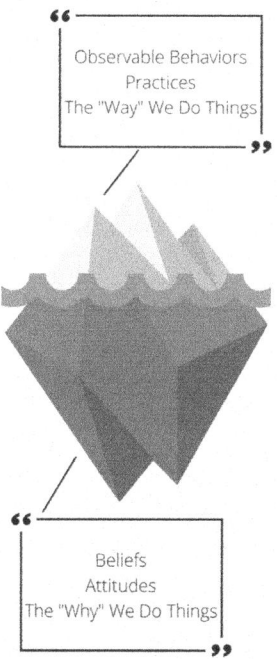

The process of cultural transformation has been likened to an iceberg. The visible part of the iceberg (above the waves) reflects existing observable behaviors and results. It represents the current reality. If one only looks at the "tip of the iceberg," failure is likely. Most of the culture is below the waves (the submerged part of the iceberg) and reflects shared beliefs, assumptions, and experiences — the "unwritten rules" of behaviors. Not understanding what lies beneath the surface can destroy chances for cultural change. Cultural shift requires changing beliefs, which is more intractable than changing behaviors.

According to Lewin-Schein, there are three stages of cultural change that will impact the ability for beliefs to be transformed: 1) "unfreezing" existing beliefs, 2) "change" processes to establish new expectations, and 3) "refreezing" to secure the new behaviors. Edgar Shein offers clarification of this model of cultural change, calling it "cognitive redefinition," stating, "If you have been trained to think in a certain way and are a member of a group that thinks the same way, how can you imagine changing to a new way of thinking ?"[3]

The characteristics of these stages resonate with my implementation experiences in building a culture of person-centered decision-making.

The "Unfreezing" Stage of Cultural Change

The "unfreezing" stage involves acknowledging the existing beliefs and the behaviors that have led to these beliefs. As a consultant, it was the norm to be confronted with beliefs that needed to be uncovered, explored, and shifted. During implementation within a large healthcare organization, the palliative care physician lead had a goal to move ACP referrals from the palliative care team to other qualified team members who would be certified in the requisite skills.

He wanted to elevate ACP conversations as a responsibility of all staff rather than perpetuate the practice of automatic referrals to the palliative care team, who were viewed as the experts in having skillful conversations about goals of care. During implementation, however, members of the palliative care team resisted this goal. They had a long history of having ACP conversations that were satisfying and, for some, consumed most of their professional time. Some believed that others did not have the competence to facilitate goals of care conversations.

"Patients don't want to talk about end of life" is another belief frequently encountered during implementation. Based on this belief, professionals avoid conversations or wait until patients "are ready to talk." Despite research to the contrary, some professionals hold the belief that "having planning conversations will take away hope." Additionally, many healthcare providers are skeptical about investing the required time and resources in a program that would increase the prevalence of advance directives. They had frequent experiences with directives that were poorly written, ambiguous, and not helpful in guiding medical decisions.

The beliefs uncovered during the implementation of an innovation are long-standing, deserve validation, and require exploration. Beliefs are formed from experiences, role modeling — or lack of role modeling — and indoctrination. Without exploration, these beliefs will serve to thwart implementation efforts. An analysis of the existing beliefs includes looking for what is valuable, what is working, and how to leverage this belief for the cultural shift.

The unfreezing stage is focused on readiness and motivation to change. People need to see that the current situation leads to dissatisfaction and that a remedy will be more satisfying. The stage of "unfreezing" includes identification of the anxiety, defensiveness, and resistance to unlearn what was previously accepted as the norm. Schein identifies eight strategies to reduce anxiety and resistance. And all must be attended to if change is to move forward:

- Creating a vision

- Formal training

- Control over the learning process

- Training includes the entire group of individuals rather than a limited few

- Training resources and safe harbors for trial-and-error

- Role models and mentoring

- Communities of Practice to provide group support for making changes

- Reward and recognition to encourage behavior change and reduce barriers[4]

To demonstrate Shein's strategies in resolving anxieties and concerns related to cultural change, let us turn back to the palliative care team who was resisting the goal of expanding resources for who would respond to ACP referrals. The lead physician had gathered data that demonstrated the time that was being devoted to ACP consultation among the palliative care staff. He created a vision that allowed them to see the advantages of a wider referral team which would result in the ability to reach all patients (not just those referred to palliative care) and allow more time for the palliative care providers to focus on the skills in which they are uniquely qualified to deliver, such as pain and symptom management.

Members of the palliative care team were invited to participate in the person-centered decision-making skills courses and become certified as Instructors who would lead skill-building activities. The mantra "ACP is everyone's responsibility" was promoted to encourage widespread participation. The palliative care practitioners were onsite to provide clinical mentoring as staff were learning new skills, role modeling, and encouraging behavior change. Lastly, this model supported the team approach to ACP rather than deferring person-centered decision-making assistance as the sole responsibility of one discipline or one specialty.

The "Change" Stage of Cultural Change

The "change" stage includes creating a new narrative that will assist in modifying existing beliefs. What would look different from the current reality? Creating this new narrative requires demonstrating, or role modeling, the desired behaviors and underlying beliefs and rewarding those who are compliant with the new behaviors.

A new narrative for an evolving person-centered decision-making culture has several compelling features. First, the creation of a vision that communicates the goal "to know and honor individuals' preferences and decisions" provides the context for a long-term commitment to quality patient care, rather than completing a project. This type of vision statement communicates a promise — a promise that serves to reduce the uncertainty that accompanies decision-making for individuals who cannot speak for themselves. This uncertainty causes moral distress for caregivers and is the source of avoidable suffering for patients. By dramatically reducing anxiety and stress for leaders, staff, and patients, confidence in the accuracy of decision-making is restored. A person-centered decision-making culture can free you to become the healers you set out to be.

Another strategy that assists to create a new narrative for person-centered decision-making is the design and analysis of small "tests of change," which are implementations of the innovation in selected sites and within motivated teams, allowing teams to learn together, practice new behaviors, and make improvements prior to wider dissemination. "Teams that find the right kinds of practices and reinforce them, time and time again, by insisting on following them, have greater influence and creativity."[5]

The RC person-centered decision-making programs provide new tools and materials that focus on asking patients "what matters to you?" versus "what's the matter with you?" They include standardized conversation guides, videos, and decision aids. New workflows are tested that help change expected behaviors.

For example, every patient on admission is asked, "Have you selected a person to make healthcare decisions for you if you become unable?" versus "Do you have an advance directive?" The electronic medical record accurately documents the patient's choice for a substitute decision-maker that steers staff to involve the appropriate individual in decision-making rather than the person who happens to be at the bedside. New and consistent language and terminology provide for improved team and patient understanding. Champions are supported to mentor the behaviors for others to role model.

As staff experience the impact of new tools, materials, and skills on patients, families, and themselves, beliefs begin to shift — beliefs about what it means to provide person-centered care. Behaviors follow, producing the desired results.

Lastly, creating a new narrative for person-centered decision-making requires communication. What are the implementation teams learning as they experience the innovation? What strategies are working; what needs to be revised? What are patients, families, and healthcare providers saying about the impact of the innovation? Stories are critical, especially during the early stages of cultural transformation when metrics are lacking. Successful team implementation serves as the catalyst for others to get on board — for others to change their behaviors.

The "Refreezing" Stage of Cultural Change

The "refreezing" stage includes setting universal performance expectations allowing for new habits to be formed. The ability to make the change permanent includes developing a new self-concept and interpersonal relationships, essentially changing beliefs and values...permanently. "Culture is a long-term game, won over multiple short-term 'sprints.' Our experience has shown that culture change in the workplace can begin quickly, with small wins to build momentum, but sustained shifts—changes that become part of the fabric of the organization—require longer-term concentrated efforts. Behavior change is, at its core, identifying behaviors to activate across different populations, then turning them into habits that embed the desired culture to support the core business strategy."[6]

This stage of culture change is a work-in-progress for most organizations. Implementation leaders are challenged with disseminating to the entire organization the strategies learned during the test of change. Creating a plan for sustainability, described in more detail in Chapters 6 and 7, is a critical step in making permanent cultural change.

Barriers to Improving the Culture of Person-Centered Decision-Making

Achieving a culture of person-centeredness is byzantine. The sheer depth and number of barriers to implementation provide fodder to understand why an innovation is abandoned or not fully disseminated. In a 2014 patient and family engagement survey of U.S. hospitals, seventeen barriers to creating a patient-engaged culture were identified. The 1457 hospitals (42.4%) that responded to the survey were asked to rate their answers to 17 questions related to barriers to the hospital adoption of patient-focused practices. More than half (51%) of respondents listed competing organizational priorities as a barrier. Other top barriers included: time to implement (42%), time available (31%), financial support (31%), and training of clinical providers in how to engage patients (25%).[7]

Not only did I grasp these barriers, but I also witnessed them firsthand as a consultant assisting with implementation of the RC person-centered decision-making programs within organizations and communities. The concerns about competing priorities and reimbursement were recurring.

Competing Priorities and Fee-for-Service Payment Model: One Leader's Observations

> I think that our organization was fragmented with multiple competing priorities. I had tangible executive support from my

vice-president, but I do not think it went any farther up into the C-Suite (high ranking executives within an organization). I think they liked the idea of our programs but were not fully aware of the importance of person-centered care and had so many other priorities that our program was not on the radar of the chief executive officer, chief nursing officer or chief operations officer. Honestly, a big barrier was the fee-for-service payment model; there was no financial motivation to change the outcomes for patients. Even during the first year of a shared-risk contract, I could not get them motivated to the importance of how person-centered care, excellent ACP, or how PCC could really improve our outcomes for the patients we are at financial risk for.

There is no escape from the leadership angst in navigating a world of competing organizational priorities. Even when an initial leadership team actively supports an innovation their progress can be disrupted when leadership turnover quickly results in a shift in priorities, funding, and resources. Leadership turnover is a universal truth and can undo months and years of implementation progress. Aligning an innovation with an existing strategic priority will decrease the odds of program disturbance when instrumental leaders leave their positions. Ensuring strategic alignment will be discussed in more detail later in this Part.

Naturally, a fee-for-service environment will challenge the implementation of an innovation that may lower hospital utilization in the last year or two of life. The fear of decreasing revenue confronts every administrator, and the evolution to a value-based payment system is slow and complicated. However, most patients who die are on Medicare or Medicaid, where payments are fixed and do not cover all hospital expenses, creating financial burden for patients.

An alternate perspective on the fear of decreasing revenue includes a commitment to being good stewards of resources, which includes striving to reduce waste in health care. Providing care that is unwanted increases financial and human burden. It is wasteful. It is also true that investing in a robust person-centered decision-making program costs money and lacks comprehensive reimbursement. The "hidden" costs of not providing this service are often overlooked or accepted as the norm. This includes long inpatient lengths of stay, resources for complex care coordination, underutilization of other services such as palliative and hospice care, and complex and frequent family conferences when decision-making uncertainty exists.

Influential leaders will prepare for additional barriers in implementing a person-centered decision-making program, to include push back from mid-level managers such as, "We didn't think it would take this much time" and "We can't train all of our clinical providers in the skills of person-centered decision-making."

Leading cultural transformation takes courage at multiple levels. It requires a commitment at the organizational level to create the vision for the future, create the systems consistent with this new vision, and communicate why a change is needed, what is expected, and how everyone will benefit. It requires commitment at the team level to experience the new behaviors and serve as the catalyst for change. And it requires acknowledgement at the individual level of those that have been transformed.

At this time, if you are still reading, you might be understandably depressed or disillusioned by the utter reality of the responsibilities, challenges, and barriers to leading the transformation to person-centered care. I think I understand, now more than ever, why an innovation is abandoned. Real results take time, resources, resilience, patience, and a whole lot of fortitude.

Leaders will need to celebrate small gains and value the signs of cultural change that slowly but surely emerge. I observed these signs with every implementation I had the privilege to facilitate. The signs that behaviors are changing, attitudes are shifting, and satisfaction is increasing are critical to acknowledge. They will fuel motivation and perseverance.

What Does a Culture of Person-Centered Decision-Making Look Like?

Throughout twenty years as a consultant, I remained inquisitive about how we could measure cultural change before, during, and after implementation. This curiosity remained unfulfilled due to lack of expertise and resources to build a measurement framework. Experiential observations of cultural change, however, consistently emerged early and throughout implementation.

In a culture that is being transformed, people start to talk and act differently. New language and terminology are used that communicates inimitable messages — messages that are person-centered. For example, advance care planning becomes a phrase that helps shift perspectives from a focus on advance directives to conversations that promote understanding. This new language is role modeled by the interdisciplinary team and allows for consistency in communicating with patients and families. Rather than checking off the admission assessment question, "Do you have an advance directive?" providers probe further. With the goal to motivate people to learn more about ACP, to move them from a stage of precontemplation to taking action, the follow up question becomes, "Have you thought about who could make decisions for you if you become unable to make your own decisions?"

Or, when physicians integrate the skills of person-centered decision-making into their consultations and real-time treatment decisions, a path to person-centered care is possible. A surgeon who was consulted to insert a peg tube for a complex patient who had lost decision-making capacity began a family discussion with the question, "Is this what your loved one would want if he could speak for himself?" Given the opportunity to reflect on this question, the family declined the peg tube insertion.

In a culture that is being transformed, people start responding differently once patient goals and values are known. An emergency room physician caring for a seriously ill patient with uncertain outcomes reviewed the advance directive and advance care planning documentation in the medical record, discovered the patient's goals and used this information to guide the plan of care: "This patient's request is to take all reasonable measures to treat his complications. We will transfer him to the ICU."

Or a neurosurgeon consulted for a patient with a severe head injury who, after reviewing the medical record documentation, offered the following advice to the patient's family: "Based on my review of your father's medical record, it appears that we should consider transferring his care to the palliative care team rather than pursue surgery."

In a culture that is being transformed, the organization implements system changes to monitor the achievement of person-centered care. As part of one organization's morbidity and mortality review, there is an analysis of whether the individual received care that was consistent with goals and values in the advance directive. Or, when conflict or uncertainty emerges, providers start asking different questions. In caring for a seriously ill patient in the ICU who had no documentation of their preferences or decisions for future medical treatment, a critical care nurse asks, "This individual was never approached for advance care planning. How did we miss the boat?"

In a culture that is being transformed, healthcare providers talk about the impact of person-centered decision-making on job satisfaction and how it has re-energized their professional purpose.

> I am a former pediatrician, retrained in adult palliative medicine and working full time in that capacity. I do the Respecting Choices conversations on this campus with adult patients and have been very happy with it. In the unexpected turn my life has taken in the past couple of years (from pediatrics to geriatrics), I am now having these conversations with families of adult patients with dementia, COPD, CHF, and renal failure. We use Respecting Choices with our adult patients extensively and very effectively. I am amazed, even after many years of experience honing communication skills with families, how useful this tool has been to help me explore the

tough questions with patients and families. —Jennifer Cohen, MD, Palliative Care, Kaiser Permanente, San Jose, CA

After experiencing the impact of facilitating quality person-centered decision-making conversations, a recurring comment from nurses, social workers, and chaplains reinforces the professional impact, "This is why I went into healthcare" and "My conversations with patients and families have forever changed."

Individual transformation is permanent. A program manager for one ACP implementation who had spent four years leading the team and promoting system-wide changes to support sustainability accepted a different position, but her commitment to cultural change continued.

> Even though I am so sad about the [ACP] team being broken up, I am hopeful for their new home and my connection to them through my new role. I hope to be an influencer for them and the work we hold dear to our hearts.

These are a few of the signs of cultural transformation that inspired and motivated me as a consultant. Without these signs, I am not sure I could have persevered. I remained confident that these signs of culture change would become self-reinforcing patterns of behavior that would gradually grow resistant to change and fuel the momentum for sustainability. I learned that it would take a bit more effort.

Leadership Recommendation #2: Create Engagement Activities

Engagement strategies must be created for the entire leadership and executive teams — those responsible for providing support, funding, and program evaluation. Education is not sufficient to maintain the level of leadership involvement for dissemination and sustainability.

To "engage" means to be committed to a cause, to participate, battle, fight, even to charm.[8] It is challenging to accomplish this level of engagement for an entire leadership team, yet it is essential for successful and early implementation.

Respecting Choices uses a variety of engagement strategies to assist organizations and communities in their understanding of the program — strategies that have been adapted for local use. Stories are one of the most effective engagement strategies, a lesson I learned from the Escape Fire.

The Escape Fire: An Early Leadership Engagement Strategy

The original 2001 four-day Organization and Community ACP course introduced the "Escape Fire" to promote dialogue on the importance of leadership engagement. The Escape Fire is a memorable true-life story.

In 1949, a forest fire broke out in Mann Gulch, Montana.[9] To manage the fast-moving fire, a team of 15 smokejumpers (ages 17-21), headed by their foreman Wag Dodge, were parachuted into the fire. The fire was moving fast, and the smokejumpers quickly became trapped. They could not outrun the fast-moving fire, as they tried to reach the top of the steep Gulch. They were trying to run up the gulch, in extreme heat with their heavy backpacks — called a "Pulaski" — full of firefighting tools. Wag Dodge knew they would all perish, that they would lose their race to the top. He created what has come to be known as the escape fire. He lit a match to create a fire in front of him. This served to burn the fuel around him so that when the fire reached him, it would have nothing to fuel its flames, and he would be safe. In the middle of his escape fire, he tried to get the other smokejumpers, who must have thought he was crazy, to join him. No one followed. All the smokejumpers died. Wag Dodge was the sole survivor.

Don Berwick, chief executive officer of the Institute for Healthcare Improvement (IHI) at the time, integrated the story of the Mann Gulch fire into a 1999 keynote presentation at the National Institute for Healthcare Improvement conference.[10] He related this story of innovation to a healthcare system in chaos. He asked a series of provocative questions: "Is healthcare unraveling?" and "How do organizations make sense in a complex world?" As in the Mann Gulch fire, in the heat of the moment, people cannot see the answer to a problem even when it is right in front of them. He challenged organizations to create their own "escape fire" to address the multiple problems of medication errors, fragmentation of care, and person-centered quality of care.

This compelling story and excerpts from Berwick's presentation were used to engage the participants who attended the Organization and Community ACP course in dialogue on an agenda topic, "The Challenge of Shifting from a Culture of Advance Directives to Advance Care Planning."

Following the video — which included the story of the Mann Gulch fire and Berwick's personal experiences with healthcare — the audience discussed the challenges within their organizations and communities in creating a more effective ACP program, reflecting on questions such as: "What are your 'Pulaski's'? Can you envision ACP as the 'escape fire'? What are your cultural barriers?"

The Escape Fire promoted dialogue and increased awareness and resonated with participants who often used this story as an engagement strategy when they returned to their organizations or communities. Through redesign efforts to condense the agenda, we eventually eliminated this engagement strategy, but not the effectiveness of storytelling.

On a personal note, I investigated how I could visit the site of the Mann Gulch fire during a consultation in Montana. I wanted to stand on the side of the hill where the Mann Gulch firefighters stood. I learned that the path to this infamous site would require an additional flight, a very long hike, and lots of time. Regrettably, I never stood at the site of the Mann Gulch fire.

Years later, when asked to speak at an ACP conference, I was introduced by an individual who had experienced the original four-day course and participated in the "Escape Fire" conversation. She recalled the dialogue and its ongoing impact on her implementation work. It had made a lasting impression that continued to motivate and inspire her efforts — exactly what an engagement activity is intended to do.

Other leadership engagement activities include interactive workshops, implementation summits, and online tools.

Leadership Engagement Workshops

Leadership engagement workshops are offered to organizations and communities prior to the decision to partner with RC for implementation of the person-centered decision-making programs. These workshops create support and enthusiasm to invest in the RC programs and implementation strategies. Half to full-day workshops are mutually designed to meet with leaders from an organization and/or community, discuss the application of the programs as a pathway to deliver person-centered care, respond to concerns and barriers, educate, create shared understanding, and create momentum for moving forward. A typical agenda includes presentations from RC faculty and organizational and community leaders and small group discussions with leadership, clinical managers, operations, steering committees, and other stakeholders. The expectation is that there will be leadership dialogue and a decision on whether to invest in the program as a pathway to meet stated goals, priorities, and resources.

The Leadership Summit

Once a formal partnership for implementation is finalized, leadership engagement becomes a priority. The commitment to implement and sustain successful person-centered decision-making programs requires leadership support at multiple levels: executive, administration, steering committee, program coordination, health professionals, and community stakeholders. A one-day consultation "summit" is organized to prepare these leaders to understand the innovation, assess readiness of implementation teams, and create supportive relationships with the leadership team. The summit includes a description of the five design elements for systems change, leadership roles in creating a vision and strategic plan, and ongoing responsibilities to support, communicate, and support innovation. Consultation is provided for design workgroups, leadership and initial implementation teams, and community stakeholders as appropriate. Unfortunately, attendance from the leadership team was limited, leaving participants with the responsibility to disseminate the information and construct other engagement activities.

Ongoing Leadership Support

The "refreezing" stage of cultural change is the hardest. This stage includes setting new performance expectations to embed permanent behaviors and standards as the norm. This stage typically occurs well after implementation partnerships have concluded. The dissemination, ongoing monitoring, and improvements continue as an organizational and community challenge.

To support organizations and communities in disseminating and sustaining program improvement, RC created new roles and networking strategies. Organization and community-specific individuals are selected as ACP and SDMSI Faculty to provide local expertise to continue to implement strategic objectives. Their responsibilities include, but are not limited to, establishing the clinical and business case for program implementation, performance monitoring and measurement, analyzing program process and making improvements, creating program reports, and conducting ongoing skills education. These individuals participate in Fellowship programs for mentoring, competence validation, and certification.

Implementation teams, Faculty, and Instructors are invited to join national networking communities to continue to learn from other teams and Faculty, sharing stories, success strategies, and barriers. The next chapter will continue to explore leadership recommendations for program dissemination and sustainability.

Chapter 6: Leadership Recommendations for Program Dissemination and Sustainability

I Won't Be Attending the Workshop

The Respecting Choices First Steps, Next Steps, and Advanced Steps programs were chosen for implementation within a healthcare organization. The decision to choose RC was influenced by an influential physician champion who collected data and completed his due diligence in recommending RC. He secured support from the chief executive officer and was chosen to be the physician lead. During the first leadership engagement when the program was introduced to over 100 physicians, nurses, community leaders, among others, the CEO arrived for morning introductions.

Immediately after the introduction, the CEO stated, "I'm sorry, but I won't be able to stay to hear this presentation," and then, over the next few years, a team of certified RC Instructors and coordinators created an advance care planning program that was well received by those who participated. Departments and clinical programs were recruited to be part of the implementation teams who would test and customize the ACP strategies. Another administrative sponsor supported the initial investment in the innovation, but after he left the organization, his predecessor was not enthusiastic, wanting the program leaders to concentrate their efforts on increasing the prevalence of advance directives.

With a lack of accountability and expectation to participate, the program struggled and lost momentum. Concurrently, another organizational executive invested in the development of a department dedicated to shared decision-making geared toward physicians. Staff were selected to be trained in the skills of shared decision-making, to create decision-making tools for patients, and to facilitate decision-making conversations with patients. Patients could be referred to this shared decision-making program by physicians. Over time, the leaders of the ACP program were laid off, and the shared decision-making program was eliminated.

Indisputably, it takes courage to lead cultural transformation. Michelle Obama has stated, "You may not always have a comfortable life, and you will not always be able to solve all of the world's problems at once, but don't ever underestimate the importance you can have because history has shown us that courage can be contagious, and hope can take on a life of its own."

Courage is the "mental or moral strength to venture, persevere, and withstand danger, fear, or difficulty."[1] This definition begins to help us understand the meaning of courage, but courage is more than mental or moral strength. I have known many people who have this internal fortitude but are unable to act, unwilling to suffer its consequences. Courage requires action and is an essential leadership characteristic in embracing cultural transformation.

This Part will explore additional leadership recommendations to support program dissemination and sustainability.

Leadership Recommendation #3: Create a Plan for Sustainability from the Beginning of Implementation

Without a formal plan for sustainability, improved outcomes that may be achieved during a small-scale initial program typically do not automatically result in lasting improvements. There is a 70% failure rate in sustaining long-term change in organizations.[2]

An examination of the factors that lead to program sustainability was reported in an article that reviewed 19 empirical studies of American and Canadian health-related programs. Five elements were identified for program sustainability:

- the ability for the program to be modified over time

- a visible champion

- consistency with the mission of the organization

- a clear perception of benefit

- support from stakeholders.[3]

The core features in developing sustainability plans are explored in a qualitative research study and report on the factors that assist with the spread of collaborative improvements.[4]

Sustainability is "When ways of working and improved outcomes become the norm," — a definition that can be applied to a person-centered decision-making innovation.[5] First, the definition acknowledges that a group of individuals have started to work in new ways. For example, people start using their newfound communication skills to promote person-centered decision-making, or new written materials are used to promote community engagement.

Second, the definition acknowledges that outcomes have improved. For example, patients and families are highly satisfied with person-centered decision-making conversations, and professionals have increased job satisfaction.

Lastly, the definition implies that permanent changes have occurred that no longer need support. For example, person-centered communication skills courses are routinely offered, and the documentation of person-centered decision-making conversations is standardized into the electronic medical record platform.

To assist leaders in designing a sustainability plan, a toolkit of 12 questions is recommended. Questions to be explored throughout implementation:

1) Is the innovation being perceived as valuable for patients, families, healthcare providers, and others?

2) What outcomes are being achieved? What data exists?

3) What is the degree of continued engagement by leaders and champions?

4) Do staff have the skills, confidence, and interest in continuing to use the new program materials, systems, and processes?

5) Is the innovation being shared and integrated with other organizational models of care?

6) Do the organizational operations support the new expectations?

7) Has the innovation helped improve the organization's strategic priorities?

8) Is the innovation still a good "match" with the organization's overall goal and operations?

9) Does the innovation fit with the needs, interests of the community?

10) What partners are available and interested in supporting the innovation?

11) What strategies for spread are acceptable?

12) What sources of funding are available?

13) To what degree is the innovation supported by government policies, surveillance systems, and reimbursement agencies?

These probing questions require leaders to think long-term, to examine what components of the innovation will be disseminated (and the ones that will not be disseminated), to decide what resources will be needed, and understand how to communicate the plan.

The previous example of the large health care system that created the program vision, "All adult patients' wishes for future healthcare needs are elicited, known, and honored," demonstrated a commitment to sustainability from the beginning. They hired a program director and related staff to achieve the aim of rapid spread and dissemination. Their initial implementation "tests of change" were rapid improvement cycles of three months. They allowed approximately 12 months of testing and then quickly moved to system-wide expectations for adoption.

Policies changed; dashboard outcomes were selected; practices were monitored, and data collected. This organization selected the program strategies that were working, adapted others to meet their needs, and abandoned some. After one year of implementation, they communicated the ongoing implementation plans for sustainability system wide, thereby demonstrating ongoing commitment to their original vision.

Leadership Recommendation #4:
Embrace the Innovation and Conduct a Cultural Assessment

It is impossible to create and communicate a compelling vision and strategic plan without a full understanding of the chosen innovation. A detailed understanding of the innovation prepares leaders to be convincing spokespeople and advocates for integrating the innovation into strategic priorities — to describe how the innovation is unique from similar programs within the organization. Leaders familiar with the evidence on the effectiveness of the innovation can use this information to influence specific audiences and naysayers. Understanding the innovation will allow leaders to support the involvement of personnel necessary to create or redesign supportive systems.

The executive in the opening story of this chapter missed an opportunity to understand the innovation, to participate in dialogue, and to contemplate strategic alignment. Regardless of his intent, he sent an overwhelming and transparent message to other members of the leadership team and participants that the innovation was not his priority.

Naturally, the group of leaders who need to understand and become engaged in the innovation must be identified. Leaders are responsible for ensuring that the right talent is hired and creating the structure and function of the teams that will be implementing the program. Simply giving someone a title without requisite responsibilities, accountabilities, authority, and resources will yield frustration, unsuccessful outcomes, and abandonment.

I also encountered (numerous times) leaders that assigned the work to a person without authority. Responsibility without authority meant the program never got off the ground. How could a social worker, who was given responsibility but no authority, ask a clinic manager, for example, to identify some of their staff to be facilitators and give them the time to do the work?

Roles and responsibilities for all members of the team must be developed at the beginning of an initiative, evaluated, and revised as appropriate.

National Respecting Choices courses have been offered one or two times per year to provide a forum for participants to learn the requisite design elements and communication in creating an effective advance care planning program. These three-day courses — offered in person or virtually — are attended by a diverse group of individuals from the United States and other countries.

For twenty years, at each of these in-person offerings, I provided a personal welcome, introduced the attendees, and asked them for their reasons for traveling to La Crosse, Wisconsin. There were typically three groups of attendees: 1) individuals from existing implementation teams, 2) teams of individuals from organizations or communities who were contemplating implementation partnerships with RC, and 3) lone individuals that had personal interest in the program or were sent by their organization to learn more.

Consistently, each of these groups expressed typical reasons for attendance. Individuals from existing teams desired information and certification but understood that their organizations or communities sent them to fortify the current team and allow for program expansion. Teams contemplating implementation partnerships were often leaders who desired to understand the work involved, resources needed, and relative evidence to be able to make a business case when they returned.

The lone individual's reasons for attending were diverse: to learn, to improve a program they were developing, to become an independent consultant, or to "jump-start" their learning in preparation for implementation. But the responses that gave me serious consternation were, "I don't know why I'm here. I was sent by my boss," and "I was told that I needed to start an ACP program when I return." These responses smacked of a lack of leadership involvement or commitment. I always worried about what would happen when they returned to their organizations or communities.

Conduct a Cultural Assessment:
What are the Strengths, Barriers, and Opportunities?

Every culture has unique characteristics. It was fascinating to observe the differences that each organization or community presented — differences that reflected their diverse populations, geography, resources, talents, resilience, and aspirations. No single implementation was the same. I learned to adjust my consultation style, strategies, and recommendations. I remained curious to learn from various leaders what they believed would work and what would not. Navigating their intuitions with my recommendations required negotiation and compromise.

A cultural assessment allows leaders to customize implementation strategies and be informed of specific challenges and barriers. "…in the absence of an honest assessment of the organization's current strengths and opportunities, its goals, practices, performance, and operational realities, without a desire to create change, and without leaders on board, PFEC [patient and family engagement care] efforts are vulnerable to becoming an afterthought in the midst of competing priorities, or a 'flavor of the month' that is abandoned when the desired results do not come quickly enough."

Armed with an understanding of the innovation being implemented, leaders can customize cultural assessment strategies. For example, professionals who live in a culture that asserts that "we are already doing ACP" will benefit from an assessment that explores and exposes this assumption. It is true that to comply with the Patient Self-Determination Act (PSDA) and The Joint Commission standards every health organization has some type of ACP activity. A deeper investigation into the meaning of the assertion that "we are already doing ACP" among healthcare providers, patients, and families will typically reveal gaps and opportunities for improvement.

A baseline examination of ACP practices typically uncovers inconsistencies, lack of standardization, and inadequate communications skills. Organizations discover that, while they may be compliant with the basic and minimum standards for ACP, the outcomes are unsatisfying and insufficient to provide person-centered care. Everyone is "doing" ACP differently. Some people utilize person-centered decision-making skills effectively, others do not. The ACP service is unreliable, not available to all patients, and not universally supported or endorsed by all members of the healthcare team.

Analysis and communication of data, concerns, and perspectives from a cultural assessment serves to motivate people to learn more about the innovation, decrease resistance to change, and pave a pathway for open dialogue for improvement opportunities. Finally, a cultural assessment provides baseline data for performance improvement and will assist in customizing the innovation to the specific strengths, goals, resources, and challenges.

Leadership Recommendation # 5:
Create and Communicate the Vision
and Align the Vision with Strategic Priorities

Create the Vision

With an understanding of the impact of the innovation and an analysis of the existing culture, an inspirational vision can be created that will guide every stage of implementation through dissemination to sustainability. "A vision is a mental picture of the result you want to achieve—a picture so clear and strong it will help make that result real. A vision is not a vague wish or dream or hope. It is a picture of the real results of real efforts. It comes from the future and informs and energizes the present."[6]

It was common for leaders to resist the creation of a vision or to connect it to the strategic priorities of the organization. At times, leaders participated in a futile or cursory exercise in creating a vision statement that was completed by a few; rather than an exploration by the entire executive branch. Organizations tended to communicate the implementation of the program but once the components were delivered, once the "project" was completed, there was incomplete dissemination.

A well-crafted vision is captivating for many reasons:

1) It tells people where you are headed. This forward-thinking will inform the barriers, the need for resources, and the set-backs likely to occur along the journey and most importantly, creating the business plan.

2) It provides motivation and inspiration to think big and accomplish cultural change, not simply implement a project and believe that is all that is expected.

3) It will help everyone persevere through the natural setbacks and frustrations of implementation.

4) It helps maintain focus to work on the big stuff and not get bogged down by the mundane.

5) It gives meaning and purpose, defining the reason why leaders are committing to innovation.

People yearn to participate in something that makes a difference. Daniel Pink's research has found that people are motivated by "...the human need to direct our own lives, to learn and create new things, and to do better by ourselves and our world."[7] This yearning to improve things that matter to us was expressed consistently by physicians, nurses, social workers, and others after experiencing the impact of PCDM conversations. "This is why I went into nursing/healthcare," and "Thank you for helping me get reenergized with my job," and "This is a professional burnout buster."

In retrospect, the inability to adequately articulate the authentic vision of the RC programs — "to know and honor individual preferences and decisions" — made it challenging for organizations to create a comprehensive vision consistent with the power of advance care planning. Instead, the following examples of vision statements demonstrated a focus on short-term outcomes, completing a "project," increasing the prevalence of advance directives, or on education:

- "Members will have POLST (portable medical order) forms completed prior to admission to a long-term care facility."

- "Patients in region xx will be educated on options for life-sustaining treatment."

- "Everyone in the xx region will receive care that honors personal values and goals at the end of life."

There were a few organizations that got it right — that understood the culture they aspired to create, as in the following vision statement:

> All adult patients' wishes for future healthcare needs are elicited, known, and honored.

The above vision is illustrative. It does not solely focus on advance care planning or end-of-life care, but *any* future healthcare need. The vision places responsibility on healthcare providers to "elicit" preferences for future care. It communicates the goal of standardization to serve "all" patients and reflects a commitment to widespread dissemination. This vision propelled the organization to invest in human and financial resources to sustain the momentum.

Communicate the Vision Over and Over

Creating a compelling vision is a noble beginning. But to provide ongoing inspiration, commitment, and behavior change, the vision needs to be communicated… over and over again. When asked to reveal what she and her colleagues had learned during the implementation journey, the director of a program implementing the RC person-centered decision-making programs included in a presentation a slide that simply said: "Communicate, communicate, communicate."

The opening story of this Part demonstrates effective communication of a vision. The executive personally delivered the message. The vision delivered a big picture of what would be accomplished: improving the way healthcare is delivered. She provided an expectation that the journey was just beginning but would not end. She acknowledged the trailblazing efforts of the early adopters. Her simple statements were inspirational and emotionally appealed to the passion, energy, and commitment to the program that was being developed.

Align the Vision with Other Strategic Priorities

Organization leaders often identify competing priorities as the number one barrier to building a culture of person-centered engagement. People experience initiative fatigue and are susceptible to dropping an initiative when the work becomes too hard or the outcomes obscure. Viewing the program as a "project" instead of an innovation will not lead to cultural transformation.

"All too often, user experience and engagement programs are created in a response to a mandatory requirement for measurement, or an organization's response to a particular set of results and/or complaints. To deliver a consistently positive user experience, it is vital that an organization's user experience and engagement programs form part of its strategic priorities."[8]

Leaders who understand their existing culture have the capacity to analyze and determine how the person-centered decision-making component can be strategically aligned with other organizational priorities. Strategic alignment will ensure the viability and sustainability of the innovation rather than run the risk of it being viewed as a project that is vulnerable to elimination. Person-centered decision-making programs share a natural alignment with a variety of organizational priorities: patient safety, population health, advanced illness management, care coordination, transition of care, and quality of the patient experience.

An exploration into the impact of aligning a person-centered decision-making program with patient safety is enthralling. The impact of this alignment extends beyond patient safety to include safety for families, the healthcare providers, and the organization. For patients, person-centered decision-making opens communication channels with families, healthcare providers, and supportive others, with a host of benefits that promote a safe environment. Initially, a person-centered decision-making approach assists individuals in exploring and discovering what matters most and provides information on benefits and burdens of treatment choices customized to match an individual's goals and values.

For most patients, participation in decision-making is satisfying and builds trust in the healthcare team. Care plans are created and documented to guide healthcare decisions. Most importantly, a person-centered decision-making culture that promises to honor healthcare decisions allows patients to receive care they want and avoid unwanted treatments. There is nothing more essential to patient safety.

A person-centered decision-making milieu promotes safety for families as well. Family involvement in decision-making allows them to provide added information, ask questions, demonstrate support, and come to understand what is most important to their loved one. A family who understands a loved one's goals and values will be better prepared to make substitute decisions if needed.

Without this understanding, substitute decision-makers bear the burden of decision-making when uncertainty exists. When goals and values are understood, families will avoid complicated grief associated with making life and death decisions. This promotes the overall safety of the community and promotes population health.

Uncertainty in making health care decisions leaves its mark on physicians, nurses, social workers, and other healthcare providers. Moral distress incurs when healthcare providers witness medical decision-making that conflicts with their values, beliefs, and perceptions of their professional roles. A recent study that examined the frequency and intensity of moral distress among physicians and nurses concluded that "Moral distress threatens the psychological well-being of healthcare providers...moral distress was also significantly linked to caregivers' intention to leave their positions."[9]

In this study, a modified distress scale was completed by 342 physicians and nurses, asking them to respond to 38 questions. Despite variability in responses, the two statements with the highest mean scores included: "Carry out medical orders for what I consider to be unnecessary tests and treatments," and "Follow the family's wishes to continue life support even though I believe it is not in the best interest of the patient."[10]

In a person-centered decision-making culture, the safety and well-being of healthcare providers is improved. When healthcare providers have confidence in an individual's informed decisions, supported by family understanding, the uncertainty in making treatment decisions abates, relieving one cause of moral distress. Without the angst of uncertainty, healthcare providers can sleep better at night knowing they have followed the expressed goals and values of the patient. Professional satisfaction improves, and burnout and turnover are minimized.

Last, a person-centered decision-making culture promotes safety for the organization. Providing unwanted care is a medical error. Providing care consistent with an individual's goals and values decreases the risks of litigation as well as organizational monitoring of sentinel events.

A person-centered decision-making program that is aligned with the strategic priorities of the organization communicates stability and commitment, ensures ongoing resources, and increases the prospect of program sustainability.

Naturally, leaders understand the importance of creating a strategic plan. However, in my experience, these plans are often narrowly focused on the achievement of short-term goals. For sustainability, the strategic plan must integrate the vision consistent with "to know and honor an individual's preferences and decisions." A vision must be activated and "come alive" with an intentional plan to tie the vision to team and individual goals and outcomes.

As a component of the strategic plan, leaders must set clear expectations for accountability. Without these expectations, behavioral change will be inconsistent, and those that take accountability will be frustrated.

**Looking for ACP Documentation is a "Nuisance":
One Leader's Frustration**

Our team spent several years improving our ACP documentation, which required nurses to review existing documentation of patient preferences and decisions as part of the admission responsibilities. We listened to the nurses and made the documentation module as user friendly as possible. I thought we had made a huge win when that module went "live."

However, mid-level managers did not support this expectation of their nursing staff as a new responsibility. The review of existing documentation rates remained low. This activity was seen as a nuisance, and "one more thing to do," rather than a professional responsibility to uncover the wishes of the patient. I often felt like it was just me pushing the rock up the hill each day with my small team.

This story exemplifies typical frustrations experienced by implementation leaders when they strive to disseminate new ways of working. In the above example, the lack of mid-level management support for employee accountability was a reason this leader eventually left the organization.

Leaders at all levels must embrace a set of expectations for all employees if the culture is to be transformed. These common expectations allow personnel to work collaboratively as a team for the benefit of patient and family decision-making. Providing assistance with person-centered decision-making is everyone's responsibility. "…the practices guide how individuals within the organization behave and interact with each other…the adoption of structured approaches for executing these practices, such as tools, guidelines, and other implementation supports, reduce variability in how PFEC is delivered provider to provider, shift to shift, and day to day."

The remaining leadership recommendations — Lead by Example and Expect Setbacks and Remove Barriers — are explored in Chapter 7.

Chapter 7: Recommendations to Lead by Example and Expect Setbacks

A Breakthrough Moment for a Palliative Care Physician

Dr. Angelo was a physician champion for the implementation of a person-centered decision-making program. Despite her extensive training in palliative care and effective communication skills, she attended and actively participated in the communication skills courses and implementation meetings. After a year of implementation, a "Share the Experience" event was organized for over 50 team members who had participated in the initial waves of implementation. Participants passionately conveyed personal experiences facilitating person-centered decision-making conversations and implementation challenges and barriers.

Dr. Angelo relayed her experience with a patient who she had taken care of for years. Despite the patient's serious illness, he was unable or unwilling to voice his preferences for future healthcare in the event of complications. Dr. Angelo emotionally revealed that she had finally had a breakthrough moment with this challenging patient. Using one of her newfound communication techniques, she uncovered the patient's fears that were preventing him from making healthcare decisions.

Leadership Recommendation #6: Lead by Example

Leaders who understand the innovation, actively engage in the implementation, and experience the impact on their personal and professional lives, have compelling real-life stories to propagate. Storytelling is an irreplaceable communication strategy to lead by example. Stories help frame the problem, the reason for the innovation, and the emotional impact of the work (or not doing the work). Stories resonate and motivate when metrics are not yet available.

The messages in the opening story were clear. If this skilled palliative care physician could learn a new skill and improve her communication techniques, then everyone could. The physician actively engaged in the innovation, understood, and embraced it. This single story was likely the motivation that some individuals needed to persevere and that others needed to join the initiative.

The development of personal skills is a powerful strategy to lead by example. Participating in person-centered decision-making conversations for a family member provides a unique opportunity to "walk the walk" and understand the imperative for system-wide improvements.

"What if my Dad was not there when my mom needed a decision-maker?"

Dr. Carole Montgomery, who, at the time was one of the administrative leads at an organization implementing RC, was personally transformed through her own example. Carole — now the executive medical director for RC — invested in PCDM activity for her mother, Ann, who was 83 years old with progressive dementia and a platelet disorder. Her father, Jerry, was dutifully taking care of Ann, transporting her for regular platelet transfusions and keeping track of her platelet count. He eventually sent an email to his physician daughter asking, "How will all of this turn out?" Ann's hematologist had attempted to allay Jerry's worries, saying, "Don't worry, Ann will be fine. You can call me anytime, and we can decide what to do." That answer did not feel comforting to Carole or her dad. Carole arranged for an ACP conversation for her and Jerry. Although Ann was unable to participate in the conversation, Jerry brought a picture of her to the conversation and introduced Ann to the facilitator. For Carole, the meeting was "transformative…. we left with clarity around [Ann's] joys and priorities and how those would form the basis for future decisions."

On reflection of what mattered most to Ann, Jerry was able to articulate her goals: to be free from being afraid, to avoid having things done to her, to be free from being in strange surroundings, and to avoid treatments that would not improve her quality of life. Several months later, Jerry had the confidence to make decisions that were aligned with these goals. Finding her unconscious on the bedroom floor, he directed the medical decisions: there would be no IVs, extensive diagnostic testing, or neurosurgical consult. He agreed to a CT scan that demonstrated a subdural hematoma with a midline shift. Ann was moved to hospice and died a week later. Dr. Montgomery poses a question at the end of this story [paraphrasing]: I am still haunted by the experience. What if my dad was not there when my mom fell? What if he could not be so assertive? What if the healthcare providers had not listened?

Dr. Montgomery told this story time and again to various audiences. It was a powerful testament to the person-centered decision-making programs being implemented. She validated the stress on family members of patients who had serious illness and were unable to make their own healthcare decisions. She personally experienced the same person-centered decision-making conversations she had asked others to learn how to deliver. Beyond the personal engagement, she reflected on the gaps that may exist for other patients and families — gaps that would go unattended without systematic implementation and integration of strategies for all.

Leading by example can be accomplished in sundry ways, to include asking employees to participate in their own advance care planning, conducting employee attitude or knowledge surveys, establishing employee ACP clinics, including an ACP activity as a component of a health prevention or wellness program, and offering opportunities for physicians and advanced practitioners to share their experiences with other peers.

**Leadership Recommendation #7: Expect
Setbacks and Remove Barriers**

Numerous implementation barriers have been introduced throughout this Part of the book to prepare leaders for the natural and recurring challenges encountered during cultural transformation. Setting the expectation that barriers will be encountered and resolved helps build resilience in the team.

While many implementations experience "bumps in the road," some were a complete surprise. I never experienced a single implementation that did not struggle or was not faced with the need to identify a barrier and regroup. Organizations that are strong and have great leaders will identify the reason for the glitches, regroup, and become stronger. The missteps will be openly acknowledged, examined, and resolved.

"View bumps as gifts that force you to regroup."

An executive of a large integrated health system whose CEO had made a financial investment in implementing the RC PCDM programs was designated as the administrative lead. The implementation team was hired and began working with the RC consultant. Within several months, concerns about the progress of the team were identified and discussed with the executive lead. It was proposed that implementation halt until there was a resolution of the following concerns: 1) the lack of clarity around the roles and responsibilities of the program leaders, 2) inadequate follow through on recommendations, and 3) lack of visible leadership support.

The executive might have been offended, been irritated, adamantly disagreed — or a variety of other off-putting reactions — and ignored these concerns. Instead, the executive listened and led the team to re-engage and develop a new plan to get back on track. An investigation into the talent and capabilities of the implementation team revealed gaps, the need to create clear roles, responsibilities, and accountabilities. There was a change in personnel and commitment to complete action plans in a timely manner. The executive vowed to increase involvement by participating in monthly consultation calls, attending onsite meetings, and getting regular updates from the RC consultant on progress, barriers, and challenges. Importantly, the executive created a communication strategy with other organizational leaders to keep the program visible to those not intimately involved.

Implementation of First, Next, and Advanced Steps ACP programs proceeded successfully. In retrospect, this leader was able to view the implementation setback as a gift that allowed the team to regroup and the leaders to become fully engaged.

Another common "bump in the road" is the realization that the work is hard, complex, and takes time. Hearing comments such as, "We didn't think it would be this hard," and "We just don't have the time," were familiar refrains. Of course, any cultural transformation will take years, requiring leaders to communicate this reality in their vision and strategic plans. Real results require real work. Cultural change is not a project. It is a long-term commitment. Leaders who understand and communicate this reality will provide reassurance to those when the work gets hard.

However, during implementation of a complex innovation, it is important to prepare for some natural inclination to withdraw and return to the familiar conditions that were not working but were familiar. This "push and pull" of cultural change is to be expected. Factors that push individuals toward change include their excitement over the innovation and diffusion strategies, such as storytelling. Factors that pull individuals from the change and cause them to resist it include habits, comfort, and group dynamics.

Even when we desire change, we may remain skeptical as it requires us to trust the process, trust others who may not have the expertise we have, and trust that we will be better off in the end. Group dynamics are a powerful factor in resistance to change. The actions of a few individuals — those who underperform or refuse to learn new skills — can thwart forward progress and will demand leadership attention and resolution. Underperformance that is tolerated for too long becomes a habit. And habits are difficult to address. There are situations that demand that leaders recognize and act against resistors who impact forward progress.

One program initiative was getting significant pushback from the clinical ethicist from the workgroup assigned to redesign the advance directive document. It was delaying the ability to move forward with implementation. The leaders listened to the concerns, provided education and rationale for the changes, and scheduled consultation time with RC faculty. In the end, the leaders had to recognize that one individual was creating unnecessary conflict. They took the issue to a higher level for support to help realign one person's views with the agenda of the initiative.

Summary

Leaders who make a promise to build a culture of person-centered decision-making must understand why this is a worthy investment, understand how to navigate the stages of cultural change, and demonstrate actions that promote program dissemination and sustainability. This Part has illustrated lessons learned from *one* leader of *one* person-centered decision-making program: sharing examples, stories, and recommendations from organizations and communities around the country.

I have witnessed profound leadership acts of courage and disruption. The theory of Disruptive Innovation describes these exceptional individuals. Disruptive innovation "exists to disrupt and refresh every part of life that is not accurately or efficiently serving people's needs. And that's why people are called to do it. They cannot stand the status quo." The Tribeca Disruptive Innovation awards are intended to applaud such leaders: "The awards focus on breakthroughs occurring at the intersection of technology and culture where frequent clashes and resistance to change impede social progress and solutions for some of the world's most vexing problems."

In 2015, Bud and I gratefully received the Tribeca Disruptive Innovation award for our work at Respecting Choices. Still, the real heroes are the multiple disruptors we partnered with from around the world that have led the implementation of person-centered decision-making at their organizations, in their communities, within their respective programs, and in their personal lives. They are the true disruptors whose actions are contagious and give us hope that person-centered care will be more than an aspiration. As Harvey Picker said to all champions of person-centered care days before he died, "Carry on."

Personal Exercises

1) What experiences have informed your leadership skills?

2) How would you describe your organization's or community's vision and strategic plan to create a person-centered decision-making culture?

3) Describe the leadership engagement strategies that you have found effective.

4) What barriers to program implementation have you experienced?

Chapter 8: The History and Evolution of the Respecting Choices Program: A Personal and Professional Journey

As trailblazers of a national program, Dr. Bernard Hammes ("Bud") and I experienced our own leadership journey, dissemination challenges, and evolution. A historical review of this journey gives context to the dynamic state of the program, exposes salient lessons, successes, and misgivings uncovered along the way, and provides a context for leadership recommendations. This is more than a personal journey. The experiences were often analogous to the challenges I observed in leaders who implemented the program within their organization or community. Naturally, the RC program and its leaders continue to learn, evolve, and adapt.

The Innovation: Why Was Dissemination Important?

After the publication of the La Crosse Advance Directive Study (LADS) in 1998,[1] Gundersen Lutheran received inquiries from folks around the country, requesting assistance and replication of the variables that had led to the success of the La Crosse implementation. People were hungry for improved advance care planning outcomes. Despite policies enacted as a result of the Patient Self-determination Act, the data on the completion of advance directives remained deplorably low. The outcomes from the LADS study were too impressive to ignore — to wonder if these results could be achieved in other healthcare organizations and communities. Many organizations and communities were focused on increasing the prevalence of advance directives.

For me, the program had more capacious hopes than increasing the prevalence of advance directives. I was drawn to the vision for advance care planning that Bud articulated — a vision that represented what I felt was missing in all the ethical dilemmas I had witnessed as a critical care nurse specialist and consultant. This vision fueled my passion to participate. To be part of a movement that would help the masses, heal wounds, relieve pain and suffering, and help me be the patient advocate I had envisioned when I went into nursing. The vision seemed so clear and simple, yet proved to be so complex.

Bud's vision for advance care planning — a vision I recanted during the presentation of his life-time achievement award at the RC National Share the Experience conference in 2018 — stretched far beyond the goal to increase the number of advance directives. The vision included novel beliefs about the power of ACP:

- ACP is more than patient autonomy, more than individual self-determination. Inherent in the very definition of "patient" is the inclusion of family as defined by each individual. We never felt compelled to include the word "family" in our definition of person-centered decision-making. It was an innate characteristic.

- ACP is focused on how we care for those we love. I was reminded of this fact every time Bud told the story of how he was responsible for making healthcare decisions for his mother, afflicted with dementia. His approach extended beyond specific decisions that were needed, such as a feeding tube, CPR, whether routine mammograms would be continued, or where his mother would be cared for. His approach was intent on answering the question, "What would a loving son do?" I heard him emotionally tell this story a hundred times.

- ACP is about the conversation, not the completion of a document. This conversation later became labeled as "person-centered" to include conversations about current as well as future healthcare decisions.

- For ACP to be effective, systems must be created or redesigned that make it easier for busy people to do the "right" thing, to change behaviors, to embed practices as the standard of care, and transform the healthcare culture.

- The ultimate outcome of ACP and person-centered decision-making interventions is to produce evidence that an individual's healthcare preferences and decisions are honored; that concordant care is delivered, which is the essence of person-centered care.

This vision of the power of advance care planning as a pathway "to know and honor individual preferences and decisions" occurred amidst a national dialogue on death and dying.

National Events that Spurred Program Disseminations

The 1990s sparked new conversations for Americans about death and dying. The Patient Self-determination Act (PSDA), stimulated by the case of Nancy Cruzan, promised to give Americans autonomy over their end-of-life decisions. Debates over physician-assisted suicide spurred controversy and dissent. In 1995, the results of the largest investigation examining end-of-life care, the Study to Understand Prognoses and Preferences for Outcomes and Risks of Treatment (SUPPORT), was published, revealing a disappointing picture of end-of-life care. This study was instrumental in launching the Robert Wood Johnson funded campaign, Last Acts, to improve care of people at the end of their lives and included the Means to a Better End report.

Each of these events, among others, provided the context and craving for a person-centered decision-making program that had demonstrated success in one midwestern community.

An Opportunity to Fulfill the Spirit of the Patient Self-determination Act?

In December of 1991, the Patient Self-Determination Act (PSDA) — an amendment to the Medicare and Medicaid Social Security Act — took effect. This federal law mandated that all hospitals, skilled nursing facilities, home health agencies, hospice programs, and health maintenance organizations institute policies that would ensure that a patient's right to self-determination in healthcare decisions be communicated and protected. Competent adults, age eighteen and older, have the right to decide what medical treatments they receive.

Specifically, the PSDA requires organizations to 1) inform patients of their rights to make medical decisions, 2) inquire if patients had completed an advance directive and documented preferences, 3) not discriminate against those that had completed documents, 4) ensure that legally valid advance directives be implemented, and 5) educate patients, staff and the community on issues related to advance directive document completion. States were required to create and implement laws on the use of advance directives and address such variables as who can be appointed as a surrogate decision-maker, and the extent of their authority to make life-sustaining treatment decisions. When the PSDA was enacted, the incidence of advance directive completion was 4-20 %.[2]

An implicit goal of the PSDA was to increase communication between patients and their healthcare providers, specifically in the area of end-of-life decision-making. However, the PSDA did not specify or allocate resources for communication skills programs, public education, the integration of preferences into clinical decision-making, the needs of the pediatric population, or how to ensure that the written advance directive truly represents an individuals' goals, values, preferences, and decisions.

Consequently, organizations focused their efforts on compliance with the letter of the law rather than the spirit of improved communication. As a clinical manager during this time, I helped develop organizational policies to comply with the PSDA. I was initially excited about the potential of this Act to promote communication and help patients receive care that aligned with their goals and values. We instituted the standard admission questions: "Do you have an advance directive?" and "Would you like information?" I quickly realized these questions would do little to support person-centered decision-making.

In their efforts to comply with the PSDA, healthcare organizations regrettably got started on the wrong foot, resulting in a culture that, for years, became fixated on a document rather than a process of decision-making. After a decade of implementation of the PSDA, the prevalence of completed documents did not substantively increase; those that were completed were incomplete, ambiguous, did not reflect an individual's goals and values, and did not assist in clinical decision-making when needed.

We saw an opportunity to fulfill the spirit of the PSDA. We believed the country was ripe for a different approach — one that would shift from a focus on a document to a process of person-centered decision-making.

An Answer to the Disappointing Results from the SUPPORT Study?

The Study to Understand Prognosis and Preferences for Outcomes and Risks of Treatment was published in 1995, the largest research study conducted on end-of-life care to date.[3] The goal of this study was to improve end of life decision-making and decrease the use of life-sustaining treatments in hospitalized patients with one or more of nine life-threatening illnesses and an overall mortality rate of 47%. The study enrolled over nine thousand patients in five teaching hospitals in the United States.

Phase I of the study collected data on the characteristics of the dying process in the stated populations. Less than 50% of physicians knew their patient's

CPR preference; 46% of DNR orders were written within two days of a patient's death; over 1/3 of patients spent ten days or more in an ICU, and over 50% reported moderate to severe pain.

Phase II of the study involved an intervention where physicians were informed of their patients' outcomes for survival and CPR; trained nurses conducted multiple conversations with patients, family, physicians, and others to elicit preferences, provide information on treatment outcomes, attend to pain issues, and improve overall patient/physician communication. This multi-million-dollar funded intervention did not improve outcomes in communication, or any other substantive metric, such as number of days in the ICU and use of hospital resources near end-of-life. The study concluded that communication alone was insufficient to change the routines of care.

I recall viewing recorded video taped conversations from the SUPPORT study's trained nurse interventionists. During one conversation with an individual with advanced heart disease, the nurse invited the individual to consider whether he wanted CPR if his heart stopped. The nurse had a wonderful bedside manner, was empathic, patient, engaged emotion and developed a relationship. However, there were notable gaps in her ability to assist the individual in making an informed decision. She did not provide information on the benefits, burdens, or side effects of CPR, nor did she elicit the patient's values.

This study revealed the magnitude of designing systems to support a person-centered decision-making culture and elevated the value of skilled communication techniques during decision-making conversations.

A Means to a Better End: Momentum from The Last Acts Campaign?

The Robert Woods Johnson Foundation launched Last Acts, a multi-million-dollar national campaign dedicated to improving communication about end-of-life, changing the culture of health care institutions, and changing American culture and attitudes toward death. Among its program efforts in 2002, Last Acts, it published Means to a Better End, a report on dying in America, spearheaded by national experts in palliative care, spirituality, pain management, and healthcare system management.[4]

The report attempted to provide a state-by-state report card on selected outcome measures such as state policies on advance directives, proportion of a state's deaths that occur at home, use of hospice, the presence of palliative care services, and the number of elderly who spent a week or more in an intensive care unit during the last six months of life. The report revealed that "...Americans at best have no better than a fair chance of finding good care for their loved ones or for themselves when facing a life-threatening illness. In most states, too few patients are accessing hospice and palliative care services, there are too few professionals trained in pain management and palliative care, and there are too many patients dying in hospitals and nursing homes — in pain — rather than at home with their families."

The report also identified statewide coalitions and partnerships in 30 states who, working to improve quality of end-of-life care, created four main goals for their activities: improve advance care planning, improve pain management, improve care coordination, and increase the demand for and access to high-quality care at the end-of-life.

The RC person-centered decision-making programs offered a pathway to assist coalitions and partnerships in addressing their advance care planning goals.

In summary, the country was ready for solutions that could address perplexing issues surrounding care at the end-of-life. I had "drunk the Kool-Aid" and naively forged ahead, believing that the power of the RC person-centered decision-making programs would be so apparent, so convincing, that it would be easily replicated across the country within five years...did I have a lot to learn.

Early Dissemination Efforts

Bud and I began the process of learning how to transfer the success of RC in La Crosse, Wisconsin, to other places in the United States and beyond. The RC program transferred to Australia in 2002, health systems in Canada starting in 2004, a German research project in 2007, and to Singapore in 2009.

In 2000, we offered the first national course, "Organization and Community Advance Care Planning," to assist participants to learn the skills of advance care planning, educate professionals and community, and design effective organization/community systems to support quality outcomes with the following program description:

> Since 1993, the La Crosse advance care planning program has demonstrated success in implementing a community program that incorporates all the area's major healthcare systems, develops effective partnerships with other professional groups and organizations, and is committed to consistent educational materials, training and practices. (Arch. Intern. Med., Feb. 23, 1998) The lessons learned, and skills enhanced from this endeavor are being shared with other interested communities and organizations.
>
> Through this curriculum, critical strategies will be presented that will facilitate the replication and individualization of the La Crosse experience. Inherent in achieving successful outcomes in implementing an organization and community-wide advance care planning program is the commitment and expertise of dedicated instructors and leaders.
>
> Through the course, participants will receive specific guidance on how to organize and teach the Respecting Choices® Advance Care Planning Course for Facilitators and how to develop effective implementation strategies for organization and community

success. For those who intend to teach the Facilitators' course in their community, an Instructor Certification component is added to ensure competency in advance care planning education. Each team or individual will have an opportunity to begin to design an individualized implementation work plan for his or her own organization and/or community.

The first two days of the Organization and Community course centered on the Advance Care Planning Course for Facilitators; day three described the leadership and systems required to create an effective ACP program and cultural change. Day four was the Instructor Course that certified participants to replicate the ACP Course for Facilitators and learn their role as mentors for system-wide change and ongoing monitoring. The objectives of this four-day program were robust and, as I reflect on them now, unrealistic:

- Complete the objectives of the Respecting Choices Advance Care Planning Course for Facilitators

- Describe the necessary system changes in implementing an organization and community-wide advance care planning program

- Discuss organizational principles of implementation

- Assess organizational barriers and develop strategies to overcome

- Develop strategies for improving professional skills in advance care planning

- Develop strategies for developing partnerships and educating the community

- Discuss strategies to manage resources and systems

- Develop continuous quality improvement strategies to monitor ongoing improvement

- Participate in the development of a specific organization/community implementation plan

- Participate in dialogue regarding personal and ethical issues relative to end-of-life treatment decisions

From approximately 2000-2005, this four-day program was offered in over 32 organizations or communities. We traveled across the United States, from small communities such as Enumclaw, Washington, to statewide initiatives, such as the Foundation for Healthy Communities.

These educational events promoted the program and assisted in "word of mouth" dissemination. Dissemination of the RC program took additional pathways, to include participation in a Last Acts initiative, onsite media visits, and collaboration with other leaders.

- A Last Acts Initiative

  A Last Acts Initiative of the Robert Wood Johnson Foundation helped to jump-start our dissemination goals. This initiative first vetted a list of programs or interventions that communities might use to improve end-of-life care. It then offered $12,000 to communities who applied and agreed to use one of the vetted programs, which included Respecting Choices.

  In a Last Acts summary of the programs that participated in this program: "Partners realized many benefits; support and reinforcement from others in the field; and legitimacy with their members and boards."[5]

- Media Exposure

Following publications and implementation experiences, a variety of journalists traveled to La Crosse, WI, to talk to local healthcare providers and community residents, observe decision-making conversations with patients and their families, and conduct interviews. These activities produced video (e.g., CBS, Good Morning America, NBC nightly news), audio (National Public Radio), and print (Washington Post, The New York Times) reports.

With confidence in what investigators would discover, these reports assisted in the independent dissemination of the impact of the program to a broad audience. We trusted the experiences that we made accessible to journalists, to include observations and videotaping of the facilitation of person-centered decision-making conversations with real patients and their families, or a reporter who went door to door in La Crosse to hear what people knew and felt about Respecting Choices.

These media outlet onsite visits were not scripted, nor did we have "control" over what they chose to report. However, I have always cringed at an ABC news report that referred to La Crosse as "The Cheapest Place to Die in America."[6] This was not the message we wanted to deliver, especially given concerns that ACP was an effort to withhold expensive treatments from patients.

- Consultation Efforts

There were multiple attempts to consult with national and international leaders interested in developing or improving their respective programs. Extensive education and consultation were provided to several groups in the U.S., Canada, and other countries. Onsite consultations were designed for leaders of other programs that included observations, sharing of tools and strategies, and recommendations.

We hoped that these collaborations might lead to partnerships where our programs would be nationally recognized and sustained. While these consultations did not always result in implementation partnerships, they continued to promote the principles of person-centered decision-making. These consultations and our recommendations advanced and improved the quality of related programs.

Program Evolution

Throughout the early years of dissemination, valuable lessons were learned that spurred program improvements, such as the creation of a compelling vision and strategic alignment, designing partnerships for implementation, strategies for leadership engagement and ongoing sustainability, and collaboration efforts.

Vision Setting & Strategic Alignment

The national interest in replicating the success of the local RC program prompted the development of a vision that was focused on advance care planning (rather than person-centered decision-making). For years, the program was marketed as: "Respecting Choices: An Advance Care Planning System that Works." This "vision" assimilated several seminal messages: the shift from a focus on advance directives to advance care planning; the need for systems to embed new practices as a standard of care; and evidence that this approach is effective.

In 2017, Gundersen Medical Foundation transferred the RC program to a newly created, non-profit 501(c)3 organization, C-TAC Innovations, which is an affiliate of C-TAC (Coalition to Transform Advanced Care).[7]

This transition provided an opportunity to communicate an updated and historically accurate vision — a vision that articulated the power of ACP as a person-centered decision-making strategy that facilitates person-centered care. A rebranding of the program was launched with a change in the tagline from "Respecting Choices: An Advance Care Planning System that Works" to "Respecting Choices: A System for Person-Centered Decision-Making that Transforms Healthcare."

The current vision and mission statements — as of this publication — are stated as follows:

> Mission: Guide organizations and communities worldwide to effectively implement and sustain evidence-based systems that provide person-centered care
>
> Vision: Transform healthcare culture by integrating and disseminating best practices to achieve person-centered care

The updated statements reflect a commitment to provide mentorship in implementing evidence-based systems, to use these systems and best practices to provide person-centered care, and ultimately, to change the healthcare culture. Despite these revised communication efforts, the program was often regrettably referred to as "the advance directive program."

The authentic vision of the RC programs, "To know and honor individual preferences and decisions," is the most compelling and enduring. It was envisioned from the beginning, when the program began as a "pilot" study in the renal dialysis unit following a series of tough decisions faced by patients contemplating the withdrawal of hemodialysis. The original description of the La Crosse RC program articulated the potential power of advance care planning efforts. The first ACP facilitator manual offered the following description:

> To achieve this goal (families knowing the patient's preferences), the program creates the opportunity and atmosphere for renal patients, their loved ones, and select staff to examine and discuss the patient's values and preferences regarding life-sustaining medical treatment at a time when the patient can participate. While this activity may lead to the signing of "living wills" or advance directives, the primary goal of the program is to deepen awareness, to increase discussion, and to improve communication.

Simon Sinek, a British-American author and motivational speaker who studied the characteristics of influential leaders, designed the Golden Circle as a framework for leaders to inspire and motivate people to change. How leaders think, act, and communicate is pivotal for organizational success. Sinek describes his observations of inspirational leaders in a communication and leadership framework he calls "The Golden Circle."

Based on biology, the Golden Circle has three rings of influence. The outer ring is the WHAT and refers to a product or service. The middle ring, the HOW, explains how the product or service is different from others on the market. The inner circle, the WHY, is what a company or organization believes. Inspirational leaders communicate from the inside out rather than the outside in. The impact of this communication strategy is based on the biology of the human brain. The HOW and WHY circles are controlled by the emotional part of the brain — the limbic system — responsible for feelings and resultant human behavior. The WHAT circle is controlled by the neocortex, responsible for language and rational thought.

In applying Sinek's Golden Circle concept to the RC person-centered decision-making programs, the WHAT is often communicated. RC is a person-centered decision-making system to help transform the delivery of healthcare. It is supported by research and practice-based evidence. The HOW includes consultation to integrate the five design elements (leadership, systems design, education and certification, community engagement, and continuous quality improvement) as the framework for building a culture of person-centered decision-making.

But the WHY is the most important. The WHY — "to know and honor individual preferences and decisions" — has always been at the heart of the program. It is the authentic vision as it explains "why" the program should be implemented as opposed to the "what" the program aims to achieve.

Strategic Alignment

For more than 18 years, the national RC program was supported by the Gundersen Medical Foundation, dedicated to medical education, multi-faceted research, and community outreach activities to improve community health. This alignment was more practical than "strategic." Still, it allowed the program to be supported long enough to demonstrate its ability to be disseminated, prove community interest, and continue quality improvement and research interests. Resources remained slim; Bud and I were a two-person team.

To improve efficiency and provide additional resources, the RC program was transitioned to the Bereavement Department, nationally recognized for its "Resolve Through Sharing" strategies that provide training and materials to improve care for patients and families experiencing loss through dying and death. This alignment allowed for shared resources and the ability to hire the first business development person and team coordinator.

Support for dissemination of a national program within a healthcare organization had benefits and burdens. The legal, marketing, and program development resources of the organization were valuable. The healthcare organization and community furnished program leaders with a "living laboratory" where new ideas could be tested prior to development and dissemination. The burdens included conflicting commitments to achieving the vision of the program as well organizational human resources regulations.

It was mutually decided to investigate the options to affiliate with an outside organization whose vision was aligned with RC and could support ongoing dissemination. In 2017, the program transitioned to the Coalition to Transform Advanced Care (C-TAC) — a coalition of national organizations from the healthcare sector, patient advocacy and consumer groups, and faith and community leaders, dedicated to ensuring that Americans with advanced illness receive care that is consistent with their values and honors their dignity. Respecting Choices is a division of C-TAC Innovations, an affiliate of C-TAC, devoted to implementing delivery systems for advanced illness.

This strategic alignment offered the promise of increased collaboration and partnerships with national organizations, initiatives, and leaders.

Implementation Partnerships

Education alone does not change behavior or result in cultural transformation. The four-day Organization and Community Advance Care Planning course exposed hundreds of healthcare professionals, community leaders, and those developing person-centered care innovations to the principles of person-centered decision-making. The program was consistently well received, but there was no follow-up to assist with implementation, and it gradually became obvious that long-term sustainability was not being achieved.

In 2002 and 2003, an informal survey was conducted of individuals from organizations and communities who had attended the four-day course in the previous years. The intent of the survey was to gain insight into follow-up actions and major accomplishments that had been stimulated by attendance at the four-day course.

This unscientific survey revealed that the majority of actions were focused on education: replicating the ACP facilitation course, employee, or professional staff in-services, and community presentations and engagement activities to include the development of written materials to increase awareness of ACP. A few organizations had worked on their internal systems, such as creating a consistent place in the medical record to store advance directives or revising an existing advance directive document.

There was minimal reporting of the development of formal implementation teams being organized to create a systematic approach to ACP for all patients. Many attempts to integrate ACP into the clinical setting were unsuccessful: "We attempted to implement ACP at the cancer care center with limited interest and results."

Despite the popularity of the four-day program, it did not result in consistent replication of the RC programs, a goal we had hoped to accomplish. ACP practices improved; systems design work began; people became more skilled at person-centered decision-making conversations. But too many organizations or communities eventually abandoned the materials and educational strategies developed or created their own programs.

A consultative approach was created to assist organizations and communities to implement, disseminate, and sustain program changes.

Respecting Choices Multi-Year Consultation Services: A Description

To assist an organization or community through the stages of implementation of one or more of the person-centered decision-making programs, a formal partnership between RC and a customer (typically an organization or community initiative) is created to support the multiple stages of change. A Senior Faculty consultant mentors and supports the designated leaders over several months or years, depending on the specific program(s) implemented and organizational goals. The terms of the partnership are negotiated to allow for customization, cultural assessment, resources, among other variables. The implementation partnerships consist of a set of services — person-centered decision-making communication certification courses, system design resources and education, community engagement materials, decision aids — and ongoing phone, email, and onsite consultation to support the implementation strategies.

The continuous quality improvement model is integrated into these partnerships, using this familiar approach to design and test implementation strategies before they are widely disseminated. These "tests of change" occur through the selection and preparation of implementation teams or sites who are assisted in designing a targeted population approach focused on creating a standard of care that is tested over a six-month period, including the collection and monitoring of process metrics. These implementation periods — or "waves" of implementation — are used to evaluate and improve the new or redesigned systems, materials, and workflows for replication and dissemination.

The structure and content of the implementation partnerships continue to evolve to meet customer needs and desire for program flexibility and to address a criticism of the RC person-centered decision-making programs, which has been its prescriptive approach to implementation. Through ongoing experience and research, greater customization is encouraged, and the implementation partnerships are mutually designed.

This "freedom within a framework" allows for the tested principles of system design to be adapted to the culture of the organization and community, its strengths, challenges, and resources. The skills-based communication certification courses remain standardized to ensure the integrity of these educational offerings, a concept like CPR or Advanced Cardiac Life Support (ACLS) certification courses. Competency validation and certification principles ensure fidelity to a consistent approach to PCDM conversations.

Collaboration

A renewed and revised commitment to collaboration continues.[8] The RC leadership team searches for opportunities to collaborate with organizations, programs, researchers, and others to promote person-centered decision-making and improve dissemination. For example, RC has part-nered with Wiser Care to increase scalability of ACP conversations: "The strategic partnership features the first-ever Respecting Choices-certified digital approach compatible with First Steps® ACP, which Wiser Care will offer to customers through its enterprise suite of online ACP experiences and tools for individuals, families, healthcare agents and care teams."

A collaboration with the Center to Advance Palliative Care (CAPC) resulted in the dissemination of the Respecting Choices online course, "Building Physician Skills in Basic Advance Care Planning."[9] Additionally, Respecting Choices and six other partners are collaborating on a three-year grant on "Building Public Engagement and Access to Palliative & End-of-Life Care for Persons Living with Serious Illness," sponsored by the John A. Hartford and Cambia Health Foundations.[10]

Through program evolution and new leadership, one objective remains constant as RC leaders continue to disseminate person-centered deci-sion-making strategies: to integrate this innovation as a pathway to person-centered care.

Part Three

Chapter 9: The Promise of System Redesign in Building a Culture of Person-Centered Decision-Making

Honoring an Individual's Request for DNR

Jonathan, a 72-year-old man with a history of heart disease, expressed assistance with advance care planning (ACP) offered during his annual physical appointment. We scheduled a First Steps ACP conversation at his convenience, and we met in the education center of the hospital clinic.

Jonathan came to the appointment alone but had reviewed the preparatory information mailed to him on choosing a healthcare agent and announced that his wife and eldest son had agreed to be his first and second choice, respectively. Jonathan had been battling heart disease for over a decade, surviving two heart attacks, a cardiac angioplasty, and several hospitalizations. He was enrolled in the Heart Failure clinic, where his medications and lifestyle were adjusted and monitored.

As we began to explore his understanding of cardiopulmonary resuscitation (CPR), he instantly stated, "I have taken care of that issue," and pulled out a necklace from under his shirt with "DNR" (Do-Not-Resuscitate) inscribed on the pendant. He had ordered the necklace from the local pharmacy, proud that he had taken steps to ensure he would not receive CPR if his heart stopped. He had not discussed this decision with his primary physician, cardiologist, or the staff at the Heart Failure clinic.

Overview

If Jonathan has a cardiac arrest in a public place and Emergency Medical Services (EMS) are called to respond, would (or should) it be considered a medical error if CPR is attempted? Do healthcare administrators, healthcare physicians and providers, care management coordinators, policymakers, and community resources bear any responsibility to ensure Jonathan's preferences are honored?

People inherently want their goals, values, and preferences to be communicated and respected. Jonathan's intent in wearing a DNR necklace was unmistakable to him, but he was unaware that system barriers would prevent his decision from being automatically honored by all healthcare providers. Wisconsin state statute requires a specific physician's order and standardized language and format for a DNR bracelet.

If paramedics saw Jonathan's DNR necklace, they would have no authority to follow the inscription, although they may be conflicted when attempting resuscitation against his expressed preference. Jonathan's care management team had not discussed or understood his CPR decision or provided information on obtaining a state-sanctioned DNR bracelet. The community-based pharmacy resources were uninformed of Wisconsin law or the impact of Jonathon's request for a DNR necklace. These system failures resulted in Jonathan's false sense of security that his DNR decision would be honored.

Unfortunately, Jonathan's situation is not an isolated event. The New England Journal of Medicine published a case report of a 70-year old man brought to the hospital unconscious, heavily intoxicated with alcohol, and with dropping blood pressure.[1] Healthcare providers ignored a DNR tattoo with his signature; in Florida, a DNR order must be recorded on a specific yellow form. The team requested a follow-up ethics consult, and after collecting further evidence of his wishes, obtained a Florida DNR order. In 2012, the Journal of General Internal Medicine reported that a team of doctors was placed in a similar position when they found a DNR tattoo on the chest of an unconscious patient.[2] They decided to resuscitate, a fortunate decision because when the man recovered, he admitted to having gotten the tattoo after losing a bet in a poker game.

The ability to know and honor an individuals' healthcare decisions is increasingly complex. It is often hindered by inadequate organization and interagency policies, federal and statutory regulations and restrictions, ambiguous, incomplete, or absent documentation systems, fragmentation of care, and the absence of a team approach to support the decision-making process. Building a culture of person-centered decision-making — and the success of the Respecting Choices program — is inextricably linked to the leadership commitment to design, and redesign, systems that make it easier for people to do the right thing; there are no quick fixes. Conversations, user-friendly documents, and public engagement campaigns alone do not ensure that an individuals' goals, values, preferences, and decisions will be known and honored.[3]

In a two-part webinar on "Advance Care Planning: Challenges and Opportunities," the National Academy of Medicine convened a panel of experts to discuss the state of ACP. Experts debated the ACP evidence base, the mixed intervention outcomes from systematic studies, and the lack of consistent metrics. They openly acknowledged the complex nature of the ACP process. Some panelists questioned the value of further invest-ment in ACP research and expressed frustration that so little has been accomplished in the last 30 years, despite the existence of various tools and interventions. In a brief but uplifting discussion of the practical steps to achieve ACP outcomes, a few speakers signaled the imperative to integrate systems that, for example, allow easier access and transparency of previ-ous conversations, clarity on decisions previously made, and document care concordance.[4]

Mildred Solomon, the President of the Hastings Center, a bioethicist and social science researcher, highlighted the necessity for increased "account-ability and obligations" of healthcare organizations to create multifaceted systems to deliver person-centered care.[5] Although there was no consensus on the core systems requisite to promote person-centered decision-making, the panelists agreed that more can be done to enhance ACP efforts.

For example, Scott Halperin, a panelist and critical care physician and professor at the University of Pennsylvania Perelman School of Medicine, credited the role of ACP in improving care concordance, stating that when goals are documented, the rate of care concordance is high. Dr. Halperin also acknowledged the need to resolve flaws in the evaluation of ACP effectiveness and inadequacies of system implementation.

Until and unless the core systems are identified, funded, regulated, and evaluated, ACP and shared decision-making (SDM) efforts will fall short of achieving their full impact in delivering person-centered care. Respecting Choices has consistently been a leader in the design, and redesign, of systems that promote person-centered decision-making, beginning in the early 1990s with the local La Crosse AD program and evolving through decades of implementation experience with organizations and communities in the U.S. and in other countries, and research partnerships.

Creating a comprehensive system that promotes a culture of person-centered decision-making is the focus of this book. Different chapters describe the various "microsystems" — leadership, education, consumer engagement, research and continuous quality improvement — that work synergistically to produce successful outcomes. In this Part, we'll dive deeper into how four specific microsystems — leadership, planning documents, medical record storage and retrieval, and the interdependence of the healthcare team — created early in the implementation of an ACP or SDM program assist in forming the building blocks for ongoing improvement and widespread dissemination. We'll conclude this Part in Chapter 14 by revisiting the opening story and applying the principles of system redesign to improve the ability "to know and honor" Jonathan's DNR preference.

While many of the microsystem examples are specific to ACP implementation, the principles are applied to SDM programs when applicable.

The Magnitude of Microsystem Design

The application of systems thinking to organizational improvement is fundamentally grounded in research and field expertise.[6] A component of systems thinking is the design of microsystems that seamlessly work to "hardwire excellence" into an organization's culture. What are microsystems, and how do they influence cultural change? Why did the RC program embrace microsystem development as the building blocks in the successful implementation of person-centered decision-making programs?

Microsystems are defined as "...a small group of people who work together on a regular basis to provide care to discrete subpopulations of patients. It has clinical and business aims, linked processes, and a shared information environment, and it produces performance outcomes. Microsystems evolve over time and are often embedded in larger organizations. They are complex adaptive systems, and as such they must do the primary work associated with core aims, meet the needs of internal staff, and maintain themselves over time as clinical units."[7]

To gather insight into how adaptive systems are designed, a Dartmouth research team evaluated 20 high performing microsystems throughout the U.S. and Canada.[8] Using a qualitative research design, the study identified nine characteristics of effective microsystems that synergistically produce positive outcomes: leadership, culture, macro-system support, patient focus, staff focus, interdependence of care teams, information and information technology, process improvement, and performance patterns. In addition, four external features—financial, regulatory, policy, and market environments (features that cannot be resolved by a single organization or community)—influenced microsystem development.

Consistent with the characteristics of effective microsystems is the emergence of "design thinking," a research-rooted practical application of the processes involved in design which includes:

- a focus on individuals (person-centric)

- the acceptance of ambiguity

- redesign is inevitable

- effective communication to make ideas tangible to stakeholders[9]

In addition, design thinking requires personal attributes of "empathy, optimism, iteration, creative confidence, experimentation, and an embrace of ambiguity and failure."[10]

The dynamic nature of design fits seamlessly with my experiences implementing the RC principles of microsystem creation. For example, the original design of the "greensleeve," a plastic folder used to store advance directive information in the medical chart, served as an effective system to communicate and transfer ACP information to allow preferences and decisions to be honored. However, this storage system was redesigned when electronic platforms provided a more effective alternative. The principle of "storing and retrieving" did not change; the means to accomplish the intended outcome needed to adapt.

The Respecting Choices program understands the power of early microsystem creation as a foundational element in the implementation of ACP and SDM programs. Microsystems communicate mutual accountability, increase professional satisfaction, result in fewer missed opportunities, produce stories of effectiveness that motivate people to continue to change, and identify areas for improvement. The four microsystems described in the remainder of this Part are not a panacea for success but illustrate the influence of standardized tools and processes to create momentum for widespread dissemination and cultural change.

Chapter 10: Microsystem #1:
Leadership Expectations to "Grow" Microsystems
That Promote Person-Centered Decision-Making

Earlier we talked about a broad range of leadership principles in building a culture of person-centered decision-making, but the indispensable responsibility for leaders to "grow" essential microsystems deserves specificity. The leadership microsystem comprises a small and dedicated group of executive-level individuals who work together to promote person-centered decision-making, linking clinical and business aims and monitoring outcomes. These leaders set the expectations for *why* systems redesign is occurring, explain how progress will be measured and reported, and communicate a plan for dissemination.

> An overarching suggestion for senior leaders is to recognize the fundamental nature and power of using microsystem-based approaches for strategic thinking, operating excellence, and deployment of change and innovation. Using this framework to design care for defined patient populations will include building the finely tuned care processes, linking them, making them safe and reliable, and removing costs while adding quality. Moreover, it will incorporate shared purpose, cooperative leadership, performance goals derived from purpose, and mutual accountability for reaching goals and outcomes aligned with purpose. —Microsystems in Health Care: Part 1 [1]

A leadership microsystem is essential to combat the confounding barriers to the implementation of person-centered decision-making programs. The

literature documents persistent obstacles to widespread ACP implementation, including time constraints, competing demands, lack of perceived
value, scalability, the extent of organizational change required, lack of
resources, and lack of an electronic reporting system, among others.[2]

For example, recent research on the implementation of the POLST (portable
medical order) program in long-term care facilities exemplifies systemic
barriers to sustainable outcomes.[3] A study of POLST implementation in
40 Indiana nursing homes revealed that, while concordance in treatment
decisions was higher for residents with POLST than without (59.3% versus
34.9%), there remained a significant number (41%) of cases where care was
not concordant. The authors note, "The decision to implement POLST in
a nursing facility requires a commitment to ongoing education, changes
to policies and procedures, and quality improvement activities as well as a
philosophical shift about the role of resident preferences in guiding care."[4]

Like ACP, shared decision-making programs face countless implementation hurdles to include the absence of standardized workflows to ensure all
patients who desire SDM assistance receive it, lack of clinician understanding, awareness, and buy-in for SDM, and lack of organizational resources
and tools.[5] Recommendations to promote reliable and consistent SDM
practices include payment incentives for conversations, certification of
patient decision aids, support for policy changes to make SDM the standard
for the informed consent process, and acceleration of accreditation and
certification requirements for SDM skills.

As new tools, policies, and practices are created, the leadership team acts
strategically to "grow" these microsystems throughout an organization
and/or community and overcome resistance to change. A person-centered
decision-making leadership microsystem:

- Provides additional resources for implementing microsystems
  at the local level, for example, in one clinical area or target
  population or segment of the community. It takes time to recruit

and engage patients in ACP and SDM conversations requiring additional staff support. Health information technology resources need support to prioritize the creation of electronic health care (EHR) improvements.

- Communicates the mission for *why* new technology, practices, and policies are being created and tested with the expectation that the refined microsystems will be utilized by all members of the healthcare team and offered to all interested and engaged patients. Sending a few people to a skills-based educational program or developing a new form is inadequate for long-term success.

- Sets the expectations for improved outcomes by selecting a few simple metrics that can be routinely monitored, reported, and rewarded.

- Remains engaged in the implementation experience. Leaders who experience the impact of ACP or SDM conversations can disseminate personal stories that motivate participation and acceptance by others.

- Investigates opportunities to expand the microsystems to a broader community, understanding that healthcare is delivered in multiple care settings by diverse individuals. Incremental change in one organization will not result in widespread cultural change that impacts patients and families as they live in communities, receive healthcare in various locations, and are counseled by many professionals and well-meaning social groups.

A Person-Centered Decision-Making Leadership Microsystem Story

In a two-part webinar series on ACP organized by the National Academy of Medicine, Dr. Nina O'Connor, Chief Medical Officer of Penn Medicine, the University of Pennsylvania Health System, provides a stellar example of a leadership microsystem committed to implementing an SDM program.[6] The ultimate mission of the leadership team was to create a "safety net" to ensure that all patients with serious illness are offered SDM conversations, exploring three questions in the creation of an initial implementation plan:

1) Which patients will be initially targeted to have conversations? Analytics were used to identify high-risk patients with serious illness, and text messages were sent to their providers to remind them to initiate a conversation. The target population's *entire* healthcare team was educated in the skills of person-centered decision-making.

2) What outcomes will be expected, measured, and reported? The leadership team focused their measurement on the number of conversations completed rather than the number of planning documents completed. The goal was that 100% of patients in the high-risk category would have a documented "goals of care" conversation, and a dashboard was created to display and monitor improvement. Once these initial outcomes are achieved, the service would be expanded to all patients with serious illness.

3) How will these organization-wide objectives be met? The team identified the tools, education, and microsystems needed to support the original goal that all patients with serious illness are offered conversations.

Dr. O'Connor's example demonstrates the type of leadership strategies necessary to "grow" microsystems, strategies that lead to widespread dissemination and the delivery of a consistent person-centered decision-making service for all.

Chapter 11: Microsystem #2:
The Design or Redesign of Planning Documents

Poorly designed and completed planning documents, such as advance directives and POLST forms, often create barriers to a system's ability to allow transparency, communication, clarity, confidence, and ability to transfer an individual's goals, values, preferences, and decisions among all sites of care. A planning document microsystem is tasked with analyzing the organization's and communities existing documents and looking for opportunities to improve their effectiveness in guiding person-centered care.

The Advance Directive

Advance directive (AD) laws were enacted to protect an individual's right to self-determination and were spurred by right-to-die cases, such as Karen Ann Quinlan and Nancy Cruzan. The original intent of these laws was lauded as a strategy to promote patient rights, assist with the documentation of goals and values, and prevent family angst over decision-making for individuals who lose decision-making capacity.[1]

But then, state-specific statutes imposed strict legal requirements and restrictions, such as detailed and ambiguous language and execution requirements, that resulted in obstacles for many adults to complete the form and physicians to use the information to provide person-centered care. Unfortunately, this legalistic approach and standardized statutory documents became the gold standard as organizations and physicians sought to avoid legal consequences.

Two decades after the passage of the Patient Self-determination Act, AD documents remain a barrier to accomplish their original intent. In a 2011 study to identify the unintended consequences of advance directive laws, the authors analyzed 51 AD documents and 21 publications, resulting in the description of several legal and content related barriers:[2]

- *Poor Readability* - Most ADs are written at a 12th-grade reading level, contain ambiguous language, and some require extensive disclosures. For example, the Wisconsin AD statute demands a full one-page disclosure titled "POWER OF ATTORNEY FOR HEALTH CARE DOCUMENT NOTICE TO PERSON MAKING THIS DOCUMENT,"[3] intimidating language that introduces the statutory form.

- *Ambiguous Language* - Terms such as "terminal," "burdens outweigh benefits," and "life-sustaining" are familiar ambiguous terms in many ADs. For example, the Wisconsin "Declaration to Physicians" — a living will type of AD — includes the following paragraph:

> If I have a TERMINAL CONDITION, as determined by a physician, physician assistant, or advanced practice registered nurse who has personally examined me, and if a physician who has also personally examined me agrees with that determination, I do not want my dying to be artificially prolonged and I do not want life-sustaining procedures to be used.[4]

The meaning of "terminal," artificially prolonged," and "life-sustaining" are fraught with varying interpretations.

Another example of ambiguity is found in the South Carolina Health Care Power of Attorney (HCPA) document that references the authority of the state's living will over the HCPA document with no direction to resolve the existence of conflicting information between the two documents.[5]

EFFECT ON DECLARATION OF A DESIRE FOR A NATURAL DEATH (LIVING WILL)

I understand that if I have a valid Declaration of a Desire for a Natural Death, the instructions contained in the Declaration will be given effect in any situation to which they are applicable. My agent will have authority to make decisions concerning my health care only in situations to which the Declaration does not apply.

- *Healthcare Agent Restrictions* - AD statutes impose varying levels of restrictions on healthcare agent designations and authority. Clinicians (physicians, nurses) and care facility personnel (social workers, nursing assistants) are often excluded as healthcare agents. When a surrogate decision-maker is not delegated, most state statutes have surrogacy laws that restrict the designation of a decision-maker. Limitations on the authority of an agent may prevent some patients from having their preferences understood and honored.

For example, the Wisconsin statutory advance directive requires the explicit permission from a patient to be admitted to a nursing facility accompanied by confusing terminology:

If I have checked "Yes" to the following, my health care agent may admit me for a purpose other than recuperative care or respite care, but if I have checked "No" to the following, my health care agent may not so admit me:

1) A nursing home Yes No
2) A community-based residential facility Yes No

If I have not checked either "Yes" or "No" immediately above, my health care agent may admit me only for short-term stays for recuperative care or respite care.

Many individuals have interpreted this statement to represent their desire not to be admitted to a nursing facility rather than giving permission for their healthcare agent to make arrangements for appropriate healthcare services.

- *Execution Requirements* - Improperly executed advance directives—absence of qualified witnesses, signatures, notarization, dates—can result in a person's preferences to be negated or offer legal "loopholes" when there is family discord or differing clinical opinions. Moreover, execution requirements for completion of a legal document present practical burdens for healthcare organizations when, for example, employees are not allowed to serve as witnesses. Organizations and communities struggle to devise creative workarounds to help complete the legal document. One small rural community enlisted the help of the fire department located next to the hospital, recruiting volunteer firefighters who were willing to come to the hospital and witness AD signatures.

- *Inadequate Reciprocity* - Reciprocity laws, the ability for an AD executed in one state to be accepted in another state, have been activated in most states, but are not fool-proof due to mandatory language and restrictions. For example, Wisconsin law requires that the authority to withdraw artificial nutrition and hydration must be explicitly documented, and if an out-of-state document does not include this requirement, this life-sustaining treatment cannot be withdrawn.

- *Religious, Cultural, or Social Inadequacies* - Most U.S. advance directives do not allow for cultural variation in decision-making authority. For example, some cultures prefer family decision-making rather than the designation of one or two healthcare agents. It is not uncommon for patients to request that two siblings share the decision-making responsibility if needed, but ADs require a hierarchy of decision-makers.

Efforts to create a universal AD to overcome the barriers to statutory laws have been attempted with varying levels of success. The Uniform Health-Care Decision Act was drafted in 1994 to simplify AD legislation, combine living will and durable power of attorney statutes, allow oral directives, and decrease execution requirements. Only a few states have adopted the act.[6] A review of state statutes on ADs revealed that, by removing some barriers, the creation of a universal form was feasible in 41 states, but insurmountable barriers existed in other states, including the requirements for mandatory forms, notices, and language.[7]

An alternative to a universal AD document is the adoption of a geographic or statewide document, created to meet statutory requirements and increase the utility of the document to assist with the delivery of person-centered care.

The La Crosse Advance Directive Microsystem

The La Crosse AD task force took a decidedly different approach to a robotic dissemination of the Wisconsin statutory form, a form that includes legalistic and confusing language, is poorly formatted, and does little to stimulate conversation about goals of care and how treatment decisions would be made. Soon after the Patient Self-determination Act of 1991, the local La Crosse AD task force designed a power of attorney-type of AD that conformed to statutory requirements in three states (where the La Crosse health system operated), but also provided consistent, common, and repetitive messages about ACP, educated the public in a uniform way to decrease confusion, increased confidence from healthcare providers in the utility of written plans, and complemented the education of those who provide assistance, such as ACP facilitators, who learn to use the document as a tool to stimulate conversations about goals and values.

The redesigned AD document, endorsed by the legal community, included more engaging and understandable language, included instructions about the importance of ACP conversations, and invited individuals to reflect on their goals of care if they were to suffer an event that resulted in a severe, permanent brain injury, described as the "Imagine This" scenario:

A sudden event (such as a car accident or illness) left you unable to communicate. You are receiving all the care needed to keep you alive. The doctors believe there is little chance you will recover the ability to know who you are or who you are with.

The value of this scenario is often underestimated or misunderstood. The outcome depicted—"little chance you will recover the ability to know who you are or who you are with"—is an outcome many people fear, being permanently kept alive in a poor cognitive state and incapable of making decisions. The scenario is not specific to a diagnosis (such as cancer) or illness complication (such as a stroke or cardiac arrest).

Rather, this person-centered "conversation starter" allows individuals to reflect upon and verbalize the level of cognitive outcome they would deem acceptable—or unacceptable. It prompts people to ask questions about life-sustaining treatment, explore their chances of a full cognitive recovery, and consider time-limited trials — among other information important to assess personal goals and values and communicate decision-making guidance to the designated health care agent.

Dr. Paul Kalanithi, a former Stanford neurosurgeon and author, wrote eloquently about living with terminal lung cancer and about his experiences as a surgeon. He was interested in understanding the goals and values of his patients prior to brain surgery, appreciating the potential consequences of a less than optimum postoperative outcome: "Before operating on a person's brain, I realized, I must first understand his mind: his identify, his values, what makes it reasonable to let that life end" (Kalanithi p.98).[8] Dr. Kalanithi died on March 9, 2015.

The redesigned La Crosse task force power of attorney for healthcare form was disseminated as the preferred AD document for the community, available at all healthcare facilities, community centers, and recommended in educational programs on ACP and ADs. Consequently, healthcare professionals were consistently exposed to this standardized document regardless of where they practiced and learned to trust its validity and clinical usefulness. The previous culture of "ADs don't work" had changed.

A retrospective study of 400 adult deaths from La Crosse County over a seven-month period in 2007-2008 demonstrated the impact of a standardized AD document. Ninety-six (96%) percent of the decedents had some type of advance care plan; all but two of the power of attorney type of documents were the La Crosse version of the Wisconsin statutory form.[9]

Geographic Uniform Advance Directive Microsystems: Examples from the Field

While the adoption of a universal AD document may have insurmountable barriers, organizations and communities implementing the RC First Steps ACP program are encouraged to create a planning document microsystem to explore the following questions:

1) What planning documents are currently in use in the geographic community (healthcare systems, community, state)?

   (a) What are the barriers to each document? This analysis commonly reveals content issues, poor organization, and confusing terminology.

   (b) Is it possible to select a preferred document for geographic use?

   (c) What education is needed to ensure the accuracy of document completion?

2) Is redesign of the existing document possible? Redesign suggestions include efforts to:

   (a) Comply with requirements of state law (notices, signatures, witnesses/notarization)

   (b) Improve document layout (use of plain language, organization, large font, introductions that provide explanations for how to complete the document, use of a cover page with name, date-of-birth, and where copies were sent)

   (c) Organize document contents (Divide it into separate sections—with easy to understand instructions—such as "the importance of conversations with a healthcare agent," "appointing a healthcare agent,"or "making the document legal." Also have the option to include a statement of desires, care instructions or limits, and to include a response to the "Imagine This" scenario described above, especially regarding organ and tissue donation, and cultural or religious beliefs and traditions.)

3) If redesign is not possible, what strategies can be employed to improve the accurate documentation of an individual's goals, values, and preferences? Examples include:

(a) Creating recommendations for how to assist with the transfer of articulated goals, values, and preferences to the existing AD, recognizing the limitations and areas of ambiguity that may exist. These recommendations can be integrated into informational guides on how to complete ADs and educational programs for those who offer assistance in ACP and AD completion.

(b) Offering a "Special Instructions" addendum as an option to add more specificity to the existing document. Respecting Choices faculty provide suggested content for creating a one-page addendum to provide documentation of an individual's goals for a severe, permanent brain injury (the "Imagine This" scenario described above), CPR preferences, and the level of decision-making leeway for healthcare agents.

(c) Creating organizational policies that permit alternative documentation options, such as an Advance Directive Letter to Physicians, the Statement of Treatment Preference form completed during a Next Steps ACP conversation, and the transfer and legitimacy of oral directives

verbalized during SDM conversations with physicians and
advanced practitioners.

Several communities and healthcare organizations implementing the RC
ACP program have used these recommendations to create an improved AD
document for geographic dissemination.

An Advance Directive Document Microsystem: Collaboration in the Minneapolis Metropolitan Area

In 2008, leaders of the Twin Cities Medical Society in Minneapolis,
Minnesota, convened representatives from over 40 area organizations to
learn about the RC ACP program and decide on the level of commitment to
sponsor a geographic implementation. Most of the senior leadership from
the metro area healthcare systems agreed to collaborate on a standardized approach to ACP, including the development of shared materials and
resources. The initiative—Honoring Choices Minnesota (HCM)—created
an AD microsystem that resulted in an improved AD—modeled after the La
Crosse AD–that was endorsed and disseminated to all healthcare systems,
the public, and in educational programs. With ongoing evaluation and
improvement, HCM continues to promote the statewide dissemination
of the uniform document–now available in several languages–along with
resources and educational information for promoting ACP conversations
and the accurate completion of planning documents.[10]

Kaiser Permanente Northern California: The Life Care Planning Document

The RC First, Next, and Advanced Steps ACP program was initially
implemented at Kaiser Permanente, Northern California (KPNC) with
a leadership microsystem that embraced the advance directive redesign
recommendations, adding creative and local program elements. For example, the revised AD document allowed them to communicate their ACP
program logo, "Life Care Planning," (LCP) directly on the AD document,

which is available on the LCP website with links to additional resources such as group ACP classes and step-by-step instructions to complete the AD.

Additionally, the KPNC AD document integrated the "Imagine This" scenario under Part 3, "My Health Care Instructions: My Choices, My Care":

---

1) Treatments to prolong life

Consider the following situation:

You have a sudden accident or stroke.

Doctors have determined you have a brain injury, leaving you unable to recognize yourself or your loved ones. The doctors have told your agent and/or family that you are not expected to recover these abilities. Life-sustaining treatments, such as a ventilator (i.e., breathing machine), or a feeding tube, etc., are required to keep you alive. In this situation what would you want?

I would want to be kept comfortable and:

☐ I would want to STOP life-sustaining treatment. I realize this would probably lead me to

die sooner than if I were to continue treatment.

☐ I would want to continue life-sustaining treatments.

Please provide any additional instructions about life-sustaining treatments. For example, you may want to state a specific time period that you would want to be kept alive if there were no improvement to your health.

The KPNC redesigned AD document served as a template for customization in other KP regions such as Colorado and Maryland, where appropriate changes—such as execution requirements—were made to meet statutory requirements.[11]

Honoring Choices Wisconsin Endorsement of a Statewide Advance Directive

In 2012, I served as the RC consultant for an ACP initiative sponsored by the Wisconsin Medical Society (WMS) to promote statewide dissemination of best ACP practices.[12] It was exciting to partner with leaders of the Honoring Choices Wisconsin (HCW) initiative to assist with the dissemination of the RC program in my home state, in order to improve ACP for my family, neighbors, and friends. The HCW initiative made a commitment to create a standardized AD form, provide consistent education on ACP facilitation, and assist participating healthcare systems in making system-wide changes to improve the culture of person-centered decision-making.

The revised AD—modeled after the La Crosse form—was disseminated throughout Wisconsin, integrated into ACP educational programs, and adopted by healthcare organizations who participated in the HCW initiative and provided access to the document on their respective websites.[13] Additionally, this HCW AD was adopted in the La Crosse community.

The HCW initiative made significant progress in the statewide dissemination of a uniform AD document—a redesigned document that resolved the barriers of the statutory form. Yet today, Wisconsinites encounter confusion when choosing an AD document. For example, the Wisconsin Department of Health Services website continues to distribute the Statutory Power of Attorney for healthcare form.[14]

The POLST (Or, Portable Medical Orders)

National POLST provides leadership in the dissemination of the essential elements of a POLST Program[15] that includes both a *process*—similar to ACP—and a *form*. The POLST form, completed as a part of ACP for those with serious illness, is a set of medical orders that directs healthcare treatment decisions, especially in emergency situations. Individual states and regions are responsible for implementing POLST programs, which has resulted in a variety of synonyms, including MOLST (Medical Orders for Life-sustaining Treatment), MOST (Medical Orders for Scope of Treatment), and POST (Provider Orders for Scope of Treatment). To become endorsed as a POLST program, states must meet the minimum program requirements, such as a single form for the state or region, among others. As of October 2020, 24 states have received endorsement as mature programs, and 21 states are designated as "active" programs—those working to achieve the minimum requirements.[16]

National POLST released a recommended POLST form in August 2019 to promote a uniform document that could be used throughout the United States, improving consistency in consumer and professional education and research activities. As of December 2020, a few states have adopted the National POLST form,[17] with several other states working toward this goal or considering adoption.[18]

The La Crosse healthcare community was the first region outside of the state of Oregon to adopt the POLST Program in 1997. Implementation of the POLST program was local to the La Crosse healthcare community and did not originate from state statute or its protections. It was adopted as a standard of care after legal liability was assessed and consensus achieved on the positive outcomes from improved documentation and portability of an individual's healthcare decisions. A retrospective review of the effectiveness of the POLST program ten years following its implementation revealed that among 400 adults who died between 2007-2008 in La Crosse County, 67% of decedents had a POLST form in their medical record. Additionally, the medical orders were concordant with POLST orders in all but two cases.[19]

Statewide adoption of the POLST program in Wisconsin has been sluggish, creating challenges in honoring preferences when patients with completed POLST plans are transferred to a community or healthcare system unfamiliar with the legitimacy of the POLST form and its ability to inform the plan of care. In more recent years, the efforts of a Wisconsin POLST initiative to meet the criteria for statewide endorsement by National POLST has resulted in the state being granted "active" status in 2017.[20]

Redesign is the hallmark of an effective system, and after more than a decade of use of the POLST program in the La Crosse community, an expert panel of users and community leaders, including religious groups, was convened to analyze content concerns and make necessary revisions. This process unearthed input from various stakeholders, promoting dialogue and eventual consensus on content revisions to the POLST form, including changing the name of the form to "Provider Orders for Scope of Treatment (POST), acknowledging the prescriptive authority of advanced practitioners."[21]

Chapter 12: Microsystem #3:
Medical Record Storage and Retrieval

Failure to Honor an Individual's Healthcare Decision

Marilyn, an 83-year-old woman with advanced dementia, was admitted to the hospital with complications from chronic obstructive pulmonary disease (COPD), accompanied by her live-in niece, who had been providing care and support for several months. The acute onset of pneumonia was compromising Marilyn's fragile lungs requiring an impending decision about intubation and mechanical ventilation. Marilyn's niece, in consultation with family, informed the healthcare team to proceed with intubation.

A few days after admission, a nurse reviewed the AD found in Marilyn's medical chart, discovering that the niece was not listed as the delegated healthcare agent. Upon notification, the legally appointed designated healthcare agent was understandably upset and reported the organization to the Health Care Financing Administration (now the Centers for Medicare and Medicaid Services, the federal agency that administers the Medicare and Medicaid programs) who issued a citation to the organization for a violation of patient rights.

The medical record is intended to convey information to improve the delivery of quality healthcare. Many readers will be intimately familiar with the paper medical record system — information intended to provide documentation for clinical, administrative, financial, and research objectives — available to one user at a time, delaying the completion, accuracy, and accessibility of relevant patient information. The emergence of the electronic health record (EHR) and health information technology (HIT) has opened unprecedented opportunities to improve patient care by eliminating transcription errors, improving accessibility and transferability, reducing storage space issues and lost records, increasing data transfer, demonstrating improved patient compliance, providing quality assurance, and reducing medical errors.[1]

To improve the quality of our healthcare while lowering its cost, we will make the immediate investments necessary to ensure that, within five years, all of America's medical records are computerized.
— President-elect Barack Obama, Jan. 8, 2009[2]

President Obama's mandate, along with federal funding and financial penalties for non-compliance, has stimulated the evolution of the EHR and the use of HIT to store, manage, share, and analyze health information, improve transparency of planning conversations, referrals, and provide decision aid support with the goal of facilitating person-centered care. Along with the EHR, HIT includes the development of personal health records, electronic prescribing, and privacy and security protections.[3]

Privacy and security concerns of the EHR have resulted in federal protection, such as the creation of the Office of the National Coordinator for health information technology and its guide of activities to reduce privacy and security risks — a guide that that includes meaningful use of certified EHRs, Medicare and Medicaid incentive programs, enforcement of HIPAA (Health Insurance Portability and Accountability Act) rules, and educational resources.[4] The Office of the National Coordinator for HIT refers to the medical record as "not just a collection of data you are guarding, it is life."

From its inception, the Respecting Choices program — locally and nationally — understood how the medical record could improve patients' lives and could assist in honoring their treatment preferences. At the beginning of the La Crosse AD initiative, when medical records were paper charts, the local participating healthcare organizations agreed on a "green sleeve" storage system: a green plastic folder to store and transfer AD documents, placed at the front of the medical chart, transferred with the patient across the continuum of care, and visible to healthcare providers to impact treatment decisions as appropriate.

Later, Gundersen Health System invested time and resources in the creation of a "homegrown" electronic ACP application that included features that made it easy to find information, such as ACP conversations, to facilitate communication among all healthcare providers and patients, ensuring that everyone is operating on the same set of facts to provide person-centered care, and to make it easier to assess care concordance. This medical record storage system was instrumental in changing the culture of person-centered decision-making; physicians started to have — and document — different conversations, using previous information to continue with decision-making and ensuring this information would be available in the future for other physicians and healthcare providers.

The initial electronic ACP application was described as follows:[5]

> Finding this application in the EMR (Electronic Medical Record) is simple. On the first page of the patient's EMR (eg., the Patient Summary page), there is an obvious link to the ACP application. Once in this application, it is possible to determine whether the patient has any type of written AD and, if so, to view this document as a PDF file. If the patient has a power of attorney for healthcare, the names of healthcare agents and their contact information are immediately in view, as is any preference about cardiopulmonary resuscitation (CPR). In addition, the application features a computer-directed system to interview a patient about ACP needs, to retrieve dictated notes involving ACP, to make referrals to ACP facilitators, and to allow facilitators and others to record notes about ACP education or interactions. This application is available to all Gundersen Health System professionals in all Gundersen Health System care settings, making it a powerful way to communicate patient preferences and ACP discussions. Thus, if planning were started at the Medical Center when a patient was hospitalized, a

facilitator at a regional clinic could access this information through our integrated EMR system when a patient returns for a referred visit.[6]

The features of this original electronic system were also available to patients, who could view their AD online, ensure it was entered into their medical record, review its accuracy to determine if revision were needed, and download a copy of the AD for personal storage and distribution to healthcare agents and family as needed.

When Gundersen Health System made a decision to implement the Epic system for EHRs, physicians and nurses insisted that the Epic platform integrate features of the homegrown system. The culture had changed. Physicians stated, "We cannot take good care of our patients unless the Epic system can function to capture and display patient preferences."[7] Eventually, many of these features were built into the Epic ACP platform based on principles that remain relevant to improve the culture of person-centered decision-making:

1) *Easy access to critical information regarding healthcare treatment decisions in all settings of care* - When planning conversations have resulted in the identification of a substitute decision-maker, the completion of documents, or specific treatment decisions, this information should be easily accessible to providers to provide person-centered care and avoid medical errors in honoring preferences and decisions.

   Finding ACP information in the electronic record has been a perpetual challenge and source of frustration to healthcare providers. In a survey of 70 emergency department physicians, only 31% reported being confident they could find ACP documentation in the EHR and only 55% felt "very/extremely" confident they could use this information in making care decisions for their patients, even though 43% of physicians reporting that they needed this information more than five times per week. Having critical information available on the "main screen" was recommended.[8]

Examples of "main screen" data include (but are not limited to) the following:

- <u>Names and contact information for designated decision-makers (healthcare agents)</u> - These are the individuals chosen by the patient to make substitute healthcare decisions when needed. Honoring this decision is consistent with an ethical and regulatory responsibility toward patient rights but also a risk management concern for healthcare organizations, as in the opening story of this section.

- <u>List of separate planning document types</u> - (AD, POLST, other) with the ability to retrieve the documents for review at all sites of care.

- <u>Specific treatment decisions made by the patient or healthcare agent</u> - For example, code status information prominently displayed in the banner bar of the EHR.

- <u>Decision-making capacity</u> - Patients with decision-making (DMC) have the right to make their own healthcare decisions. The assessment and documentation of the loss of DMC must comply with state statute and clinical criteria. The electronic platform can assist with required documentation of DMC and the frequency of reassessment.

2) *Provide structured opportunities to review and update healthcare decisions* - Creating systems for regular review of healthcare decisions serves to resolve AD document completion inaccuracies, identify changing goals and values with illness progression, edit contact information, and update specific healthcare decisions. Opportunities to review and update healthcare decisions include:

- Review of ADs prior to entry into the medical record - As noted above, there are many barriers to the accurate and thorough completion of an AD. A review process provides an opportunity to correct inaccuracies and resolve potential ambiguity or misinterpretation by healthcare agents and healthcare providers seeking to determine a person's preferences. The goal is to enter into the medical record an AD document that is complete, accurate, thorough, including clearly written statements of goals, values, and beliefs. This review process can reveal other concerns for resolution. In reviewing an AD, an ACP coordinator was alerted to the following plea: "My husband is abusing me physically and I am scared. I don't know where to turn." The ACP coordinator transferred this information to the patient's provider for confidential follow-up.

- Improve the admission review process - Specific to ACP, federal law requires organizations to assess for the existence of an AD on admission to a healthcare facility, but a more robust guided admission review process can go beyond the minimum requirements. The simple question "Do you have an AD?" does little to assist with person-centered decision-making.

As a component of a quality improvement project at Gundersen Health System, a revised set of nursing assessment questions was integrated into the electronic ACP application in a decision tree format based on the patient's responses. For example, if the patient has an AD in the medical record, the decision tree prompts the nurse to open the AD and review the accuracy of the information provided, such as the name and contact information for the health-care agent or the documentation of a CPR preference.[9]

Implementing this new assessment review required nursing time and initially was met with resistance. However, this resistance changed after the first few weeks of implementation when several outdated ADs were identified that led to referrals for assistance with document updates. In addition, nurses became immediately aware of specific patient treatment decisions, such as DNR, that prompted physicians to confirm the patient's request and write a corresponding medical order. This systems change was instrumental in supporting the ACP role of the nurse as a member of the person-centered decision-making team.

Additionally, POLST plans must be reviewed upon admission to a healthcare facility to assess the patient's (or healthcare agent's) understanding of treatment decisions, resolve inaccuracies and incomplete document completion, and convert specific decisions to the organization's guidelines for writing medical orders.

- Review of AD information during annual physical appointments - As a component of preventative healthcare, a simple question during routine annual healthcare appointments, "Have you reviewed your AD within the last year?" could encourage patients to request a copy of their AD or prompt the healthcare provider to make a referral to an ACP facilitator for a document revision. At Gundersen Health System, an ACP review or discussion must be completed annually for patients 55 and older. The review is reflected in a dictated note that is automatically tagged and integrated into an ACP section of the EHR.[10]

3) *Create documentation guidelines* - Documentation guidelines include standardized conversation templates for ACP and SDM conversations, the value and utility of oral directives, and systems that allow transparency of an individual's goals and values specific to current or "real-time" healthcare decisions.

Standardized documentation templates - Typically, there is incomplete guidance on documentation standards for ACP and SDM conversations. For example, the Joint Commission standard on

AD documentation of discussion only requires a response to the following data point, "Was documentation present in the medical record of a one-time discussion of advance directives/advance care planning with a healthcare provider?"[11]

Standard conversation templates available in the EHR make it easier to document the essence of planning conversations, record key information for others to use, streamline "handoffs" to other team members, identify appropriate referrals and education provided, and document decisions made.

- Guidelines on the value of oral directives - One of the unfortunate outcomes of the emphasis on the completion of planning documents, such as ADs, DNR forms, and POLST forms, has been the loss of critical information gleaned from planning conversations — conversations that evolve over time, in a variety of settings, and are influenced by factors such as readiness to participate. If a patient makes a DNR decision in consultation with his/her primary physician during a clinic visit and then is subsequently admitted to the hospital in critical condition, this planning conversation should be transparent and used to make person-centered decisions, regardless if this decision has been documented in an advance directive or POLST form.

Oral directives may not be universally accepted or honored by physicians and healthcare organizations, even though they may be the best evidence of a person's treatment preferences. Organizational policies can clarify the value of an oral directive as a clear expression of an individual's goals and decisions and provide direction on how these oral expressions can be communicated to the entire healthcare team.[12]

- Transparency of goals of care - When the healthcare team assists patients in making treatment decisions aligned with their goals and values, the rationale for such decisions provides valuable information for the entire team. Efforts to standardize the documentation of goals of care will increase transparency for all members of the healthcare team and form the basis for future person-centered decisions.

4) *Embed decision-support features* - The electronic platform can provide easy access to a variety of resources to support a patient's decision-making process.

- Referral system - ACP and SMD conversations may reveal an individual's need for additional information or the expertise from another member of the healthcare team. An electronic referral system makes it easy for these referrals to occur in a timely manner and ensure their transparency.

- Standardized checklists, predictive tools, and guidelines to motivate and encourage healthcare providers to utilize best practice alerts - Early in the implementation of the home-grown electronic ACP platform, guidelines were posted on topics such as "How to initiate an ACP conversation" and "Assessment of Decision-Making Capacity" that served to remind, educate, and reinforce best practices.[13]

- Integrate prompts to initiate conversations - Electronic triggers can prompt healthcare providers to initiate or continue planning conversations.

- Educational resources - These include ACP information, AD forms, and certified decision-aids.

As HIT evolves, the EHR will afford many other opportunities to improve person-centered decision-making, the pathway to person-centered care.

Chapter 13: Microsystem #4:
A Person-Centered Decision-Making
Interprofessional Team

In a culture of person-centered decision-making, *everyone* bears responsibility to "know and honor" an individual's goals, values, preferences, and decisions. Promoting person-centered decision-making is not a centralized activity, reserved for one discipline or for "just in time" decisions; it is an environment cultivated by an interdisciplinary team.

Teamwork is integral to the delivery of *any* quality healthcare service. "Team-based health care is the provision of health services to individuals, families, and/or their communities by at least two health providers who work collaboratively with patients and their caregivers — to the extent preferred by each patient — to accomplish shared goals within and across settings to achieve coordinated, high-quality care ."[1]

The delivery of person-centered care — and its corollary, person-centered decision-making is increasingly convoluted, especially for those living with chronic and serious illness who are touched by primary care physicians, specialists, advanced practitioners, nurses, rehabilitation specialists, pharmacy, and a host of others. Each encounter has the potential to foster an individual's decision-making skills for both current *and* future care and treatment.

Creating a person-centered decision-making interdisciplinary team ensures a culture where everyone "wins":

- Individuals receive care from multiple experts in their respective fields. Each member of the team is encouraged and expected to deliver care that matches their expertise. No single person can meet the needs of an individual faced with health care treatment decisions, especially those with chronic and serious illness. An ACP facilitator, for example, may begin a planning conversation with a patient about CPR, but will use this intervention to help the patient identify questions, concerns, and expected outcomes to be discussed by the primary physician, advanced practitioner, or specialist.

Likewise, patients referred to a cancer specialist to discuss treatment options may benefit from a follow-up referral to another team member — a social worker or ACP facilitator — for further exploration and creation of a written plan. Or a patient who is contemplating withdrawal from hemodialysis will be assisted in making this decision with the help of palliative care specialists to understand the management of symptoms of the dying process.

In a recent editorial that casts skepticism on the value of ACP, the author states: "First, goals of care conversations require sophisticated knowledge of prognosis, disease and associated comorbidities, and treatment outcomes — knowledge that most patients, families, and advance care planning counselors do not have."[2] While this statement may be true in some situations, it signals a physician-centric perspective that disavows the knowledge and timely contributions of other members of the team who can assist an individual in building capacity for person-centered decisions.

- There is timely provision of information to assist with decision-making. Patients enjoy multiple opportunities to be supported and educated about healthcare decisions through their relationships with physicians, nurses, pharmacists, chaplains, social workers, and other members of the healthcare team. These relationships allow for timely and efficient communication of information to foster the decision-making process.

Consider the respiratory therapist providing care in the pulmonary rehabilitation program who, as a member of the interdisciplinary team, responds to patient queries and concerns about their last hospitalization and wonders if intubation and mechanical ventilation are inevitable for the treatment of future respiratory failure. Using a certified decision aid — vetted by the healthcare team — the respiratory therapist can begin providing information on the options for airway management, identify specific questions for exploration with a physician, and create a follow-up plan.

- There is accountability to transfer an individual's goals, values, preferences, and decisions across the healthcare community, thereby improving continuity of care.

- Patient satisfaction is prioritized. An individual who receives coordinated and consistent information from the entire healthcare team may feel better understood and supported in their healthcare decisions, experience less confusion, and feel more satisfied with their overall healthcare. "...patients who think their care team works well together tend to report better experiences and feel safer, research has shown. Experts from patient experience and healthcare consultant Press Ganey revealed that patients perceive their care as higher quality when they perceive their providers as all working well together."[3]

- There is increased ability to honor healthcare decisions. When the entire interdisciplinary team is accountable for improving person-centered decision-making, they become active participants in creating a plan of care that is aligned with the individuals' goals, values, preferences, and decisions and employs systems to ensure the plan is honored.

Designing the Person-Centered Decision-Making Interdisciplinary Team

"Given this complexity of information and interpersonal connections, it is not only difficult for one clinician to provide care in isolation but also potentially harmful. As multiple clinicians provide care to the same patient or family, clinicians become a team — a group working with at least one common aim: the best possible care — whether or not they acknowledge this fact. Each clinician relies upon information and action from other members of the team. Yet, without explicit acknowledgment and purposeful cultivation of the team, systematic inefficiencies and errors cannot be addressed and prevented."[4]

An interdisciplinary team approach to person-centered decision-making will not magically appear; it must be designed. In fact, without a defined approach, harm and medical errors may occur. As in the opening story, members of Jonathan's healthcare team did not take responsibility for exploring his preferences for CPR, understanding his decision for DNR, making recommendations for systems to honor this decision — a Wisconsin state-sanctioned DNR bracelet and POLST form — documenting his decision and associated rationale in the medical record, or identifying other planning needs Jonathan may have in managing his serious illness. Without an interdisciplinary approach to person-centered decision-making, Jonathan may receive care that is unwanted and is a medical error — an error that no one took accountability for.

To better define the characteristics of interprofessional team-based care, Mitchell and colleagues reviewed the literature, interviewed health care teams for refinement of team-based principles and identified five synergistic core principles that make up "teamness": the creation of shared goals, clear roles, mutual trust, effective communication, and measurable processes and outcomes.

How could the principles of "teamness" apply to the design of a person-centered decision-making interprofessional team?

The Person-Centered Decision-Making (PCDM) Interprofessional Team: The Author's Proposed Framework

1) *Shared Goals* - Establishing shared goals for person-centered decision-making will require a reexamination of ACP and SDM outcomes beyond the completion of documents or assistance making a specific treatment decision, although both are important. An important goal of ACP and SDM is the activation of decision-making behaviors, such as increased knowledge, perceived ability to make decisions, readiness to participate, and ability to initiate planning conversations with healthcare agents and other family members.[5] These behaviors transcend the completion of a document or a decision to accept or reject a proposed treatment. Therefore, the shared goals of a person-centered decision-making interdisciplinary team may encompass the following:

We will provide person-centered decision-making assistance to individuals, patients, and families in order to 1) design an individualized approach to decision-making that respects the individual's knowledge, readiness to participate, and religious, cultural, or personal beliefs, 2) help people reflect on, identify, and communicate their goals, preferences, and decisions for healthcare, 3) complete documentation that reflects SDM conversations and actionable decisions, 4) institute standards and policies to ensure plans are honored, and 5) gather evidence of team effectiveness.

---

2) *Clear Roles* - The roles of a specific team will vary based on resources, care delivery setting, and commitment to creating PCDM competencies. For example, in one healthcare organization, the

policy on Advance Care Planning defines multiple team roles for physicians, nurses, social workers, chaplains, and volunteers. A community-based team may consist of a priest or minister, parish nurses, and volunteers. A clinic-based team may include the physician or advanced practitioner, medical assistants, nurses, and volunteers—for example, the spouses of clinic employees. Once the team is defined, specific role expectations are defined in job descriptions, competency education integrated, and ongoing performance improvement established.

3) *Mutual Trust* - When team roles are defined, members can be expected to recognize and respect the complementary perspectives and skills of the entire team. All members have a moral, ethical, and legal responsibility to assist individuals in designing personalized plans. Members share a respect for patient advocacy and shared decision-making and are accountable for each other's practice.

4) *Effective Communication* - All members of the team will receive standardized education in person-centered decision-making communication. Members of the team will have access to and utilize consistent materials to assist individuals in making healthcare decisions. Decision aids will be reviewed and adopted for use by the entire team. A team referral system is created to allow easy access to other members of the healthcare team and to determine who will receive specific requests, what information needs to be collected, and how best to meet the needs of the individual seeking assistance. Documentation will provide transparency for each member's contribution to patient decision-making to streamline effective "handoffs" to other team members.

5) *Measurable Processes and Outcomes* - As discussed in the research Part, there is wide variability in choosing the outcomes that reflect person-centered decision-making. While goal-concordant care is perhaps the ultimate outcome to achieve, there are multiple

outcomes to select to measure the effectiveness of an interdisciplinary team approach to person-centered decision-making, including the frequency and quality of documentation of planning conversations, the number of referrals to team members, patient satisfaction with planning assistance, the frequency of use of certified decision-aids, and the quality of communication among team members.

In addition to the five principles of highly effective interprofessional healthcare teams, Mitchell and colleagues identified personal values of honesty, discipline, creativity, humility, and curiosity that impact team effectiveness. Honesty improves mutual trust, discipline promotes consistent behaviors, creativity encourages problem solving, humility acknowledges that mistakes will be made and that there are "things I don't know," and curiosity promotes ongoing improvement.

A Story of the Value of an Interdisciplinary Team Approach to Person-Centered Decision-Making

An organization investing in the implementation of the RC (Respecting Choices) Shared Decision-Making in Serious Illness (SDMSI) program began the initiative in a "chronic coronary occlusion" outpatient clinic coordinated by a physician's assistant (PA). The clinic serves patients who are contemplating their options — procedures or surgeries — to manage their diagnosis and prevent further complications from coronary obstructions. According to the PA, "real-time decisions are made at every appointment." The SDMSI program offers a semi-structured "conversation guide" to assist individuals in making real-time healthcare decisions.

Part I of the SDMSI conversation is focused on understanding "what matters most" to patients and includes an exploration of 1) the patient's understanding of their medical condition(s), identifying gaps in information (such as complications to be expected or prognosis), 2) hopes for the current plan of care, 3) living well (factors that give life meaning), and 4) outcomes that would be unacceptable.

Part II of the SDMSI conversation uses this information to guide patients in making a specific treatment decision that aligns with their identified goals and values. Part II requires education on the benefits and burdens of treatment options, prognosis, the integration of decision aids when available, and an analysis (and at times, recommendation) for a treatment option that best meets the person's identified goals. The entire conversation may take 30 minutes or more, which the PA verbalized as a significant implementation barrier in this clinic.

The coordinator for the SDMSI program decided to experiment with an idea, proposing that an RN member of the team facilitate Part I of the conversation, gathering information and making a "handoff" to the PA for Part II of the conversation. The PA — well-known for her communication skills and effective patient relationships — was skeptical that this team-based intervention would be of value but agreed to "test" the approach with two patients.

After observing the RN's facilitation, the PA asked if she could stay and see *every* patient that day. In evaluating the "test," the PA estimated that she spent 20-30 minutes less time in decision-making conversations with each patient, and more importantly, she discovered that Part I of the conversation made her realize that the procedure she had planned to offer one patient would not help the patient meet his goals. The approach changed the PA's understanding, approach, and eventual recommendation.

The PA displayed several values of an interdisciplinary approach to person-centered decision-making:

- Honesty ("I don't think this approach is any different from what I already do.")

- Discipline ("Maybe the RN has something to offer.")

- Creativity ("Let us give this a try.")

- Humility ("The information the RN provided helped me reset my treatment recommendations for a patient.")

- Curiosity ("I would like to observe Part I of the conversation.")

In summary, there are many advantages of a person-centered decision-making interdisciplinary team, but it requires design and reevaluation. Naturally, adopting this approach will require acceptance by all members of the healthcare team rather than a few motivated champions. There may be resistance to working differently, resistance that must be acknowledged and resolved. As in the above story, the PA's resistance to the team approach was best overcome by experimentation and gaining practice-based evidence of the effectiveness of a proposed strategy. With practice, experience, and leadership expectations, trust and communication among the entire interdisciplinary team improves, and patients are better served.

Chapter 14: Honoring an Individual's Request for DNR Revisited

In a culture of person-centered decision-making, Jonathan's story would look different:

Jonathan is a 72-year-old man with a ten-year history of heart disease and recently enrolled in a heart failure clinic where modifications were made to his medications and lifestyle habits. In addition, person-centered decision-making conversations were initiated by a member of the heart failure care management team to assist in determining his goals, values and preferences for both current and future treatment decisions.

Jonathan's wife and eldest son, his chosen first and second healthcare agents, respectively, were invited to participate in an ACP conversation and creation of an advance directive. During the ACP conversation and exploration of the CPR decision, Jonathan had several questions about his CPR outcomes that were referred to his cardiologist. Armed with accurate information, Jonathan made a decision not to be resuscitated if his heart suddenly stopped.

The team's social worker assisted Jonathan in securing a Wisconsin approved DNR bracelet, completion of his advance directive document, and discussed the healthcare agents' concerns in honoring Jonathan's decisions. Jonathan's ACP conversation and CPR decision was documented in the medical record and understood by the care management team, who assured Jonathan that he would continue to receive ongoing care and support to manage his heart disease.

Within a culture of person-centered decision-making, Jonathan's story looks much different. Jonathan's care management team initiated planning conversations as a component of quality heart failure clinic services, working together to help Jonathan receive information he needed to make a decision about CPR. Documentation of his CPR decision was reflected in the advance directive and medical record storage and retrieval micro systems created. Jonathan's healthcare agents were included in planning conversations to prepare them for a future decision-making role and lastly, this person-centered decision-making experience would prepare Jonathan and his family to assume an integral role in future treatment decisions.

Summary

This Part describes experiences and exemplifies designing or redesigning four specific microsystems in building culture of person-centered decision-making. There are undoubtedly other systems that are important; including those described throughout this book. Until and unless there is consensus on, and support for, the core systems that support person-centered decision-making, cultural change is not sustainable; ACP and SDM efforts will not reach their full potential in helping to deliver person-centered care. Who will take responsibility for developing this consensus? The Joint Commission? The Centers for Medicare and Medicaid? Other regulatory agencies?

Moreover, healthcare leaders and organizations must assume accountability for creating microsystems that synergistically work to hardwire excellence in person-centered decision-making.

ACP is right for patients and clinicians, but health systems have to do their part for it to have real impact. Health care systems need to develop a system-wide infrastructure that promotes quality ACP for all individuals as a standard of care. Such an infrastructure includes a process for proactively addressing ACP with patients and their families, reviewing earlier conversations to provide coordinated care, and ensuring an efficient and effective medical record that makes it easy to document and access prior discussions and decisions. Even the best ACP conversations will not result in goal-concordant care in a system that is ill equipped to honor patient preferences. This need cannot be met through specialty palliative care alone or by relying solely on physicians. These goals are lofty and challenging in our complex chaotic health care system. This does not make them wrong.[1]

Personal Exercises

1) Identify and examine the advance care planning documents in your organization and community. What did you learn?

2) What gaps exist in your organizations' system for storing, retrieving, and updating planning conversations and documents?

3) Describe your current role as a member of a person-centered decision-making interdisciplinary team. How effective is this team in meeting patient's decision-making needs?

Part Four

Chapter 15: The Promise of Education and Certification in Building a Culture of Person-Centered Decision-Making

So, You're the One They Have Sent to Kill My Mother

As the on-call consultant of an organizations' clinical ethics team, I responded to an ethics consult from a medical resident to "help a healthcare agent make a Do-Not-Resuscitate (DNR) decision for her seriously ill mother." The patient was unresponsive and had completed an advance directive naming her daughter as her substitute decision-maker. In discussion with the medical resident (after clarifying that my role was *not* to get patients to make specific decisions), the healthcare team was frustrated. They were caring for a seriously ill patient who, in their medical opinion, was unlikely to survive her current medical crisis.

They had attempted a few "unproductive" conversations with the daughter to help her understand that cardiopulmonary resuscitation (CPR) was not likely to be successful and that her mother's underlying medical condition was untreatable. In reviewing the medical chart, I found cryptic documentation of these conversations, including statements such as "She [the daughter] is being unreasonable and unrealistic and is demanding CPR." In preparing to meet with the daughter, the nursing staff informed me that she had not left her mother's side in several days, refusing to go home. They worried about her health and mental state.

Upon entering the patient's room and introducing myself as a member of the ethics consultation team, the daughter responded ardently, "Are you the one they have sent to kill my mother?"

Overview

Imagine the possibilities. What would it mean if all healthcare professionals were competent in person-centered decision-making (PCDM) communication? Imagine if every healthcare professional were equipped with the knowledge, skills, behaviors, and judgment to assist patients and families in making healthcare decisions aligned with their goals and values? Now imagine all members of the patient's healthcare team working together to achieve the ultimate goal of person-centered decision-making, the provision of person-centered care.

Imagine if you were a patient reaping the benefits of this teamwork. How would it feel to have this level of decision-making support — to have the care team asking consistent questions, documenting individual and ongoing conversations in the medical record, providing information in an unbiased manner and, in the end, creating plans and decisions that are in line with what matters most to you, are that are understood and honored by the healthcare team and your family? I simply cannot imagine how an organization can aspire to a mission of person-centered care without this commitment to communication excellence.

Person-centered decision-making communication skills make a difference in how patients understand information, make medical decisions, develop trust in healthcare professionals, and express satisfaction with the patient and family healthcare experience. As the opening story depicts, unskilled conversations can cause harm.

This Part will make the case that, despite the barriers, it is time for national certification standards in attaining competency in PCDM communication, the core attribute of person-centered and family-oriented care. To support this national dialogue, the author shares her twenty years of experience creating, testing, and improving the Respecting Choices PCDM communication programs, Advance Care Planning (ACP), and Shared Decision-making in Serious Illness (SDMSI).

Four foundational principles are described in the evolution of these programs: competency-based education (Chapter 17), program delivery adaptations (Chapter 18), instructor certification (Chapter 19), and organizational and community commitment (Chapter 20). Chapter 21 illustrates the power of PCDM communication competency through selected personal stories in facilitating tough conversations. This Part will conclude by revisiting the Opening Story, emphasizing the harmful effects of unskilled conversations, and summarizing the imperative to create a culture of PCDM communication competency.

Barriers to Standardization and Certification in Person-Centered Decision-Making Communications Skills

The pathway to standardization and certification in person-centered decision-making communication is arduous, complicated by real and alleged barriers. Regrettably, these barriers are often perceived as burdensome and unsurmountable. Acknowledging and attempting to resolve these barriers was, and remains, integral in the design of the Respecting Choices ACP and SDMSI communication courses.

Clinician lack of self-awareness of personal barriers to effective communication - Clinicians often lack self-awareness of personal barriers to communication, which results in reluctance to participate in activities to improve their skills.[1] Clinicians may have maladaptive beliefs that justify this reluctance believing that "patients really don't want to talk" or that decision-making conversations will "take away hope." Many clinicians have experiences with conversations that have gone poorly, have resulted in intense emotional reactions from patients and families, or in condemnation from a superior. Each barrier exacerbates the others. With lack of skill and confidence, conversations are avoided, experiences in navigating challenging emotions are not gained, and most importantly, patient and family decision-making needs are not met.

Lack of consistent standards, definitions, or nationally sponsored certification programs - Communication skills programs exist, but each curriculum has differences that make it challenging for organizations to decide which programs to use and disseminate. Existing programs vary in their defined expectations for competency, terminology, target audience, length, requirements for certification, costs, and effectiveness.

Tension and controversy on who should be accountable for facilitating person-centered decision-making conversations - Who is responsible for facilitating PDCM conversations? Which health professionals or community advocates should be targeted to receive communication skill education? The lack of support and endorsement for an interdisciplinary approach to PCDM leaves a gap in continuity of care for patients and families. Without a team approach, accountability is often deferred to someone else.

Communication competencies are not consistently valued in the clinical setting - While it is essential for clinicians to be competent in CPR or to be able to institute the most up-to-date stroke protocol, how healthcare providers communicate with patients is often accepted as a matter of personal choice or ability. Historically, proficiency in communication skills among healthcare professionals has been chastely considered an "art." It is alleged that nurses, physicians, social workers, and others are either born with suitable communication skills or will magically learn them through role modeling of other clinicians or by attending educational seminars.

Harm caused by poor communication skills is "invisible" - As the opening story depicts, unskilled conversations can cause medical errors, leave patients and families unsatisfied, and healthcare staff distressed. The lack of consistent measures to monitor communication skills allows the consequences of unskilled conversations to remain invisible and therefore, unresolved.

The lack of financial or regulatory incentive - At the system level, healthcare organizations have no financial or regulatory incentive to invest in communication skills education. In fact, the costs of this education may be highly scrutinized, and administrators may seek the least expensive strategy to this education, despite evidence of effectiveness.

Inadequate systems to support a culture of person-centered decision-making - Systems barriers — explored in this book — make it difficult to build a culture of person-centered decision-making such as inadequate documentation platforms that allows transparency to sensitive and important conversations among the interdisciplinary team and ability to impact decisions and the plan of care.

Lack of research on communication skills program effectiveness - Research on the effectiveness of communication skills programs is lacking. Participants may rate communication skills programs helpful and satisfying, but do these programs affect behavior change in the clinical setting? Do these programs result in improved PCDM conversations for patients and families?

There are capricious expectations, education, and ongoing monitoring of clinicians' communication behaviors and outcomes. Clinicians are often left to their own means to figure out how to navigate decision-making conversations with patients and families. "Thus, the majority of clinicians now in practice learned to communicate on the job, without a curriculum, explicit role modeling, or learning techniques backed by evidence."[2]

These barriers underscore the painfully slow dissemination of standardization and certification in person-centered decision-making communication competency. In the chapters that follow, you will learn how the RC programs were intentionally designed to promote and increase the dissemination of a standardized and replicable curriculum.

Chapter 16: Setting Standards for Person-Centered Communication Education and Certification: It is Time

It is long past time for change. The attainment of communication competency to support person-centered decision-making deserves the same level of education, competency assessment, and ongoing monitoring as *any* other clinical procedure that is focused on the delivery of quality patient care. The attainment of competency in person-centered decision-making will not happen accidently or by individuals pursuing isolated training programs; it will require national standards, organizational commitment, and a well-orchestrated interdisciplinary team devoted to person-centered care.

The phenomenon of unreliable, ineffective, unavailable, and underfunded PCDM communication programs for clinicians is in stark contrast to the tireless investment by organizational leaders in the expectations for clinical staff to demonstrate and maintain competencies in an exhaustive list of job-related procedures, techniques, and institutional policies.

Critical Care Competency-based Programs

I experienced this organizational investment in clinical competency first-hand as a clinical nurse specialist in critical care. To ensure the provision of quality patient care, I was responsible for the creation of competency-based programs to attain and maintain the clinical competence of the nursing staff. This explicit organizational commitment to clinical competency was profound; eleven clinical nurse specialists were charged with the same responsibility for other areas of patient care, supported by a robust team of nurse educators.

The critical care competency-based program was multifaceted. Nurses were expected to:

- Successfully complete a three-week critical care course that was jam-packed with information: heart, lung, and neurologic anatomy and physiology, physical assessment, the body's response to injury and insult such as septic shock, and the interpretation of 12-lead electrocardiogram (one of my personal favorites). Enumerable skills were demonstrated: how to analyze arterial blood gases, and the accurate collection of data from a Swan Ganz catheter, and critical thinking scenarios were integrated to promote analysis of questions such as "What would you do if you spotted a new bundle branch block on the ECG (electrocardiogram) monitor?" or "If you suspected septic shock, what assessments and data would support this suspicion?"

- Actively participate in the completion of a unit-based preceptor program. A clinical expert mentored each nurse through selected patient assignments, observing demonstrations of a long list of technical skills and context-specific clinical judgments. The mentorship program extended from three weeks, for an experienced nurse, to up to three months, for a new graduate. Preceptors were required to complete a program in mentoring strategies, performance evaluation, and creating improvement plans. This "buddy" system allowed for inexperienced nurses to learn from experts, to examine their nursing actions, and to receive immediate feedback on their skills and performance. Preceptors could observe and provide guidance on the critical thinking decisions of novice nurses as they experienced real-world application. Staff were expected to comply with critical care policies and procedures that were developed under the guidance of nationally recognized standards of the American Association of Critical Nurses (AACN), who offers certification (CCRN) as a critical care nurse.[1] Resources were dedicated to support CCRN certification for nursing staff, recognizing that this board certification demonstrated to patients, employers, and the public that a nursing competency is consistent with national best practices in caring for critically ill patients.

- Demonstrate ongoing monitoring and maintenance of defined ICU competencies through regular in-service education, daily round observations, annual skills simulations, and performance evaluations. Individual improvement plans were designed for nurses who struggled to attain competency.

This massive investment in the clinical competency of the ICU staff was undoubtedly expensive but never scrutinized or deemed unnecessary. According to the American Federation of State, County, and Municipal Employees (AFSCME), the orientation of a new graduate nurse will cost around $50,000 to teach and retain.[2] A comparable investment does not typically extend to ensure an interdisciplinary team incompetent in the skills of person-centered decision-making.

In my role as a RC consultant engaged in program implementation at a large medical center, I was challenged by an administrator to justify the cost of sending employees to a day-long communication course. "This is a huge commitment of time and human and financial resources," he stated. I agreed and offered the counter argument. "As leaders, we don't question our commitment to sending people to CPR and ACLS (Advanced Cardiac Life Support) certification and recertification courses, even though these services impact a small fraction of our patient population. Why do leaders question the investment in effective ACP communication — a service that benefits all patients and their families?"

An organization's investment in the clinical competency of its staff stretches far beyond orientation and preceptor programs. Organizational competency expectations are incentivized by aspirations to achieve national accreditation through standard-setting programs such as the American Heart Association and The Joint Commission.

Advanced Cardiac Life Support (ACLS)

Advanced Cardiac Life Support (ACLS) certification is the putative national standard for competency in emergency management for clinicians in critical care environments; maintenance of certification is a condition of continued employment. Created and disseminated by the American Heart Association, ACLS certification comprises an assortment of competency-based educational strategies.[3] The program has clearly defined outcomes for high-quality CPR and high performing teams. It also has a blended learning component via a self-directed online program (typically completed in 6-7 hours), followed by hands-on classroom skills, which are another 5 hours of sessions using dramatizations, simulations, animations, mega code cases, and other activities to integrate ACLS knowledge with expected skills. The classroom skills sessions are led by certified Instructors who reinforce skill achievement.

As ACLS certification became an organizational benchmark, CPR outcomes improved, and best practices safeguarded. Prior to ACLS certification, emergency code situations were chaotic. As a member of these pre-ACLS code teams, the chaos was palpable. In response to an overhead "code blue" page, multiple people would arrive at the bedside, some to participate and others to observe (and often get in the way). There were no assigned roles or protocols. If several physicians arrived, contradictory orders were simultaneously shouted, leaving the team to wonder who was in charge. Without evidence-based standard protocols for emergency care, each code situation resulted in different orders, drugs, and outcomes. The code team was typically left with the uncertainty of the impact of our efforts. We did not know what worked or what did not. We received no organized feedback for improvement.

I was relieved when ACLS certification arrived on the national scene. Organizational practices and expectations shifted. The organization supported my certification as an ACLS Instructor, and we proceeded to certify all critical care staff in these national standards for emergency care.

Educational budgets afforded time and resources for recertification efforts. Organizations instituted code blue committees for the review of all emergency situations, compliance with ACLS protocols, and clinical outcomes.

The Joint Commission

The Joint Commission accredits United States healthcare organizations and programs and sets forth competency standards for employee orientation to assure consumers that the staff can deliver safe, quality healthcare.[4] Each organization defines the specific competency expectations and timelines, but typically includes key content in the areas of: safety (fire, infection control, emergency response, active shooter); organizational practices (work schedules, patient rights, codes of conduct, privacy); and more specific competencies based on the needs of each population, the types of procedures conducted, conditions or diseases treated, and the kinds of equipment it uses. The documentation of competency assessment is focused on specific knowledge, technical skills, and abilities required to deliver safe, quality care.

For accreditation, each organization participates in onsite survey activities that examine the organization's requirements, compliance with evidence-based guidelines, standards of practice, and regulatory requirements. Onsite surveys are repeated every three years. The Joint Commission also offers specialty-types of certifications, such as its Comprehensive Cardiac Care certification, a collaboration with the American Health Association that include competency expectations in the areas of cardiac rehabilitation, heart failure, diagnostic cardiac catheterization, and arrhythmia management.[5]

As an independent entity, The Joint Commission determines which standards to set for measuring compliance, relying on extensive input from healthcare professionals, experts, and consumers (among others), with the focus on quality care and safety. In our early years, Bud and I approached The Joint Commission with a recommendation to define specific competencies for advance care planning. Although The Joint Commission supports efforts to improve "patient-centered communication" and its Health Equity portal provides resources (monographs, videos, podcasts) on communication strategies, we never received interest in further discussion on our recommendation to promote competency in ACP conversations.[6]

Why has such wide-ranging investment in clinically related skill development and certification of healthcare professionals *not* transferred to person-centered decision-making communication skills, despite endorsement from national organizations, professional societies, and creators of communication skills programs?

The National Academy of Sciences has called for mandatory communication skills training, and the World Health Organization's publication on Palliative care lists the importance of acquiring skills in communication, decision-making, management of pain and symptoms, and bereavement care, among many others.[7] The American Society of Clinical Oncology published consensus guidelines,[8] based on the literature, on recommendations and strategies for communicating with patients with cancer and their families.[9]

Although the path to national standardization and certification in person-centered decision-making communication competency remains tortuous, it is time for national guidance. What definition of competency will guide national standardization? Who determines the criteria for person-centered decision-making competency? What is the educational path to achieve certification? How will ongoing competency be monitored and improved?

The Development, Evolution, and Dissemination of the Respecting Choices Competency-Based Person-Centered Decision-Making Communication Programs

While there are no simple answers to these questions, the remainder of this Part offers one pathway to standardization and certification in PCDM communication; a pathway that has been created, tested, and improved by the RC program for over twenty years. While not perfect, this pathway and its experiences can contribute to the emerging national dialogue and consensus on a standardized pathway going forward.

As the RC director of program development, I was the proud leader of a team that was passionate about creating programs to improve participants' competency in PCDM communication competency and the patient experience. This programmatic pledge resulted in ongoing evaluation and evolution. We got some things right and some things wrong, but never doubted the investment in curriculum enhancement. Each revision represented the results of testing from previous versions, the assimilation of new knowledge and skills, input from customers, users, and Instructors, and the integration of novel teaching strategies. Throughout two decades of program evolution, four overarching concepts remained foundational:

- Competency-based education (Chapter 17)

- Program delivery adaptations (Chapter 18)

- Instructor certification (Chapter 19)

- Organizational and community commitment (Chapter 20)

The following description of these foundational concepts are laced with personal observations, experiences, and examples, but are intended to be instructional, insightful, and promote dialogue among national organizations, and others regarding standardization and certification in PCDM communication.

Chapter 17: Competency-Based Educational Concepts: The Respecting Choices Experience

Competency-Based Education: The Foundation

The first Respecting Choices PCDM communication program was titled "A Patient Education Program on Advance Directives" but soon modified to an "Advance Care Planning Facilitation Course" to emphasize the importance of the conversation over the completion of a document. Although the Respecting Choices ACP and SDMSI courses have evolved over time and are more appropriately categorized under the rubric of "person-centered decision-making" communication programs, the original goal — the attainment of competence in PCDM communication — was, and continues to be, a priority. Integrating the meaning of competency and competency-based education has been the bedrock in the evolution of the RC communication courses.[1]

"Competency can be defined as the application and demonstration of appropriate knowledge, skills, behaviors, and judgment in a clinical setting. Competency is not merely the product of completing required courses, nor is it measured simply by successfully passing a test or completing a checklist. Rather, competency is confirmed when knowledge and skills are accurately applied at the bedside, and appropriate behaviors and judgments are consistently displayed in practice."[2]

Competency is more than a one-time skills-based evaluation; it must be assessed over time and in the real world. A clinician may possess the knowledge to perform a skill but lack the attitude or judgment to apply this knowledge appropriately in a clinical context. Competencies are focused on performance, are observable and measurable, and use standards that are assessed by expert judgment from those in the field.[3]

Using this robust definition of competency, Respecting Choices embraced competency-based education (CBE) as its structured approach to teaching and learning the "knowledge, skills, behaviors, and judgment" that an individual must attain to be deemed competent. While CBE is not a new phenomenon to improve performance, it encounters program design chal-lenges.[4] A critical step in designing CBE programs is the identification of 1) clearly defined knowledge, skills, behaviors, and judgment competencies, 2) flexible and various strategies focused on how to attain each competence, and 3) evaluation options that demonstrate competency attainment.

While no national consensus exists to define the CBE requirements for competency in person-centered decision-making communication, Respecting Choices embraced the challenge of creating a CBE approach in the development and evolution of its ACP and SDMSI communica-tion courses.

The Respecting Choices Competency-Based Educational Components of Person-Centered Decision-Making Communication

Absent national standards, the RC program forged ahead to identify the "knowledge, skills, behaviors, and judgment" required to attain competency in PCDM communication. The selection of these CBE components was initially based on a history of diverse implementation, experiential learning, and emerging research on the outcomes of the RC program.

With dissemination of the RC communication courses, this internal process was fortified by customers, clinicians, experts, and patient feedback. Expert advisory boards were convened, composed of content experts, experienced facilitators, and instructors, to formally provide feedback and input on all aspects of program revision to include the list of competencies and teach-ing strategies

The resultant competencies and certification processes were never accredited by a national organization or sponsor. For years, the following "certification" disclaimer was included in the introduction to each RC communication course:[5]

The term "certification," as used in Respecting Choices® educational programs and products, means that Gundersen Health System issues a certificate upon fulfillment of the following elements:

Completion of a specified Respecting Choices educational program with standardized content and processes.

Successful demonstration of skills associated with the specified program; and

If applicable, an 80% or higher score on a written examination associated with the specified program.

The Respecting Choices certification programs are not credentialed by a national accreditation body.

Following is a description of the knowledge, communication skills, behaviors, and judgment competencies designed for the Respecting Choices CBE programs in PCDM communication:

Knowledge Competencies for Person-Centered Decision-Making Communication

Determining the core knowledge required to achieve competency in person-centered decision-making communication is arduous. Without national standards, opinions from experts in the field vary, and curriculum content is inconsistent. Respecting Choices PCDM program defines three categories of knowledge competency:

- Baseline (or core) knowledge that includes clarification of terms, such as advance care planning, shared decision-making, person-centered decision-making, person-centered care, advance directives, health care agent, as well as knowledge on the role of the interdisciplinary team in person-centered decision-making.

- Baseline (or core) knowledge required to facilitate more complex PCDM conversations, such as for individuals with serious illness, to include the trajectory of chronic illness, risks of complications from disease progression, and the benefits and burdens of life-sustaining treatment.

- Context-specific knowledge includes organizational and community practices or policies, statutory guidelines on completing written advance directives and POLST forms, and access to resources to support PCDM. Context-specific content also includes knowledge that reflects sensitivity to the culture, ethnicity, and religious or spiritual beliefs of the community.

Communication Skill Competencies for Person-Centered Decision-Making Communication

The ultimate goal in attaining competence in person-centered decision-making communication skills is to assist individuals in identifying "what matters most" and how they can make healthcare decisions that are aligned with their goals, values, and beliefs. This goal is achieved through communication skills that integrate understanding of adult learning principles, motivational interviewing, the doctrine of informed consent, narrative ethics, and the ethics of caring relationships.[6]

Respecting Choices has defined three categories of communication competencies for person-centered decision-making 1) Exploratory communication skills, 3) General communication skills and techniques, and 3) Stage of Planning specific communication skills.

1) *Exploratory Communication Skill Competencies* - The skill of exploration is fundamental to person-centered decision-making, to learning the patient's story. What do patients understand about their health care situation, complications, and decisions they are being asked to consider? How have past experiences, such as previous conversations or hospitalizations, influenced current goals and values? What does "quality of life" mean to the individual, and what hopes do they have for their current medical plan of care? What barriers to planning and decision-making exist? These questions exemplify the power of exploratory communication skills to gather information, uncover gaps in information, resolve fears and barriers, and develop a trusting relationship.

For patients with serious illness, exploration assists in assessing their understanding of their health condition on five dimensions: identity, cause, timelines, consequences, and curability/controllability. According to the Common-Sense Model of illness representation, these dimensions must be understood by the patient and the provider before adding new information.[7]

2) *General Communication Skill Competences and Techniques* - General communication skills and techniques emerged as applicable competencies for *any* PCDM conversation — competencies intrinsic to promote dialogue and reveal an individuals' goals, values, and beliefs. General communication skills complement and add value to exploratory skills. For example, the communication skill of exploring words and phrases is priceless and one of my personal favorites. Clinicians are frequently exposed to phrases such as "I don't want to be a vegetable," or "I don't want to be a burden," and make

181

assumptions about their meaning. Exploring these phrases helps validate meaning, correct assumptions, and allows the patient to verbally express goals and values that will serve to guide their decision-making process.

In addition to general communication skills, communication techniques, such as remaining value-neutral and utilizing "ask-teach-ask," demonstrate attention to the "behaviors" of a person competent in PCDM communication. For example, the "ask-teach-ask" technique assists in assessing an individual's understanding of information central to making person-centered decisions. This technique demonstrates a willingness to clarify misinformation and improve understanding of medical information.

Competency in PCDM communication includes the ability to understand one's personal values and biases and their potential impact on patients and families. Respecting Choices emphasizes the importance of remaining "value-neutral" as a communication technique to avoid the purposeful or inadvertent transfer of personal bias or judgment on an individual's decision-making process.

The opening story demonstrates the harm that can occur when clinicians impose their personal values and biases within PCDM conversations. Distrust of the healthcare professional results in feelings of abandonment and dissatisfaction with care. Remaining value-neutral can prevent avoidable suffering for patients and healthcare professionals.

3) *Stage of Planning-Specific Communication Skill Competencies* - The initial CBE course in person-centered decision making was developed and disseminated as ACP, a process that assists individuals in making future health care decisions. However, ACP is not a "one size fits all" intervention. The Stages of Planning approach to ACP (First Steps, Next Steps, and Advanced Steps) was created to customize the

decision-making process to an individuals' stage of illness, risk of complications, and anticipated treatment decisions.

- <u>First Steps (FS) ACP facilitation</u> includes communication skill competencies designed to motivate individuals to participate in the planning process, assist in the selection of a healthcare agent, provide instructions for goals of care in the event of a severe and permanent brain injury, and complete a written plan that reflects the individuals' goals, values, and preferences. The target audience is adults who have not started or engaged in a planning process.

- <u>Next Steps (NS) ACP facilitation</u> targets individuals living with a serious illness, actively engaged in treatment, but experiencing complications that may result in an unacceptable outcome, as defined by the individual. Specific communication skill competencies for NS planning includes exploring hopes for the current plan of care, past hospitalizations, understanding of potential complications, goals, and values in potential situations where complications result in unacceptable outcomes, and creating plans that reflect this decision-making process.

- <u>Advanced Steps (AS) ACP facilitation</u> is for individuals at risk of a life-threatening complication due to serious illness, advanced age, or frailty. Specific communication skill competencies include understanding of illness progression and exploring treatment preferences using the POLST process and its system for converting decisions into medical orders.

- <u>Shared Decision Making in Serious Illness (SDMSI)</u> is different from the Stages of Planning ACP competencies that are geared toward helping patients make *future* healthcare decisions. In 2019, the Shared Decision Making in Serious Illness communications course was designed for physicians and advanced practitioners to assist patients in making *current* healthcare decisions aligned with their goals, values, preferences, and decisions. Specific communication skill competencies include helping patients understand the trajectory of their serious illness, complications, and prognosis, evaluating the benefits and burdens of specific and proposed treatment options, and creating a plan to honor the patient's current treatment decisions.

Once competencies and curricula are defined, a variety of program adaptations can be designed.

Chapter 18: Program Delivery Adaptations: From the Classroom to Virtual Learning Platforms: The Respecting Choices Experience

Inherent in an effective competency-based education (CBE) approach is the flexible delivery of program content, an ongoing challenge faced by the Respecting Choices (RC) program in its quest to provide scalable and time efficient strategies to deliver its PCDM communication courses. Program delivery adaptations have evolved from the more traditional classroom education to online modules, blended learning strategies, and-spurred by the Covid-19 pandemic of 2020 — the virtual platform.

From Classroom Presentations to Blended Learning

The 1999 version of the Respecting Choices ACP for facilitators course included a two-day classroom agenda, ideally separated by one week to give learners time to absorb the information, conduct an organizational assessment, practice, and return with questions and concerns for discussion. It included a combination of didactic information mixed with group discussion, problem-solving scenarios, and practice role-play exercises. During practice role-plays, experienced facilitators would observe and offer feedback, perceived as supportive, but not competency-based.

This traditional face-to-face educational program — although popular with existing customers and participants — was unsustainable. A decision was made to create a new, blended learning approach that would consolidate knowledge competencies and decrease classroom time. An effective blended learning curriculum uses technology to engage learners, creates an organized classroom culture that role models expected behaviors, and designs intentional and purposeful activities that are well understood by the learners.[1]

Initially, the backlash from traditional classroom Instructors was hefty. In sundry conversations, customers lamented the loss of classroom time devoted to discussion and problem solving, worried the effectiveness of the existing course would decrease, and begged us to resist making significant changes in content. The course restructuring was challenging, but with experience, represented new opportunities to support the outcomes of competency-based education.

Online Curriculum

As a component of the blended learning program restructuring, it was necessary to create a cadre of online educational courses to provide background knowledge, introduce communication competencies, and provide critical thinking scenarios to apply the defined competencies in the real world. Creating an online component to a blended learning curriculum assists in the delivery of core knowledge in a self-directed, flexible manner. Less experienced learners can spend as much time as they need to absorb the information; more experienced learners can progress more quickly.

For experienced Instructors, accustomed to the traditional face-to-face curriculum, the impact of the online curriculum was groundbreaking. It transformed the classroom experience for participants, Instructors, and me. Learners arrived at the classroom environment better informed, engaged, and armed with questions and observations gleaned from the online experience. Participants (well, most of them) were eager to practice their newfound skills in the classroom setting. During initial testing of the online curriculum, approximately 200 participants provided positive feedback after completion. Moreover, during introductions at the classroom component of the course, participants often reflected on the impact of the online course:

- A social worker confessed that a large part of her role was to "get patients to complete advance directives," and she was personally incentivized as the number of completed documents increased. Expressing distress over previous conversations she had with patients, she stated, "I will never go back to that type of intimidation again."

- A nurse, grateful that she was invited to participate in the course, stated affirmatively, "Completing the online course affirms the reason I became a nurse: to help people, to understand what is important to them. Thank you for giving me new energy to continue in my role."

- A palliative care physician stated, "I have these conversations with patients everyday," but admitted to learning about the skill of exploring words and phrases — a skill he had neglected and was eager to bring back to his communication strategies.

- A participant who discovered new skills in the online course that gave him confidence to "try them out with a few patients" and experienced their effectiveness.

Initially, online courses were created to support each stage of planning (FS, NS, AS), and separate courses on "Basic ACP," and "the Role of the RN in ACP." During program evolution, a distinct communication skills module was created to introduce all learners to the general communication competencies (for example, listening, remaining value-neutral), competencies germane to any person-centered decision-making conversation.

In 2019, a three-module course on basic ACP for physicians was added to the online education library. While specific to the role of physicians and advanced practitioners in advance care planning, the core knowledge and competencies are consistent with other PCDM curricula.

The online courses have allowed the dissemination of consistent content on ACP and competence in person-centered decision-making communication strategies. To receive certification in ACP (FS, NS, AS) or practice in SDMSI conversations, participants may attend a classroom or virtual course that reinforces and supports the attainment of competency in PCDM communication and offers a pathway to certification.

Blended Learning

Creating a blended learning curriculum requires more than moving knowledge content to an online delivery platform; it requires a careful analysis of strategies to consistently integrate the defined competencies throughout the interactive program. A blended learning curriculum requires intentional strategies to reinforce all criteria for competency: the application and demonstration of appropriate knowledge, skills, behaviors, and judgment in a clinical setting.

The positive outcomes of the blended learning approach have confirmed that not all learning is online. To the contrary, "...all of these evidence-based studies concluded that student achievement was higher in blended learning experiences when compared to either fully online or fully face-to-face learning experiences."[2]

The RC blended learning curriculum includes an assortment of intentional classroom (and now virtual) strategies designed to enhance the attainment of the defined competencies for person-centered decision-making communication:

1) *Communicate course competency expectations.* - Merely attending a classroom or virtual course is insufficient for achieving competency. Many learners are familiar with the traditional face-to-face approach to education: simply show up, sign an attendance list, and receive documentation of compliance. As an Instructor, on several occasions, I experienced the "deer in the headlights" look from

participants who were shocked they would be expected to actively participate in role play exercises. Or participants who had no idea why they were attending the course relaying that "my supervisor told me to come."

Participants attending the RC communication skills courses are informed of the competency-based approach and certification requirements prior to registration through email instructions, web-based posting of certification requirements and course agendas, and supervisor support. A necessary component of pre-course preparation is clarification of organizational expectations for practice, certification, and integration of competencies post-course.

2) *Engage learners through pre-course activities.* - An array of activities can prepare participants for the in-person or virtual course experience and certification expectations, to include publication of the competency expectations, completion of online curriculum, viewing video demonstrations, shadowing an experienced clinician facilitating conversations, receiving sponsorship from a supervisor, department lead, or administrator, and completing pre classroom exercises.

For example, as a prerequisite to the First Steps ACP Facilitator course, participants are asked to complete a "practice" advance directive document. Feedback from this experience is shared in the classroom. Consistently, participants learn valuable lessons about their personal biases, gaps in understanding their advance directive document instructions, how difficult it is to document preferences and decisions, or how they learned that their husband or partner was not interested in being a health care agent. They swiftly learned that telling others they should complete an advance directive is easier said than done.

Asking participants to investigate their organizational practices is another effective engagement activity. How are PCDM conversations documented in the medical record? Is there a pool of resources for individuals who desire assistance with advance care planning? What palliative care resources are available? What is the policy on suspension of a DNR during surgery? How are ethics consultations accessed?

3) *Create tools to assist with competency demonstration.* - To reinforce the acquisition of the selected competencies and to create a practical tool that could be used during future conversations, the identified communication skill competencies are formatted as open-ended questions and organized into ACP (FS, NS, AS) or SDMSI conversation guides. Pocket versions of the conversation guides give practical tools to support consistent conversations and behavior change. Communication skill competencies are organized into one-page checklists and used for evaluation of skill achievement in role-play exercises, simulations, and ongoing clinical mentoring and certification.

4) *Demonstrate expected communication competencies.* - The creation of live or video demonstrations allows learners to observe experienced clinicians using the conversation guides and to illustrate defined competencies. Live role-play demonstrations are scripted for consistency among Instructors. Video role-play demonstrations include edited conversations from real patients or from simulated conversations using actors and scripts.

These examples highlight the demonstration of competency in the real world, promote critical thinking, and are valuable for ongoing review, refresher courses, and other educational objectives.

5) *Create practice role-play scenarios for demonstration of communication skill competencies.*- The opportunity to practice the newfound

communication skill competencies in a mentored environment is one of the most effective strategies for feedback and competency attainment. Well-crafted role-play scenarios simulate real conversations with individuals and their families, provide examples of common themes that arise during such conversation, and allow learners to critically think about how to respond to questions and concerns. The role-play scenarios are broken down into small components with discrete competencies that can be more easily integrated. Competency checklists provide a structured and measurable tool to provide consistent feedback and identify specific areas for competency improvement.

Experienced clinicians and certified Instructors are responsible for observing role-play demonstrations and giving feedback.

Critical Thinking-An Inherent Aspect of Competency

Lastly, competence includes the application of judgment, the ability to apply the requisite knowledge and skills in the real world. RC chose to use the term "critical thinking" to represent the judgment competency. The concept of critical thinking has fascinated me from the beginning of my nursing career, stemming from the wise mentoring of one of my favorite nursing instructors who would never give a straight answer to students' questions. She would respond to a question by asking more questions. Her response of "What would you do, Linda?" was frustrating because, as a novice nurse, if I knew the answer why would I be asking the question? However, this role modeling encouraged me to question my actions, challenge the obvious, and help others realize the value of critical thinking.

The application of critical thinking was omnipresent in my role as clinical nurse specialist in the critical care environment. Novice nurses often struggle with this application. When mentoring a novice nurse through the collection of an arterial blood gas sample, I witnessed her inability to attend to the entire patient encounter.

She was following the "procedure" perfectly: using aseptic technique, proper collection tubes, and technical requirements. In the middle of the procedure the patient, who was admitted with a heart attack, complained of "that funny feeling in my chest." The novice nurse, absorbed in her procedure, ignored the patient's complaint, saying, "You'll have to wait until I am done with this lab work." Naturally, I intervened to attend to the patient's chest pain, but the situation afforded a teachable moment to reflect on the value of critical thinking in all clinical encounters.

Critical thinking is different from solving a problem, or having the correct answer to a clinical question, or resolving a specific dilemma using a defined protocol. "Critical thinking is that mode of thinking, about any subject, content, or problem, in which the thinker improves the quality of his or her thinking by skillfully analyzing, assessing, and reconstructing it."[3]

I have a fondness for this definition of critical thinking but adopted the more simplistic explanation that was easy to remember (although I may have inadvertently borrowed it from someone else). Critical thinking is thinking about your thinking to improve your thinking. Critical thinking is not about being an expert, but about grooming your expertise. A critical thinker desires to be informed, to have an open mind about differing opinions, to understand, to have self-confidence in reasoning abilities, to honestly admit to one's own biases and prejudices, to be flexible in determining alternatives to any course of action, and to be willing to change one's own mind when new and reliable information presents itself.[4]

During the creation of the online component to the ACP facilitator courses, we searched for a learning management platform that would include critical thinking exercises. Unwilling to succumb to a curriculum that would only focus on the passive transfer of information and unable to find a platform that fit our needs in this area, we negotiated the ability to customize an existing template. Rather than settle for post-course exams, or multiple choice questions, we integrated a host of clinical case studies modeled from real life situations, asking participants to put themselves in these situations and respond to "what would you do if" and "what would you say" and "what consequences do you see?" The online platform does not allow for open discussion, but highlights the skill of critical thinking, or using judgment in the application of a stated competency.

Critical thinking can (and must) be effectively role modeled by a competent Instructor — described in the following chapter — and infused into the classroom and mentoring experience.

The Virtual Course Platform

The Covid-19 pandemic of 2020 created a new challenge for RC faculty and Instructors to continue to disseminate the familiar and popular blended learning curricula. RC leadership and faculty quickly responded and converted all the RC PCDM programs to a virtual platform, maintaining the CBE program contents described above. This adaptation allowed for the continuation and dissemination of valued education and competency in PCDM communication. RC Instructors were offered ongoing support by RC faculty in delivering the virtual courses, learning from each other, and sharing tips and strategies. The expansion of, and demand for, virtual course offerings continues at the local and national levels. Covid-19 specific educational materials were created and distributed through the RC website free of charge.

As social distancing became a mainstream strategy to prevent the spread of Covid-19, the need arose to develop expertise in telephonic or video ACP facilitation. The RC faculty responded by disseminating telephonic ACP resources, including a virtual ACP webinar series and critical thought leadership presentations.

In my role as RC consultant, I maintained a co-investigator role with a study entitled, "Reducing Disparities in the Quality of Palliative Care for Older African Americans through Improved Advance Care Planning (EQUAL ACP)," a study that included the delivery of an in-person RC First Steps

ACP intervention for people with chronic illness.[5] Due to the pandemic, recruitment for the RC arm of the study was halted. Together with RC faculty and the study team, we created telephonic ACP guidelines for the interventionists that allowed study recruitment to resume.

Respecting Choices maintains its ongoing commitment to program delivery adaptations that will continue to disseminate competency-based PCDM communication courses.

Modular Course Offerings

There are undisputed and distinct differences in the Respecting Choices PCDM courses (FS, NS, AS ACP and SDMSI), such as the knowledge needed to help patients make specific treatment decisions, the role of the physician and advanced practitioner in providing prognosis information, or the completion of an advance directive. However, core knowledge and communication skill competencies are similar.

The repetition of competencies among these four programs has proven to be frustrating for participants that desire certification with multiple target populations. Requiring learners to attend multiple courses with overlapping content is time-consuming and expensive. A modular approach to PCDM communication competency offers many advantages.

- **The delineation of baseline (or core) communication skill competencies** - A defined list of baseline competencies expected of all healthcare clinicians or community facilitators would assist to standardize communication and continuity of PCDM conversations for patients and families.

- **The adoption of an interdisciplinary approach to PCDM communication** - The delineation of a baseline (or core) list of PCDM communication skill competencies provides a unique opportunity to support the interdisciplinary, improve understanding of each team member's concerns and contributions to PCDM conversations, and promote collaboration. Those who engage in decision-making conversations should not be working in isolation from others on the team. A competent clinician could assist in setting the stage for more specific conversations with the physician, exploring fears and concerns. For example, a nurse may initiate the exploratory phase of a communication competency by assessing what is known about the decision (e.g., advance care planning, implantable defibrillator), provide information as needed, and collect more specific questions for the patient's medical team (What are the odds of CPR working with my specific medical condition?). Through exploration, other issues or concerns may be elevated that do not directly impact the specific decision but influence the patient's quality of life and overall care plan.

- **Specific PCDM communication modules (NS, AS, SDMSI) focus on more complex conversations** - Some modules address more complex communications, such as those with the seriously ill, and would integrate the specific knowledge required to facilitate these conversations.

In summary, a modular curriculum to attain competency in PCDM communication would guide the development of an organizational or community approach to consistent program materials, teaching strategies, measurement, and organizational expectations, and ongoing monitoring for the maintenance of competency in PCDM communication.

Chapter 19: Certification of Instructors as Teachers, Role Models, Mentors, and Organizational Resources: The Respecting Choices Experience

"Facilitators of communication skills training should have sufficient training and experience to effectively model and teach the desired communication skills and facilitate experiential learning."[1]

Creating a cadre of national Instructors has proven to be an indispensable component in the standardized dissemination of the Respecting Choices PCDM communication curricula. Instructor education, mentoring, and certification is a worthy investment, and although there are no national guidelines for those that teach communication skills, the American Heart Association's ACLS program provides a national exemplar.[2]

To become an ACLS Instructor, individuals must first meet minimum criteria for acceptance into the program: 1) have a valid provider card in ACLS, proving competency in ACLS certification, 2) apply and be accepted by a local ACLS training center, which ensures collaboration and communication for ACLS related courses, 3) complete the classroom Instructor course successfully, 4) participate in an ACLS course with a certified faculty member, thus receive monitoring of teaching skills in the real world of classroom teaching. Once the Instructor candidates meet these criteria, they are provided a complete set of course materials and can join a learning community of ACLS Instructors for ongoing learning and sharing of teaching experiences.

Instructor Certification

The Respecting Choices Instructor certification program follows a similar pathway as the ACLS model.[3] Instructor candidates are required to:

1) Garner organizational or community support for participation and a complete an Instructor agreement that defines role expectations

2) Attain certification in the program they desire to teach, for example, First Steps ACP or SDMSI. This certification can be attained at a local course, taught by certified Instructors, or by attending a regularly scheduled national course

3) Attend a national or local "design and implementation" course that demonstrates an understanding of the systems that must be created to improve the outcomes of PCDM

4) Successfully complete an Instructor certification course

5) Teach the related course curriculum within six months

6) Obtain recertification as defined by RC

Once these criteria are achieved, the Instructor is given access to all course materials, access to an online store, and the opportunity to join a network of Instructors who meet regularly to share experiences, concerns, and seek solutions to current challenges.

The Instructor certification course is vital to the ultimate effectiveness of the Instructor candidate as a teacher, mentor, critical thinker and evaluator, and ongoing organizational resource. Instructor candidates are mentored to practice novel teaching strategies that promote learner engagement, critical thinking, and the attainment of competency.

The Instructor as Teacher and Critical Thinking Role Model

Instructor candidates are probed to examine their teaching style — a necessary examination for Instructors to role-model critical thinking skills. Many individuals teach the way they have been taught, often adopting a 'sage on stage' veneer.[4] A "sage on the stage" approach to teaching is aligned with more traditional educational approaches where the teacher is the expert, owns all the information, and has all the "right" answers. Instructor candidates are asked to adopt a "guide by the side" approach that describes the teacher as a facilitator of learning, actively involving participants in meeting their individual learning needs, and encouraging learners to think for themselves, discover solutions… to think critically.

The "guide by the side" approach allows the Instructor to role-model critical thinking strategies in the classroom and demonstrate the application of judgment in PCDM. As an Instructor, I would often begin a course with the following: "I hope you leave here today with more questions than when you started. There is a ton of expertise in this room, and I am excited about what we can learn from each other." I understood that I was not the only expert in the room.

In helping patients make decisions aligned with their goals and values, there are often a range of acceptable solutions. Critical thinking (judgment) is essential. Consider your response to the following question from a course participant:

"Is it OK to give my personal opinion when helping patients make treatment decisions?"

A "sage on stage" response might immediately say "no" to this question, reminding participants that their role is to remain value-neutral and not impose their own values on the autonomy of the patient. However, a "guide by the side" approach would encourage critical thinking about this question with all participants, offering such responses as, "What are the consequences of giving your opinions?" and "What message might that send to patients?" and "Are there situations where giving one's opinion might be appropriate?"

Both "sage on stage" and "guide by the side" approaches are useful. There are times when an Instructor simply needs to provide a correct answer. For example, in response to the question, "Can three siblings be chosen to be primary healthcare agents?" the answer is obviously "no." And it redirects the participant to understand their state statute on advance directives.

We never figured out how to consistently evaluate the critical thinking abilities of participants within the in-person or virtual classroom setting. This evaluation seems more fitting for the clinical or real-world setting. However, Instructors who role-model critical thinking expose participants to the range of acceptable responses and ideally promote the application of this skill in future situations.

A stellar example of the role of the Instructor in promoting critical thinking is the elevation of the communication technique to "remain value-neutral" in person-centered decision-making communication. The following classroom examples highlight opportunities to elevate the impact of value-laden words and statements during PCDM conversations:

- On more than one occasion, during a classroom discussion on strategies to initiate the CPR decision, an enthusiastic (and sometimes well-respected) clinician would offer his or her approach to initiating the CPR conversation as follows, "I simply ask, 'Do you want CPR if you are already dead?'" This statement threw me back in time to my clinical days when I observed coercive conversations — conversations I think the daughter in the opening story must have been exposed to. CPR videos were shown to patients that demonstrated intubation and patients flying off the bed during defibrillation. Or, physicians telling patients, "If you were my mother, I certainly wouldn't want you to have CPR," or "Do you really want us to break your ribs and puncture your lungs like I've seen several times?" I have facilitated hundreds of CPR decision-making conversations that helped patients make an informed decision and never once had to resort to coercion or threats.

- During participant introductions, I would often ask each person to list one communication skill they would like to improve, or one they found unusually challenging. During one introduction, a participant proudly announced, "I'd like to learn how to help patients not make bad decisions." I almost laughed aloud at her open and honest disclosure.

- Or the participant who challenged the standard of offering CPR to anyone over the age of 80. Of course, the participant was only 22 years old with minimal patient care experience.

These value-laden statements are opportunities for teachable moments. As an Instructor, the path to least resistance would be to pretend that you did not hear the statement and simply move on to the next course agenda. But, not responding delivers a message to everyone else in the room that value-laden statements are condoned or even preferred. Instructors can role-model critical thinking responses that promote self-reflection, for example, asking for participant reactions and reflections on a value-laden statement, exploring the rationale behind the statement, offering alternative strategies, and at times, simply agreeing to disagree.

A final illustration of the use of critical thinking is a riveting experience with a chaplain who attended an ACP course, and believed the RC program was promoting the withholding or withdrawing of artificial nutrition and hydration. His concern was expressed forcefully in the classroom setting as follows:

Respecting Choices is promoting the withholding and withdrawing of basic food and water. That is not consistent with the values of my faith. Life at all costs should be sustained. Food and water are basic care and should never be withheld or withdrawn. Respecting Choices should not be advocating any other position, and I would not participate in this kind of decision with anyone.

This emotional expression presented a host of teachable moments for the Instructor. Responding with "everyone has a right to their own opinions and values" would be the least preferred approach. While there are many alternatives, the Instructor team began by acknowledging his emotion and faith tradition values. Concerned that others in class held similar views about Respecting Choices, the Instructor asked if others held this view.

Although most of the class had not made this assumption, the question normalized the concern. It acknowledged that patients may have a similar concern or misconception and that facilitators may need to identify fears and concerns and provide clarifying information.

A more urgent issue was the dilemma of awarding him certification. A facilitator's role is to remain value-neutral, not value-less. We discussed the tension that may exist for some facilitators who had strong beliefs and values and the options they could choose during conversations that conflicted with this, such as referring a person to a facilitator that did not share value conflicts.

This situation highlighted the communication technique of "remaining value-neutral" integrated into the PCDM and Instructor certification courses, recognizing preparation for conflict resolution in the classroom setting and role-modeling appropriate responses.

Awarding Facilitator Certification

Instructors may choose to evaluate individual competence in the classroom-or virtual platform- and award certification through the completion of standardized competency checklists used to measure minimum competence. Classroom certification is daunting, probably impossible, and certainly not optimum.

With program evolution, it is recommended (but not mandated) that certification not be awarded in the classroom, instead assessed post-course after allowing time for practice and ongoing mentoring. Instructors typically have an organizational role that provides ongoing observation, practice, mentoring, and the creation of improvement plans as needed.

The Instructor role is a basic tenet for the dissemination of standardized PCDM communication competence and certification. However, without organizational commitment, an Instructor's influence on communication outcomes is limited.

Chapter 20: Organizational Commitment to Competency in Person-Centered Decision-Making Communication

The original RC competency-based communication programs were popular and in demand by national and international organizations and communities. Bud and I traveled the country offering facilitator certification and design and implementation ACP courses. The impact of these onsite courses was short-lived.

Without system changes and leadership support to indoctrinate the newfound competency expectations, implementation teams became frustrated and disillusioned. Simply providing education was not fulfilling the RC mission to build a culture of person-centered decision-making. The imperative to build leadership support for sustainability resulted in the design of RC consultation services to assist with implementation of a more comprehensive system described throughout this book.

I often wondered why an organization or community would invest in PCDM competency without a plan for sustainability? One of the greatest disappointments in my role as a consultant helping organizations implement the RC program was when organizations abandoned their initial efforts to improve PCDM, abandoning the educational curriculum and resources for sustainability. I continue to think about these experiences and what I could have done to change the outcomes.

Through these early years of implementation, we openly acknowledged that achieving competency in person-centered decision-making communications was more than a personal improvement activity — but an organizational mission to deliver person-centered care. A strategic commitment to developing interdisciplinary competence in PCDM communication serves to convey the values and priorities of healthcare professionals and the environments in which they provide care. "Because competency-based education begins with a careful consideration of the competencies desired in the health professional workforce, it provides a vehicle for integrating the health needs of the country with the priorities of the profession."[1]

An organizational and community commitment to PCDM competency extends far beyond the classroom, the completion of an online course, or a certificate of completion. The real learning occurs in the clinical setting, where novice practitioners receive mentoring and feedback on the application of their skills in specific situations. These skills are reinforced by other clinicians who have attained competency and serve as stellar role models to reinforce expected behaviors. Competencies serve to improve the work environment, increasing job satisfaction when employees see consistent behaviors among their peers. Ultimately, competencies serve to improve patient care and safety, including the avoidance of medical errors and harmful conversations.

Demonstration of Commitment to Communication Competency

Organizational and community leaders can demonstrate their commitment to widespread dissemination of competency in person-centered decision-making communication in several ways:

- Link the person-centered decision-making curriculum to the overall strategic goal of providing person-centered care. It is not enough to devote a few resources for a few individuals. How will the vision of competency in PCDM communication be disseminated to the entire organization and community?

- Dedicate resources to support the attainment and maintenance of PCDM competency. As with ACLS certification, competency in PCDM is supported through access to certified Instructors, clinical experts, and the financial resources for ongoing maintenance of competency.

- Revise organizational policies to support an intradisciplinary approach to PCDM; define specific competencies in job descriptions for all appropriate staff.

- Create a cadre of competent clinical mentors to support the application of PCDM in the real world through role modeling conversations, mentoring novice clinicians, assessing the maintenance of competency, and gathering information on the outcomes of PCDM interventions.

- Design or redesign organization and community systems (described earlier in this book) to support PCDM decision-making outcomes, to include electronic platforms for documentation, transparency, portability, and accountability for PCDM conversations, and the design of out-of-facility systems capable of honoring individual's treatment preferences.

These organizational and community promises are hefty but consider the consequences of an unskilled team of individuals who interact with patients and families every day, influencing their decision-making process and behaviors. As in the opening story, unskilled conversations cause harm, resulting in medical errors, patient and family dissatisfaction, and moral distress for healthcare clinicians and other patient advocates.

Chapter 21: The Power of Person-Centered Decision-Making Communication: Lessons From the Field

Creating, testing, improving, and teaching the Respecting Choices PCDM curricula to thousands of clinicians was a privilege, an honor, and a learning experience, but I yearned to experience person-centered decision-making in action — to personally facilitate conversations with patients and their families. I had a craving to learn, test the impact of the strategies we had created, demonstrate personal competence, and infuse teaching strategies from real-life stories, questions, emotions, and concerns into classroom discussion. Scheduling time to facilitate these conversations also fueled my desire for patient contact, something that I missed since leaving the clinical arena. More personally, I wanted to provide a service to my friends and family.

The conversations that follow made a difference in my professional and personal life. I became a more credible instructor, program designer, and overall better person. These conversations became a constant reminder of the reason I was doing this work. This work to improve person-centered decision-making. Even when entering conversations as a stranger, I learned the power of providing hospitality which, in the words of Henri Louwen, is "…. the creation of a free space where the stranger can enter and become a friend instead of an enemy. Hospitality is not to change people, but to offer them space where change can take place."[1]

The following stories were selected to represent common themes that bubble up when patients, families, and facilitators enter the hospitality space. The stories exemplify the challenge of PCDM conversations and the competence required to engage strangers, patients, and loved ones in emotional dialogue, deal with resistance to planning, resolve fears and concerns about treatment decisions, and soothe the decision-making burden for healthcare agents. A special thanks to those who have given their permission to include their stories and to those who wish to remain anonymous.

A Planning Conversation With My Sons: Practice What You Preach

Prior to attending the classroom component of the First Steps ACP communication course, participants are asked to attempt to have a planning conversation with someone they love. I quickly understood that I needed to complete this same expectation. I was motivated by a presentation I attended by William Colby, the attorney who brought the tragic story of the Cruzan family's struggle to make decisions for their daughter to the public's attention and then to the United States Supreme Court.[2] During his presentation, he relayed his struggle to get a family member (his wife, I believe) to engage in advance care planning, but she resisted. He finally resorted to intimidation, saying, "How can I go about the country talking about advance directives if I can't get my own family to do this?"

Mr. Colby's struggle was a common theme: how to engage in planning conversations with those we love. To better understand this struggle, I initiated a planning conversation with my three sons. At the time I was a single parent, and my boys were 20, 17, and 14 years old. Given these ages, it was my eldest son, Joshua, who could serve as my healthcare agent. To my surprise, the first family conversation lasted a couple of hours. As a clinical nurse specialist in ICU and a member of the ethics committee, I had often talked about real-life ethical dilemmas of my patients at the dinner table or after coming home from a particularly distressing day. I wondered if these previous conversations would make it easier to talk with my sons.

My sons were open and engaged. After some discussion about what mattered most to me and how I would want decisions to be made if I was unable to make them for myself, my middle son, Cory, sighed and said, "Whew, I'm glad that I don't have to do this job." The boys had questions. Some related to my goals and values, others more obscure. Joshua wondered if he would need the consensus of his brothers in making decisions. Where would I want to die? If something happened to me, would they live with their dad full-time? What would happen to my worldly possessions?

This initial conversation also spurred humorous comments about what they might want for their future. Cory immediately wanted to talk about what clothes he would like to wear if he died — high-top socks and shorts, of course — and how he would want to be remembered as "lost at sea."

The conversation had a lasting impact. When Joshua was in college, he gave a speech about advance directives and the importance for young adults to select a surrogate decision-maker. When Cory turned 18 years of age, and we gathered for Mother's Day, he announced, "Now that I'm 18, and older and wiser, I think it is my turn to be your healthcare agent, Mom." When Joshua and Cory married, they both understood the importance of completing their advance directives and talking to their spouses about healthcare decisions.

This conversation helped me gain experience with initiating conversations close to home. While the "task" of completing an advance directive was completed, I learned how conversations among those we love take time and often generate unrelated concerns that require family attention. These conversations are tender, intimate, and enduring. Each conversation makes the next one a bit easier.

I Can't Imagine a Life Worse Than What I am Living:
A Conversation with a Seriously Ill Woman and Her Husband

During the development of the Next Steps (NS) ACP intervention, communication strategies were created to help patients with serious illnesses reflect on their current situation and express their hopes for the future. This novel type of planning conversation would be the subject of a research partnership with the University of Wisconsin school of nursing. During our pilot investigation and the fine-tuning of the conversation guide, I conducted several conversations with patients with end-stage renal disease and heart failure.[3]

During one conversation, I met Dorothy and her husband, Tom. Dorothy was a 76-year-old woman with advanced renal disease who had been on hemodialysis for five years. Dorothy's health had declined in recent months. Her long-standing diabetes had created peripheral vascular complications. She was fast losing her eyesight and could no longer walk. Tom needed to help her eat, bathe, and perform other activities of daily living.

Our ACP conversation was scheduled during her four-hour dialysis treatment. She was lying in bed, Tom on one side and myself on the other. It was in a four-bed hemodialysis ward, and although the curtains were drawn, I was acutely aware that other clinicians were curious and listening. Dorothy openly grieved the significant losses she was experiencing from her progressive illness, stating, "I can't imagine a life worse than what I am living."

Through the sadness, there was an eagerness to talk and to be heard. At the end of the conversation, Tom left the room, and as I was saying my good-byes, Dorothy asked me to do one more thing for her. "Will you go tell my husband that I am ready to quit dialysis? I just cannot tell him myself. I don't know what he will do if he is not taking care of me." Understanding her angst and inability to reveal her secret desire to Tom directly, I honored her request.

I found an emotional and weary Tom in the waiting room. Given the conversation we had just completed, he acknowledged his awareness of Dorothy's depth of suffering and was not surprised at her request to stop dialysis, stating simply, "Do you think she could wait to stop dialysis until spring? It is very lonely here in Wisconsin in the winter." Tom's request was honored.

This conversation helped me grasp the complexity of living with serious illness for the entire family. Caregivers desire to make life easier but may not fully understand their loved one's pain and suffering. Both caregiver and patient have individual goals, concerns, and hopes that may be kept secret for fear of disappointment or rejection. I learned that patients and caregivers need and welcome assistance navigating the profound and complicated care decisions as illness progresses. This tough conversation gave me confidence to interact with future patients and their families. Experience makes a difference.

But He's Doing So Well: A Healthcare Agent's Initial Reactions to Planning Conversations

Another couple in the NS ACP pilot study was a 55-year-old man with a diagnosis of heart failure who was accompanied by his wife, who was a nurse and his healthcare agent. The man had recently entered the heart failure program, had experienced a decrease in symptoms, improved medication management, and a renewed quality of life. He willingly talked about his hopes for continued progress but crept into a discussion of how his goals and values might change if he experienced complications if his medical condition worsened.

His wife began to cry. She was upset and perhaps a bit angry. She had invested in his progress, helping him with his diet, exercise, and medications. "I want him to continue to be positive, to not think about the bad things that may happen. This is not the kind of conversation we should be having." I secretly wanted to run out of the room. What damage had I caused? What do I do now? Instead of running, I took a deep breath and acknowledged her fears, concerns, and her notable love for her husband and his well-being. Turning to the patient for his perspective, he responded with empathy for his wife's concerns: "I really want and need to have this type of conversation, but I can wait until my wife is ready." They agreed to end the conversation at that time (an event that rarely happens) and take time for further reflection.

I learned a vital lesson that I would share with others for years to come. These conversations are not about me. They will proceed at their own pace if we listen and respect the journey that both individuals are traveling in their quest to live as well as possible with serious illness. Before this experience, I may have attempted to advocate for the husband and support his desire to talk, but they were a team that respected their individual values and need to pace the planning process on their own terms. For some, planning conversations take time. Although we had not accomplished "my agenda" for this conversation, I left with the confidence that a seed had been planted and relationships secured.

Making Life-Sustaining Treatment Decisions in Real Time: I am That Mother

What does it actually "feel" like to make healthcare decisions for a loved one? For years, I had planning conversations with strangers, helping them explore goals and values, advocating for what matters most to the individual, and helping the family hear their loved one's preferences. But what does it actually *feel* like to make life-sustaining treatment decisions in real time... for someone you love?

Previous conversations had given me a glimpse into this reality. After listening to a mother express to her daughter a clear vision of what she would (and would not) want if she suffered complications from her illness, the daughter's eyes welled up with tears, saying, "I am not surprised by what my mother is saying. It just feels very different hearing her say it. It makes it real."

The reality of decision-making became real for me when my son was admitted to an ICU with a serious medical condition. I was traveling when I was notified, miles away from his hospital bed. Over the ensuing twenty-four hours, his condition worsened.

I received a phone call from the critical care fellow assigned to my son's healthcare team. Due to significant seizures, high fever, and respiratory decline, he was placed into a medically induced coma. He was now on a ventilator and on continuous EEG (electroencephalogram) monitoring.

"We are concerned about brain damage," said the critical care fellow. He wondered when I would be coming to the hospital as I was listed as an emergency contact. During this phone call, I remember asking a bunch of questions, but cannot remember any of the answers.

I made the journey to the hospital in a nearby state with my best friend, Flo. It was a long, painful ride but started to prepare me for what to expect when I arrived. Given my background, I immediately imagined the worst-case scenario and started contemplating the types of decisions that might need to be made. What if my son did not wake up? What if he did awake but suffered permanent brain damage? Who would make decisions? How would my ex-husband respond? What were the advance directive laws in this state?

On the way to the hospital, I called my colleague Bud, who investigated the statutory laws of the state where my son was hospitalized. I received vital information. This specific state had a surrogacy statute that, absent a written advance directive, defers decision-making first to the parents if the person is not married, and then to others as defined in a formal hierarchy of potential substitute decision-makers. Despite my relief in this provision, I was aware that my ex-husband and I would need to reach consensus, an event that rarely occurred since our divorce years earlier. Bud also informed me that the assigned decision-maker, according to this state's statute, would have wide authority to make life-sustaining treatment decisions, including the withdrawal of the ventilator and a Do-Not-Resuscitate order.

These statutes were different than the Wisconsin versions that I had become intimately familiar with. Case law in Wisconsin did not give surrogates the authority to remove life-sustaining treatment for a non-decisional patient without specific evidence of the patient's wishes or a specific diagnosis of persistent vegetative state. At first, this statutory information was a relief, but then the reality of having wide authority to make life-sustaining treatment decisions for my son hit me. Would I have the responsibility of ordering a withdrawal of life-sustaining treatment for my own son? At an intellectual level I could understand. But I was now the mother.

Arriving at the hospital late that night, the RN assigned to my son gave me a medical update and asked who the designated decision-maker would be as he was obviously unable to make his own decisions. I informed her that I was an ICU nurse, somehow believing that my experience would influence this designation, yet knowing that I could not unilaterally make that decision. A family meeting was scheduled for the following morning with the ICU intensivist, a woman whose image and person-centered approach is forever etched in my memory.

The ICU intensivist arrived at the family meeting alone and sat down with me, my son's father, and my friend Flo. She started the conversation with an overview of the medical situation with a gentle but firm explanation that the prognosis was uncertain. My son may not awake, he may have brain damage if he did survive, and the family may need to make life-sustaining treatment decisions. She then paused and asked one simple question:

"Tell me about your son. What is he like as a person?"

And she listened patiently to our reflections. This simple question framed the entire hospital experience for me. Recanting our responses today remains emotional. For the next fifteen minutes, we shared our perspectives on my son's life: his intelligence, zest for travel and diverse experiences, physical abilities, and pursuit of a profession in history and research.

As I offered to be the surrogate decision-maker for my son, there was no dissent from my ex-husband. That decision then spurred a discussion of the potential decisions that may need to be made if my son did not improve or was unlikely to be able to live the kind of life we knew he had enjoyed. The physician stated that she would honor our decisions to remove life-sustaining treatments if that proved necessary but wanted more information and time for a thorough evaluation.

Through the tears of that conversation, I felt myself hovering above everyone else in the room. Looking down at them, I wondered, "Was I really that mother who was able to make a decision that would end my son's life?"

Fortunately, my son recovered, and although I escaped the immediate decision about withdrawing the ventilator, the reality of what I may have decided weighed on me for months. My young adult son had not completed an advance directive. He did not have a chance to choose which parent he would want as his decision-maker. Would I have made the "right" decision if I ordered the removal of the ventilator? Is that what my son would have wanted? How long would he have wanted to continue life-sustaining treatment? The uncertainty lingered for months after his physical recovery. I now understood the long-term suffering caused by uncertainty I had observed with other families. This was a small slice of what I had been asking people to think about for themselves and for their loved ones.

I recalled a presentation on the role of a healthcare agent that I had conducted with a small interactive audience. One man revealed that, years prior, he had ordered the removal of a ventilator from his seriously ill father, who died shortly thereafter. With great emotion, and in front of complete strangers, he wondered if he had "killed his father." He admitted he had entered counselling for severe depression and now wondered if the decisions he made for his father contributed to his feelings of despair. The pain and suffering of uncertainty can have long-lasting impact.

While this experience affirmed the consequences of the work I was doing, it gave me a renewed sense of empathy for families who are asked to make life and death decisions in real time. Reflecting on the opening story of the daughter who was asked to make a DNR decision for her mother, could it be that she was uncertain? Was she spared from making a decision she would have to live with for the rest of her life? Healthcare agents may make decisions that others disagree with. Family relationships can be torn apart.

I also realized that most families in similar situations to mine did not have my background or resources to navigate new information and decision-making options. What would they be feeling on this long ride to the hospital? Who would help them once they arrived? Would they be approached by an ICU physician with person-centered decision-making competence like the one I encountered?

An Enduring Conversation Among Strangers: The Art Loomis Story

Art Loomis…one of my favorite memories of ACP conversations is one that elevated Mr. Loomis to the status of Respecting Choices' most infamous video star. Art and his son, Greg, gave permission for our planning conversations to be videotaped and used in our communication skills programs. His stardom persists, and thousands have learned about person-centered decision-making conversations from this video exemplar.

Art had completed an advance directive naming his son, Greg, as his healthcare agent. Art's medical conditions had progressed, however, and they were invited to participate in a Next Steps planning conversation to help Art talk about specific decisions he would want Greg to make if he were to suffer complications from his illnesses that resulted in unacceptable outcomes. They understood this would be a sensitive conversation. Still, they agreed to be videotaped, to meet with a stranger (me), and give permission for the video to be edited and shared with others for teaching purposes.

I met Art and Greg fifteen minutes prior to the beginning of the conversation. Art arrived in his high-top socks and shorts, but having left his hearing aid at home. I needed to talk more loudly than normal and repeat questions. In addition, the physical space was a bit stiff, despite our efforts to make it look homey, and Art and Greg were surrounded by three cameras, bright lights, the cameraman, microphones, and me (the stranger).

Despite the awkward climate, a relationship among strangers was quickly established. Art was genuine and openly revealed his fears, hopes, and some surprising decisions. We laughed. Art shed tears over his feelings for his grandchildren. His son, who thought he knew everything about his dad, revealed his renewed and improved understanding in a personal testament to the power of the conversation:

> The conversation was eye-opening for me. With a third-party present, I learned things I never knew about my dad…what became very clear…he did not want to go to a nursing home — he considered it a 'kiss of death.' He did not want a drawn-out death. That meeting triggered multiple follow-up conversations with my father. The last few years of his life we had more father-son talks than we did for the first sixty years of my life.[4]

In the conversation, Art revealed that he had made a DNR decision that was a surprise to Greg. A decision that required more planning if his decision not to be resuscitated would be respected. Art's medical record indicated he did not want CPR if his heart stopped while on dialysis, but Art clarified that he would not want CPR under any circumstances and had assumed that this was understood by his healthcare team. He had not thought about what would happen if his heart stopped while he was on the golf course, in church, or with his family.

I explained the DNR bracelet system in Wisconsin, a medic-alert type of bracelet that would always be worn and would instruct emergency personnel not to attempt CPR. Barely getting the words out of my mouth, Art said, "Where do I get one of those?" and "I should have one of those."

With a plan created to follow up on his DNR request, Art and Greg were visibly relieved. Art looked at Greg and said, "Now you will know what I want." Greg realized the importance of this specific decision, recalling a story of one of his friends who "should have had this figured out" but had a heart attack and emergency personnel attempted resuscitation where "the body was working but everything else was gone and it [withdrawing life support] was a tough call."

A few years after this conversation, Art collapsed in the parking lot of the kidney dialysis center. He was transferred to the emergency department (ED), where tests confirmed a massive stroke. His physicians believed he would survive but would have significant cognitive and physical disabilities. He would no longer be able to take care of himself. In Greg's words:

> ....my brothers and I gathered and discussed the wishes Dad laid out....we all knew he did not want life-sustaining treatment. The decision was not up to us. Our father made it very clear what he wanted in advance[5]

Life-sustaining treatment was stopped in the ED. Art was transferred to hospice care and died two days later.

This early experience affirmed the enduring power of conversations — conversations whose full impact may not be realized for years. Skillful PCDM conversations do not only result in written plans, but they open channels of communication, strengthen relationships, and spare families the angst of making the "right" decision for loved ones. The conversation highlighted the importance of ongoing conversations with healthcare agents, family, and the healthcare team to clarify decisions and update previously created plans. It also dispelled concerns that intimate conversations can be effectively facilitated by strangers.

Art wore his DNR bracelet with pride. A year after our conversation, Art and Greg agreed to talk about the ACP conversation with visitors from Germany who came to La Crosse to learn about the Respecting Choices program. Art proudly displayed his DNR bracelet, and Greg affirmed his confidence in making future treatment decisions that would support his dad's life and preferences.

Of Course, I Would Not Want CPR:
Facilitating Family Conversations

Closer to home was an experience with my mother-in-law, Evelyn. I met this special lady when she was 88 years old. We became friends, spending time together and creating memories. She filled a gap in my life as I had been estranged from my own mother for years.

I had gained an appreciation for her values and priorities. She had a zest for life, loved to dance, enjoyed seeing her son Craig's band perform, and cherished family time. She was fiercely independent, living in her Madison home for over fifty years, a three-level home with a big yard full of flowers and memories. Her husband died when he was only 61 years old, and Evelyn never remarried. She had one true love. She thought other men only wanted "a nurse or a purse" and she was neither.

In joining the family, I built relationships with her son Tom and his wife Suzanne, who lovingly looked after this special lady. Learning that Tom was designated as her healthcare agent, I felt compelled to gently open the door to inquire what he understood about Evelyn's goals and values for life-sustaining treatment. I treaded cautiously into this conversation as I did not have a long history with this family, and I wondered, "Would Tom think I was being intrusive? Would he think I was trying to influence Evelyn's decisions? Would the family be angry that I was initiating a sensitive subject?"

Tom listened respectfully as I explained the importance of a planning conversation with his mom, choosing to focus on CPR as a specific decision. I explained the glidepath that would occur if Evelyn's heart were to suddenly stop, and a plan to honor her wishes was not developed. I gave him information and a few ideas to begin the conversation with his mom.

Eventually, Tom seized an opportunity. They had gone to church and listened to a sermon that talked about planning for the future. This opened the door to a conversation about CPR, and to Tom's surprise, Evelyn was quick to reply, "Of course I would not want that." She had thought about it, had a firm opinion, and believed everyone in the family understood.

We proceeded to get Evelyn a Wisconsin-approved DNR bracelet that she proudly wore for the rest of her life. Her granddaughters improved the look of the metal bracelet by creating a pearl band. I was relieved that a decision that Evelyn assumed the family understood was now out in the open.

For me, initiating conversations with strangers is often easier than with those that I love. With strangers, it was my job, and I could introduce myself as a member of their healthcare team. I could emphasize that planning was part of good healthcare. With my family, however, I had trepidations. I feared I would be perceived as overstepping family boundaries or risk damaging relationships.

Being an advocate for my friends and family has been part of my personal mission. I have hosted a few gatherings that have been lovingly (although inaccurately) labeled as "end of life" parties where I walked people through the steps in advance care planning, answering their questions, and encouraging them to reflect on their goals and values and talk to their family. These conversations were gifts that kept on giving.

A Video Conversation on Planning for Future Healthcare Decisions: Observations of the Nudge

One of the early criticisms of the Respecting Choices approach to facilitating planning conversations is the time and resources to conduct them in person. Although the official telephone guidelines for ACP conversations did not emerge until the Covid-19 pandemic of 2020, we had many experiences facilitating these conversations through video and telephonic modalities.

During one of our explorations with a company that was interested in acquiring the RC program, we were challenged with helping the decision-makers understand person-centered decision-making. We decided to demonstrate a

First Steps ACP conversation for Ben — one of the administrators — and his wife via videoconference. Both individuals were in my visual field, allowing me to observe their reactions throughout the conversation. When asked the question, "What experiences have you had with family or friends who have been seriously ill?" Ben immediately informed me that he was only thirty years old and, thankfully, had not had these kinds of experiences.

This is a common initial response. I noticed his wife nudging his arm and giving him a glance. I asked the question again, hoping this would give him more time for reflection. Saying nothing, his wife gave him a second nudge, which I openly acknowledged. Commenting on this observation gave his wife permission to probe Ben and ask, "What about your father?" Ben lowered his head and proceeded to tell an amazing story of his father's chronic illness, the lack of conversation, and the stress of family decision-making. This was exactly the motivation they needed to understand the importance of the ACP conversation.

Face-to-face conversations are captivating, but we have learned that conversations can be effectively facilitated through video and teleconferencing. This experience also affirms the power of including family or loved ones in conversations, sharing and remembering experiences, identifying fears and concerns, and learning together. Having group conversations can allow people to gently "nudge" each other along in the planning process.

The Conversation Opened My Eyes to What My Mom Wanted: A Daughter's Experience

Annie's mom had advanced lung disease. Annie and her mom fought daily over her mom's desire to continue to smoke, straining their relationship. In Annie's words, "We were at each other's throats."

A colleague of mine, a palliative care licensed clinical social worker, facilitated an NS ACP planning conversation between Annie and her mom that permanently improved this strained relationship. Following is Annie's reflection of that pivotal planning conversation:

> As far as the conversation, I wouldn't change it for anything. The good, the bad, the ugly. I would not trade it because it opened my eyes to see what my mom wanted. It helped mend a broken relationship between the two of us. A light bulb went on... I get it now. Why am I fighting with her when she just wants to live the best she can instead of longer? To see her happy with her cigarette and cup of coffee, that made me happy. To see the smile on her face, that was enough. We were no longer at each other's throats. I learned what was important to her: to have her cigarette, her cup of coffee and to never be alone. It was hard to hear my parent say that she did not want CPR, and other things, when I selfishly want her to be with me. It's hard to follow your parents' wishes.

The caregiver journey is not easy. Charged with the responsibility to take "good" care of loved ones, caregivers follow the recommended medical plan of care and strive to maintain a stable condition. Caregivers are often willing to do whatever is needed to keep their loved one alive if possible. This planning conversation allowed Annie to hear her mother's voice for the first time. It may not have happened without the help of a skilled communicator.

This story exemplifies the importance of including healthcare agents and other family members in person-centered decision-making conversations. Annie was now prepared to make substitute decisions for her mom, prepared to honor her mother's goals and values, and honor her DNR decision. Annie would not be making decisions based on her own values or desires. There would be sadness, but no uncertainty, as the decisions would be her mother's, not her own.

Chapter 22: So, You're the One They Have Sent to Kill My Mother Revisited

So, You're the One They Have Sent to Kill My Mother: The Harmful Impact of Unskilled Conversations

As the opening story depicts, unskilled conversations have consequences for patients, their families, and the healthcare team.

The healthcare agent had been harmed. Upon entering the patient's room, and then for over one hour, I listened to her describe the reasons for her angst and anger toward the medical team. She had felt their bias that CPR should not be attempted, their frustration over her disagreement with their medical opinions, and eventually, she felt their abandonment. She no longer trusted the healthcare team. It was no surprise that she would not leave her mother's side. Her own health was in jeopardy.

After my apology for her experience, we explored what she knew about her mother's goals and values. What would her mother decide if she could hear all the medical information being presented? The daughter was adamant that her mother would want to keep fighting. She would want every chance to live, even if the chance were small.

At the end of this conversation, I assured her that the healthcare team would support her decision about attempting CPR. Of course, I had discussions with the medical resident and attending physician about this decision. Both listened obligatorily, disagreed, and angrily walked away.

The patient had a cardiac arrest soon thereafter, CPR was attempted, and the patient died.

Unskilled conversations endanger patient safety with their potential for decisions that are not aligned with the patient's goals and values and damage the patient and family experience with the healthcare team by destroying trust in the healing relationships. Lastly, unskilled conversations reflect on the values of the organization and may have a lasting impact on professional job satisfaction.

Personally, I was embarrassed for my peers who, perhaps unwittingly, had unnecessarily imposed added stress for the daughter in fulfilling her role as substitute decision-maker, in loving her mother. I was disappointed in the reaction of the medical resident and attending physician to the results of my conversation. They complied with my recommendation to attempt CPR but were clearly upset that my consult had not resulted in a DNR order.

Over time, as part of his teaching responsibilities in the medical humanities department at Gundersen Lutheran, Bud Hammes created a competency-based program for medical residents to assist them in acquiring the skills of helping patients make a CPR decision.

These skills included exploration of goals and values, providing information, and promoting understanding. The competencies and strategies were aligned with the previously developed design elements of the communication skills programs. This program proved to consistently improve the residents' communication skills, who role-modeled these skills in the clinical arena. Moreover, patients and families reaped the benefits of person-centered decision-making conversations.

Summary

Imagine the possibilities. What would it mean if all healthcare professionals were competent in person-centered decision-making (PCDM) conversations? Imagine if every healthcare professional was equipped with the knowledge, skills, attitudes, and judgment to assist patients and families in making healthcare decisions aligned with their goals and values? Now imagine all members of the patient's healthcare team working together to achieve the ultimate goal of person-centered decision-making, the provision of person-centered care.

Imagine if you were a patient reaping the benefits of this teamwork. How would it feel to have this level of decision-making support? To have the care team asking consistent questions, documenting individual and ongoing conversations in the medical record, providing information in an unbiased manner and, in the end, creating plans and decisions that are in line with what matters most to you and are understood and honored by the healthcare team and your family? I simply cannot imagine how an organization can aspire to a mission of person-centered care without this commitment to communication excellence.

Despite the barriers, it is long past time for consensus on national standards and certification for person-centered decision-making communication skills. It is long past time for organizational leaders to set and monitor consistent expectations for PCDM outcomes.

Ideally, the delineation of PCDM communication competencies would be undertaken nationally, for example, by convening a consortium of experts who are commissioned to identify and publish core person-centered decision-making communication competencies that would apply to all healthcare professionals.

A cadre of PCDM communication competencies would be created, ranging from the minimum or baseline expectations for all employees, to more complex PCDM competencies — such as essential competencies when caring for patients with serious illness and their families or when individuals lose decision-making capacity. This is akin to the expectations that all clinicians become CPR certified, and those working in critical care settings additionally become certified in Advanced Cardiac Life Support (ACLS).

The return on this level of organizational investment extends far beyond a single, competent PCDM conversation or the ability to create and honor one plan that is aligned with a person's goals and values. The return on investment is building a culture of person-centered decision-making for everyone.

Personal Exercises

1) Can person-centered decision-making communication skills be taught? Why or why not?

2) List the person-centered communication skills you possess. How did you learn them? What skills would you like to improve?

3) Describe the prevalence and quality of person-centered decision-making conversations in your organization or community.

4) What have you learned from having planning conversations with patients and/or families? What would you do differently?

Part Five

Chapter 23: The Promise of Community Engagement and Education in Building a Culture of Person-Centered Decision-Making

Assisting Miss Sara in Making Healthcare Decisions

Miss Sara was a 72-year-old woman with advanced heart failure who agreed to participate in an advance care planning (ACP) conversation. Miss Sara had two hospitalizations in the preceding six months for increasing angina and shortness of breath, necessitating a few days of mechanical ventilatory support during the most recent episodes. During our ACP conversation, we explored her goals for living well, and her hopes and fears. She was tired of managing her illness and uninterested in another stint on a breathing machine.

She had little understanding of her treatment options in the event of illness complications — including cardiopulmonary resuscitation (CPR) — and was interested in learning more. We developed a list of questions she intended to discuss with her cardiologist, a trusted physician with whom she had a long relationship. During her medical appointment, her cardiologist discouraged her from worrying about potential complications, saying, "You are doing just fine, Sara. Please focus on staying as healthy as possible." With these words of encouragement from her well-meaning and trusted physician, Miss Sara was not interested in further conversation, expressing confidence that her cardiologist would take "good" care of her.

Overview

This part of the book is dedicated to the African proverb, "Oran a azu nwa," which means it takes a community or village to raise a child.[1] Only by communities working together will social change occur. Improving the person-centered decision-making (PCDM) behaviors of an entire community is no easy task. It demands partnerships among individuals, patients, families, caregivers, healthcare organizations and staff, media, groups with shared interests, and religious and ethnic groups.

This Part first explores the meaning of community, followed by a discussion of the distinction between education and engagement, emphasizing the importance of community engagement campaigns that require consistent and common messages delivered throughout an organization, in the settings where people socialize, in the written materials distributed, in the media, and by healthcare employees (Chapter 24). Next, an ecologic perspective is described that lays the foundation for the interaction between, and interdependence of, five levels of influence for behavior change: intrapersonal (Chapter 25), interpersonal (Chapter 26), organizational (Chapter 27), community (Chapter 28), and public policy (Chapter 29). Each chapter is accompanied by personal experiences, stories, and application to person-centered decision-making.

Chapter 30 chronicles experiences implementing the Respecting Choices ACP programs in healthcare systems and communities across the U.S. and other countries, reflecting the assimilation of diverse cultural, ethnic, socio-economic, and religious values and beliefs. This Part will conclude by revisiting the Opening Story and how it would look different in a culture of person-centered decision-making.

The Meaning of Community

Community means different things to different individuals. How community is defined will persuade the targeted engagement and education strategies designed to improve the culture of person-centered decision-making.

A launching definition of community is "…a group of people with diverse characteristics who are linked by social ties, share common perspectives, and engage in joint action in geographical locations or settings."[2] Still, a community is more than a collection of individuals. A sociologic construct embraces the relationships and interactions between members, mutual expectations, beliefs, and values as an inherent descriptor of a community.[3]

This Part — indeed the entire content of this book — welcomes the broadest possible definition of community focused on spreading person-centered decision-making behaviors throughout all facets of a community. It includes individuals (those with illness and those who are healthy), families (as defined by the individual), caregivers, groups with shared interests (disease support groups, faith affiliations, senior social centers, disability advocates), healthcare organizations (hospitals, clinics, nursing homes, assisted living facilities), healthcare staff (physicians, nurses, social workers, chaplains), media (newspapers, social networks, radio, television), schools, worksites, government agencies, and cultural and ethnic identities (African American, Hmong, Hispanic).

Unsurprisingly, these varied facets of a community bear unique characteristics requiring distinctive approaches to education and engagement to improve person-centered decision-making behaviors.

Chapter 24: Community Education is Different Than Community Engagement

It is a notorious fact that education alone does not change behavior, but attaining knowledge is a laudable goal that may accelerate progress toward transformation.

The discrepancy between education and knowledge is instructive. "Education is the process of facilitating learning, or the acquisition of knowledge, skills, values, beliefs, and habits. Knowledge is a familiarity, awareness, or understanding of someone or something, such as facts, information, descriptions, or skills, which is acquired through experience or education."[1]

Knowledge, therefore, is the end-product of education. As a process, education can be more effectual if it plainly identifies the specific knowledge goals it intends to impart. Three types of knowledge goals are defined below, with application to person-centered decision-making:

1) *Education to Promote General Knowledge*

   The dissemination of general knowledge as a single modality strategy is important, but incomplete to promote behavior change. For example, education to increase the public's knowledge of the signs of an impending stroke has been designed with the desired outcome that people will immediately call 911. However, research has demonstrated that people with more knowledge about the warning signs of a stroke are not more likely to call 911 than people without this knowledge.[2]

Perhaps a more memorable example of the propagation of general knowledge is the "Got Milk" campaign. The commercials and advertisements were engaging. We all remember the milk mustaches on pictures of Superman, Batman, and celebrities like quarterback Brett Favre (for all of us Green Bay Packer fans). Ninety percent of Americans were familiar with the slogan "where's your mustache?" Although there was a two percent increase in milk consumption in California, the origin of the campaign, nationally, there was a decline in yearly consumption from 23.0 gallons per person in 1995 to 20 gallons per person in 2011. Despite the fact that the campaign ultimately did not change behavior, it continued for 20 years simply because it was popular, catchy, and memorable.[3]

More specific to the content of this Part are the three-decade-long educational campaigns to increase the prevalence of advance directives, a tool for person-centered decision-making. Since the origin of the Patient Self Determination Act of 1991, efforts have proliferated to inform people of their right to make their own decisions and create a legal document. Providing general knowledge through the dissemination of written information in the form of booklets, pamphlets, and one-day awareness events (such as National Healthcare Decisions Day) are understandably "feel good" activities and persist in communities across the country.

While most Americans understand their right to complete an advance directive, the prevalence of completion remains low. An analysis of 150 studies on the prevalence of advance directives among U.S. citizens between 2011-2016 revealed that, among 795,909 people in the combined studies, 36.7 percent had completed documents, including 38.2 percent of those with chronic illness, a high-risk population.[4]

The dissemination of general knowledge will be more beneficial if augmented by education that increases awareness and improves skills.

2) *Education to Increase Awareness*

Educational efforts to increase awareness may cause behavior change if they emphasize a personal connection with the information, asking people to reflect on: "What's in it for me?" and "What difference will it make in my life?"

Well-crafted messages through written information, videos, or online programs can set in motion the process of personal self-reflection. As a component of the community engagement campaign designed in the mid-1990s by the La Crosse AD (advance directive) task force, written information and videos disseminated messages that helped shift people's understanding of ACP as a communication process versus the completion of an AD document. For example, a short planning guide explores the value of ACP conversations and asks thought-provoking questions to promote kitchen table dialogue.

A video interview, "Carol Goodman's Story," was recorded that captured the pain and agony Carol experienced when forced to make life-sustaining treatment decisions in a crisis situation for her mother with advanced illness who was unable to speak for herself. Carol describes her lack of knowledge about what her mother would want, the inability to consult with family, and her grief over making a Do-Not-Resuscitate decision. Carol's emotional plea of "No one should be put in this position," exemplifies the perpetual burden of making life and death decisions for a loved one.

Although the video's hairstyles and clothing are outdated, it continues to be effectively used as an engagement strategy in Respecting

Choices (RC) programs, highlighting the rationale for including healthcare agents in ACP conversations and elucidating the decision-making dilemmas that, unfortunately, persist today in healthcare organizations around the world. Organizations and communities implementing the RC program have used these exemplars to create context-specific materials that resonate with their respective communities.

Written materials can foster awareness of individual goals and values. Respecting Choices has designed decisions aids for people with serious illness (like heart or lung disease or cancer) facing a specific treatment decision such as breathing support or tube feeding for artificial nutrition.[5] Beyond describing the treatment and its benefits and burdens, these certified decision aids include the self-reflection question, "Which option best matches your values?" to assist in making individual decisions that are aligned with what matters most.

Tailored education offers an additional incentive to increase awareness and motivation to change behaviors. "Tailoring is a process that uses assessment to derive information about one specific person, and then offers change or information strategies for an outcome of interest based on that person's unique characteristics."[6] Tailoring includes asking questions, discovering individuals' goals, what they know, do, or do not want to know, and how to make decisions most urgent to their current health situation or illness trajectory.

A brochure cannot deliver tailored information. The Respecting Choices CPR fact sheet provides information on CPR to include current research-based outcome statistics.[7] However, recognizing that an individual's specific CPR outcomes vary based on their healthcare situation, the fact sheet emphasizes the gravity of receiving tailored information from a personal physician who can provide more specific recommendations and predictable outcomes. The fact sheet urges individuals to create a list of questions to be discussed with a provider prior to making a CPR decision.

Stories of patients with serious illness who have not engaged in person-centered decision-making activities thrive in the clinical arena despite the sundry opportunities that exist throughout the trajectory of patient care to tailor information, increase awareness, and contribute to proactive and individualized healthcare decisions. For example, Carol Goodman's mother had a chronic illness and had frequent encounters with healthcare providers — yet no one had initiated a conversation about her preferences for CPR, leaving her family unprepared to honor her decision.

The husband of a friend of mine was diagnosed with stage 4 lung cancer. He successfully weathered experimental immunotherapy and lived well for the better part of two years. Although aware of his rights, he had not completed an advance directive but did tell his wife he would not want CPR if his heart were to stop. Inevitably, he experienced a medical crisis without a plan for how aggressively he would want to be treated. His complication began with a urinary tract infection that resulted in septicemia.

These events were frightening for my friend who witnessed her husband's declining mental status and inability to make his own decisions, requiring her to act on his behalf. He was hospitalized, where antibiotic therapy was successful. His healthcare practitioners had consistently provided stellar medical care and offered palliative care options. But no one provided tailored education related to his lung cancer or explored his preferences for anticipated complications, such as "What type of treatment do you want if you have breathing difficulties? What actions should your wife take in an emergency if you are at home and your heart stops?" Faced with the memory and sequelae of the recent medical emergency, this couple became motivated to learn the skills to develop a more specific plan for future healthcare decisions.

Tailoring information may also begin with an assessment of a person's capacity for engagement. Judith Hibbard's Patient Activation Measure is an assessment tool to assist in designing education based on an individual's readiness and ability to change behaviors, or their stage of activation.[8]

3) *Education to Develop or Improve Skills*

Like my friend and her husband in the above story, once people have general knowledge and increased awareness, they often need assistance to devise plans that reflect their goals and values.

What are the skills necessary to actively participate in person-centered decision-making? Often, the skills for ACP are reduced to the technical aspects of how to complete a legally valid advance directive, filling in boxes, signatures, dates, and witnesses. The completion of this technical exercise may confer a false sense of security that an individual's goals and values have been sufficiently documented and that others will be prepared to "know and honor" their healthcare decisions. The indispensable skills of exploring one's goals and values, asking questions, choosing (and preparing) a qualified healthcare agent, and communicating one's preferences to family and healthcare providers are often neglected.

Recently, I updated my advance directive using the Wisconsin-specific power of attorney for healthcare form, adding an addendum that includes healthcare decisions for specific situations, such as complications from injury or illness that result in functional and cognitive decline, providing detailed guidance in decision-making for my healthcare agents. Most advance directive statutes include the option to add information in the form of "special instructions" or "additional information."

After revising my AD, I arranged a lunch date with my two sons — designated as primary and secondary healthcare agents — to review the information, field questions, and address ambiguities about their respective decision-making roles. They expressed several concerns:

> "Will the doctors and nurses agree with our decisions? Will they give us any 'push-back'?"

> "What does 'less than 80% chance of surviving a complication' (a goal in my addendum) really mean? Who would be providing that information?"

> "What does it mean to withdraw life-sustaining treatment after it has already been started?"

> "What if other family disagree with our decisions?"

Perhaps these questions were informed by a lifetime of familiar family conversations. Perhaps I just have smart sons. Nonetheless, the example reveals the value of preparing agents for a future decision-making role; preparation essential to remove the uncertainty surrounding surrogate decision-making. Moreover, the preparation of healthcare agents has additional benefits. The conversation with my sons strengthened relationships as they discovered the power of supporting each other in making healthcare decisions and clear communication with other family members — including my husband, who was not selected as my healthcare agent.

An ACP community engagement campaign, therefore, will require skills beyond the technical completion of an advance directive. Skills in exploring personal goals and values and talking to and preparing

loved ones for a future decision-making role are requisite to effica-
cious planning. Naturally, these skills can be role modeled during
facilitated face-to-face conversations, but they can also be illuminated through intentionally designed online tutorials, video demonstrations, and social media activities.

What are the decision-making skills for patients with serious illness
facing *current* treatment decisions? Consider patients contemplating
high-risk cardiac surgery, experimental immunotherapy for stage
four lung cancer, or options for dialysis with impending kidney
failure. Faced with preference-sensitive treatment decisions, many
patients with serious illness will not automatically assume an active
decision-making role. Patients are familiar with the more pater-
nalistic approach to informed consent, where the expert provides
information on the treatment or procedure, its risks and side effects,
and its alternatives. Patients have become acclimated to a subordi-
nate role to health professionals who impart personal opinions with
comments such as: "If I were you..." or "If you were my mother..."

Patients with serious illness will benefit from healthcare providers skilled in shared decision-making behaviors. For example, in
contemplating a treatment decision, introductory comments from
healthcare providers such as, "I am here to help us make a decision together," versus "You have a decision to make," immediately
confers a sense of mutual participation. Patients will need help with
other skills in person-centered decision-making, reflecting on their
goals and values as a critical factor in weighing the benefits and
burdens of a proposed intervention, identifying questions about
treatment decisions, and conferring with others to assist with treatment decisions.

In summary, educational efforts to provide general information, increase
awareness, and provide skills can collectively make a difference in improving the health of the community. These educational efforts, however, must

be complemented by activities that increase the ability for individuals to use their newfound knowledge to improve person-centered decision-making behaviors.

Community Engagement to Foster Person-Centered Decision-Making Behaviors

Community engagement is the process of working collectively to promote the well-being of a diverse population, prompted by "social animation" opportunities to organize and mobilize participants, catalyze social change, and promote a healthier environment. For me, the concept of "social animation" depicts a spirit of liveliness, partnership, and enthusiasm.[9]

Community engagement campaigns focused on improving person-centered decision-making for a diverse population requires multi-level strategies, such as tailored education for individuals, targeted messages for like-groups, coordination with mass media, public policy, and consistent organizational policies. Education can increase knowledge, awareness, and skills for engagement, but individuals must see these messages activated throughout their community.

> Engagement is a two-way street...What is needed is alignment between what patients read about and what they can expect from their care...They need engagement to be modeled, and they need their care team to meet them where they are, acknowledging that there is an engagement continuum and there must be on-ramps and entry points at various engagement levels. - Harnessing Evidence and Experience to Change Culture: A Guiding Framework for Patient and Family Engaged Care [10]

Many PCDM (patient-centered decision-making) engagement strategies have been confined to one target population: patients and families. Of course, patient and family engagement, defined as "...patients, families, their representatives, and health professionals working in active partnership at various levels across the health care system — direct care, organizational design and governance, and policymaking — to improve health and health care," is of paramount importance, but engagement activities must extend far beyond this target population.[11]

Don Berwick, a physician champion in healthcare improvement, advocates the need for an overarching framework for engagement, or "chain of effect for quality" required to deliver person-centered care that includes the environment (community, region, state), the organization (health system, hospital, nursing home), the micro-system (clinic, ward, emergency department) and the experience of care (bedside, exam room, home).[12]

While this multi-level engagement framework is functional, James Conway from the Institute for Healthcare Improvement believes something is missing in this description: "Although each of these activities in its own right adds to understanding and improvement, collectively they could be far more powerful if built across levels on common threads or principles. For example, advance care planning, access to the hospital chart, access to help and care around the clock, honoring patient wishes, and experience surveys achieve their real potential only if the activities at one level (environment, organization, microsystem, experience of care) are reinforced at the other three levels."[13]

This multi-level framework for community engagement is supported by the diffusion of innovation theory: "the process by which an innovation is communicated through certain channels over time among the members of a social system." This theory acknowledges that diffusion occurs in different settings and requires diverse strategies.[14] Innately, patient and family engagement activities are important but cannot be implemented in a vacuum. They must be actualized through coordinated organization and community efforts.

The opening story of Miss Sara is an example of the type of fragmentation that can occur without attention to the consequences of uncoordinated engagement activities. As Miss Sara's facilitator, I was successful at helping her better understand her choices for future medical care. She became informed and motivated to explore her options and identified questions to discuss with her cardiologist. She was willing to take a step forward in the process of person-centered decision-making. However, the engagement strategy was not understood by the central partner in her care, her cardiologist. I did not inform the cardiologist of the purpose of the facilitation nor alert him to the questions he might expect from Miss Sara. Moreover, his perspective was to shield and protect Miss Sara from the fear and anxiety of future complications.

The principles of community engagement described herein provide a foundation for understanding the Respecting Choices recommendations in designing an effective PCDM community education and engagement campaigns, recommendations fostered by the ecologic perspective further explored in the remainder of this Part.

Chapter 25: #1 The Intrapersonal Level of Influence on Behavior Change

Engaging Communities in Person-Centered Decision-Making: An Ecological Perspective

What does an "ecologic perspective" for community engagement mean, and why is it important? The ecological perspective emphasizes the interaction between, and interdependence of, five factors of influence in behavior change: 1) intrapersonal or individual factors; 2) interpersonal factors; 3) organizational factors; 4) community factors; and 5) public policy factors.[1]

The design of well-intentioned engagement activities has consequences. The ecologic perspective provides an overarching framework to understand these consequences, offering a rationale for developing a range of community engagement strategies. The theory offers explanations for why an organizational policy may hinder a person's ability or willingness to change their behaviors or how people are influenced to change — or not to change — by those in their social group.

The ecologic perspective exposes incongruencies within the community in promoting behavior change. For example, during the initial phases of program implementation, RC provides consultation on the existing written materials on ACP and Ads. Typically, this examination reveals conflicting information about Ads that contributes to community confusion about the planning process. Or information-laden 20-page booklets are disseminated that include everything a person would ever want to know about future planning decisions rather than designing smaller pieces that convey information about a specific topic, such as CPR, and disseminated based on the decision-making needs of the individual.

The ecologic theory illustrates the importance of creating decision-making tools that are utilized and understood by all members of the community. During early implementation of the RC program in the La Crosse community, leaders made a decision to revise the statutory advance directive, a document littered with legalistic and confusing terms. A new document was created to support person-centered decision-making, helping individuals understand their choices, reflect upon their treatment options, and document goals and preferences.

However, this document was not the community norm; it represented a drastic change that could cause individuals and organizations to be cautious about using a non-statutory form. With foresight, the task force submitted the new document to legal experts for review, compliance with state law, and endorsement. Without this vetting process, the dissemination of a novel person-centered decision-making engagement strategy would have been thwarted. Instead, the new document became widely popular and eventually adopted throughout the state. Leaders in other RC implementations have replicated this approach for their communities.

> Interventions often focus on changing patient factors, such as knowledge or motivation, without addressing organizational and societal barriers to engagement. Although highly motivated patients may become engaged without clear opportunities and invitations, the vast majority of patients will not. - Patient And Family Engagement: A Framework For Understanding The Elements And Developing Interventions And Policies.[2]

The ecologic perspective is a constructive foundation for the various community engagement activities described in the remainder of this Part. The following section will explore the intrapersonal level of influence on behavior change.

1 The Intrapersonal Level of Influence on Behavior Change

The intrapersonal level of influence to change behavior includes an individual's knowledge, attitudes, beliefs, and personality variables. Efforts to modify this basic level of influence are typically focused on the design of motivational strategies.

There are several theories that lay the foundation to understand human behavior and motivation — theories which can be used to create engagement strategies for person-centered decision-making. Initially, nursing education exposed me to a common theory of motivation: Maslow's Hierarchy of Needs. The original version of the theory described a five-tier model of human needs-physiology, safety, love and belonging, esteem, and self-actualization-depicted as a pyramid with the claim that needs at the bottom level of the hierarchy must be satisfied before people will be motivated to achieve higher level needs. The theory has been expanded to seven levels with an evolution on how it can be used to motivate people to change, but the concepts remain and have been described by newer theories.[3]

Although outdated, Maslow's hierarchy explains the opportunities for engagement in person-centered decision-making. For example, those at the bottom of the hierarchy who are in physiologic crisis-such as those admitted to a hospital for an acute illness-will not be open to examining their advance directive needs on admission. Yet, this is exactly the question patients are asked at the most unpropitious time.

More modern theories of behavioral psychology include the Health Belief Model, the Stages of Change (Transtheoretical Model), the Theory of Planned Behavior, and the Precaution Adoption Process. Although beyond the scope of this Part, each theory postulates that while knowledge is important, it is insufficient to change behavior. People are more inclined to change behavior when they perceive their self-interest will be served.[4]

Creating strategies that motivate people to change is complex. "If we are moving to a value-based world, we need a very different kind of science to deliver health. We need the science of developing more blockbuster drugs of engagement and the science of understanding what enables engagement. It is largely the science of human motivation and the art of design that seek to understand human needs and motivations."[5]

Respecting Choices uses a variety of concepts to increase participation in person-centered decision-making, such as motivational interviewing, the stages of illness model, an ethics of caring relationships, and an updated version of the doctrine of informed consent.

Motivational Interviewing

Motivational interviewing is a counseling technique that appreciates how difficult it can be to change behaviors. Motivational interviewing helps individuals self-discover and resolve ambivalent feelings about embarking on a behavior change.

According to Stephan Rollnick, co-founder of Motivational Interviewing (MI), "Interest in learning MI is probably borne of frustration in conversations about change that do not always go well: the more you try to insert information and advice into others, the more they tend to back off and resist. This was the original insight that generated our search for a more satisfying and effective approach. Put simply, this involves coming alongside the person and helping them to say why and how they might change for themselves."[6]

The engagement activities offered by MI are incorporated as a fundamental component of the RC approach to person-centered decision-making. Through facilitated conversation guides, written materials, online tutorials, and video demonstrations, Respecting Choices seamlessly integrates several MI strategies:

- Acceptance: Meeting people where they are and offering to walk alongside them.

- Evocation: Listening to and exploring the individual's story. This narrative approach is a valuable strategy to assist individuals in gaining insight into their barriers, goals, values, and beliefs.

- Attentiveness: Being fully present with individuals and their families.

- Asking Questions: Using open-ended, non-leading questions that promote dialogue and allow people to reveal their understanding, gaps in knowledge, fears, and concerns.

- Affirmation: Taking opportunities to acknowledge the individual's perspective and insights.

- Reflective Listening: Using restating, paraphrasing, and asking, "anything else?" to promote discussion.

- Summarizing: Identifying themes that emerge. Asking, "What did I miss? Did I get it right? Anything you would like to add?"

- Elicit: Asking about experiences with family or friends who were seriously ill and what was learned. By exploring what individuals learn through these experiences, they often discover their own barriers, discrepancies, and express their own need to change. MI calls this "change talk."

- Asking Permission to Share Information: "Would you like to learn about the success of CPR?"

- Values Clarification: Exploring what is most important to live well.

- Assessing Readiness to Make a Decision: Creating specific plans for next steps (talk to your doctor, your agent, your priest). MI calls this "sustain talk."

Stages of Illness

The Respecting Choices First, Next, and Advanced Stages of Planning (described in Part Two) supports person-centered decision-making as an ongoing process that helps individuals engage in planning by gearing the motivational approach to their stage of illness. Healthy adults or those who have never been exposed to planning are rarely motivated by the recommendation to complete an advance directive.

Rather, they may become engaged if they first understand the value of ACP for all adults who need to plan for an unexpected accident or injury. They may become engaged if the focus is on how to choose a healthcare agent and how to begin a conversation. These small steps will lead to increased understanding and confidence in continuing the process over time.

Once individuals experience a serious illness and its related complications, they are often motivated to participate in more specific planning. This motivation can be integrated into chronic disease management protocols as a standard of care. Disease-specific group education, such as cardiac rehabilitation or diabetes management, can integrate ACP as a component of standardized patient and family care.

An example of the integration of the staged approach to ACP into the routines of care occurred at a cancer center of a large healthcare system. The care team adopted a standard that all patients admitted to the cancer center would be offered ACP services by the team's social worker, regardless of the patient's cancer prognosis. This one invitation to participate yielded a 48% acceptance of the planning service. Several months into the patient's cancer treatment, as a routine component of the cancer center's critical pathway for those with complicated or unresolved cancer, the primary physician or advanced practitioner offered patients and their families another opportunity to participate in ACP for this vulnerable population.

An Updated Approach to the Doctrine of Informed Consent: Begin with Goals of Care

Virtually all states recognize, either by express statute or common law, the right to receive information about one's medical condition, the treatment choices, risks associated with the treatments, possible outcomes, and prognoses.

In 1972, the American Medical Association (AMA) incorporated the concept of informed consent in its Patient's Bill of Rights movement, and almost all state versions of patient rights include provisions related to informed consent.[7]

Naturally, the doctrine of informed consent obligates the need for communication between an individual intending to make a medical decision and a physician. The Respecting Choices approach to informed consent advocates that, when possible and appropriate, the process *begins* with understanding the individual's goals and delivering tailored information as appropriate. This approach requires a hefty design shift in the informed consent procedures as providers are accustomed to following the more traditional process of providing treatment information, alternatives, and risks, and *then* exploring patient goals and perspectives.

An ACP conversation with a patient with advanced heart disease included the exploration of his preference for CPR if his heart stopped. First, our conversation included exploration of his goals and values. He had been hospitalized three times in the past six months, including lengthy episodes on mechanical ventilation. Each hospitalization left him weaker and less able to do the things he enjoyed. Prior to his mother's death, he observed frequent transfers from the nursing home to the hospital in attempts to treat her bouts of respiratory failure from chronic obstructive pulmonary disease (COPD).

Through these experiences, his goal was to avoid future hospitalizations, accepting the consequence that he may die. With this explicit goal identified, he understood that attempting CPR and the requisite need for hospitalization would not be consistent with what mattered most to him. His goals determined his decision about attempting CPR rather than a detailed informed consent discussion describing CPR, its risks, benefits, and alternatives.

Chapter 26: #2 The Interpersonal Level of Influence on Behavior Change

The interpersonal factors that influence behavior change include family (as defined by the individual), friends, and others who comprise a person's social identity and support.

Consistent with the interpersonal level of influence, Respecting Choices ascribes to the ethics of caring relationships as a core concept in facilitating person-centered decision-making. An ethics of care, often depicted as feminist ethics and introduced by the work of Carol Gilligan, "…is focused on how to respond to the needs of others in complicated real-life scenarios."[1] Juxtaposed to an ethics of justice, which uses rules to make rational and consistent decisions that apply to everyone, the ethics of care is focused on context, relationships, and views human beings as interdependent. As we care for one another, our understanding of what is right and wrong is changed. Rules do not always fit the situation.

For example, some view advance care planning only as a rights-based phenomenon, focused on supporting patient autonomy and self-determination. This narrow view is devoid of the importance of interpersonal variables that often trump self-determination. This concept has assisted in the acceptance and implementation of the Respecting Choices program in diverse cultures around the world — described in Chapter 30 — that value family relationships over self-determination.

In employing an ethics of care framework, Respecting Choices urges the active recruitment and involvement of "family" in all aspects of person-centered decision-making. This begins by exploring an individual's definition of "family," avoiding assumptions of which individuals are most important in decision-making. Person-centered decision-making conversations are crafted to engage family members in learning about their decision-making role, truly understanding the goals, values, and preferences of their loved one, identifying fears and concerns, and exploring their commitment to support their loved one's healthcare decisions by asking, "Now that you understand your loved one's decisions, can you honor them?" and "Do you have additional questions?"

The involvement of family in planning conversations has additional upshots. Family members can provide valuable information that the individual may have forgotten, or simply wants to avoid discussing. Family will often remind patients of the illness symptoms, hospitalizations, complications, and communications with other members of the healthcare team. In addition, family may identify the need for additional resources or social services, assist in helping patients understand information, and complying with follow-up recommendations, referrals, and resolution of questions and concerns.

Family members comprise many of the millions of caregivers who are focused on keeping loved ones with serious illness as healthy as possible. Families and caregivers need education in developing skills to participate in planning, discovering their capacity to support and honor loved one's decisions. Respecting Choices has created an information card for healthcare agents that explains the roles and responsibilities of surrogate decision-makers. This educational strategy helps to prepare healthcare agents for planning conversations and understanding of advance directives.[2]

Family involvement in PCDM conversations reaps benefits for patients, healthcare providers, and the overall health of the community.

Don't You Think They Should Be Asking Me?

While scheduling an ACP conversation with the family of David, a 78-year-old patient with advancing dementia (assessed as unable to make his own healthcare decisions), we discussed who should be invited. It was determined that David's son, the designated healthcare agent, and wife would attend. We explored the option and consequences of including David, who lived at home with his caregiver wife, was physically capable, and who continued to be socially active in family dinners, playing games and doing light housework. The wife and son agreed to have David attend, giving him the option to listen and participate (although they had doubts he would talk).

During the introduction, I explained to David that I would be asking questions that would be directed toward his son and wife but that he could participate whenever he wanted. For the first 25 minutes, David sat silent, appeared to be listening, and undisturbed by the conversation that was focused on his healthcare decisions. However, one question sparked his interest. When asked, "What fears or concerns do you think David has?" David raised his hand, waiting for permission to speak. "I heard them talking in the kitchen the other night about where I might have to live if I get sicker. Don't you think they should be asking me about this?" We smiled and acknowledged his fear. The son and wife agreed to include him in future conversations regarding his living arrangements.

A Letter to My Family

An ACP conversation with Mrs. Sukie resulted in clarification of her goals and values about the type of interventions she would want if she suffered complications from advanced lung disease. Mrs. Sukie was living in a long-term care facility and desired the opportunity to meet with me and discuss her options. Her son and designated healthcare agent attended.

During the conversation, the son expressed concern about his nine siblings, who were sprinkled across the country. "What if they disagree with the decisions my mom wants me to make?" We evaluated the options for communicating the essence of the ACP conversation to the entire family to assist them in understanding her preferences and support the son she has selected to be her healthcare agent. Mrs. Sukie requested help drafting the letter for her family to ensure it represented her most salient values and decisions. Once completed, Mrs. Sukie sent the letter along with a copy of her advance directive to all siblings with the request to call if they had any questions or concerns.

Chapter 27: #3 The Organizational Level of Influence on Behavior Change

Change is more likely if the expected behaviors are reinforced by organizational rules, regulations, policies, informal structures, and staff actions. A warm message in an admission packet — "We provide personalized care" — will not promote person-centered decision-making. Individuals will benefit if behaviors are role modeled through the culture of the organization and in the behaviors of the employees.

Other chapters in this book detail the specific elements of organizational change required to support a culture of person-centered decision-making: leadership, education in person-centered decision-making, systems design, and quality improvement and research. This section specifically explores the organizational responsibility to motivate behavior change among its employees — those who have opportunities every day to role-model person-centered decision-making.

For example, what are the attitudes, beliefs, and actions of healthcare workers in your organization toward advance care planning? If a patient asks a nurse, doctor, or chaplain, "Do you have an advance directive?" what will the answers reveal?

A 2013 published report of a study of U.S. oncologists revealed that only 59% had completed an advance directive. Those who had not completed documents reported either a lack of time or no reason. While the activity of completing an advance directive had direct impact on the families of these physicians, it also had a significant impact on the physician's ability to have more routine conversations with their patients and assist them in completing advance directive documents.[1]

The behaviors of healthcare workers communicate messages to patients that may influence their behaviors. In the article "Why don't health care workers (HCW) universally embrace one of the greatest medical advances: Vaccination?" the authors make a case for creating a campaign to change behaviors of healthcare workers regarding their own vaccination practices, citing a study in Florence Italy that reported low vaccination rates for healthcare workers specifically for mumps, varicella, and pertussis.[2]

Using the Health Belief Model, the authors warn that education alone will not change the behaviors of healthcare workers. Rather, motivational strategies must include exploring the value of vaccination for healthcare workers' families and support and encouragement from supervisors, co-workers, and physicians.

Engaging healthcare workers in community campaigns on person-centered decision-making occurs through many avenues. Participants attending the RC facilitator certification courses are asked to complete a personal "practice" advance directive and attempt to initiate an ACP conversation with a close family member or friend as a prerequisite for attendance. These activities expose participants to the technical aspects of completing an advance directive, their goals and values about life-sustaining treatment, and the challenge of opening a conversation with someone they love. This increased awareness impacts the participants personally and gives them an appreciation for the planning they are asking others to do.

Employee orientation programs that include a brief overview of the importance of ACP, existing materials, and organizational resources prepare healthcare workers to advocate for planning activities, answer questions and concerns, and assist with the creation of personal advance care plans. Many RC teams begin their ACP initiative by focusing on their own employees as the initial target population. A large hospice organization I consulted with insisted that every employee become prepared and knowledgeable in ACP by attending a facilitator course. Employees were asked to begin to create a personal planning process before they rolled out their ACP services to patients and families.

In preparation for cataract surgery, a simple and normally uncomplicated procedure, I reviewed the preoperative instructions packet and was thrilled to discover a description of the importance of advance directives and a list of recommendations for completion. This simple event was a trigger for me to review and revise my advance directive. I made updates and proudly brought a copy with me to the surgical appointment. However, I was disheartened to learn that the admissions clerk did not want a copy of my advance directive or the name and contact information for my healthcare agents, saying, "We just need your signature that we gave you this information." I lamented this organizational failure and lost opportunity to demonstrate commitment to advance care planning.

An organization that does not engage its staff in person-centered decision-making will leave a noteworthy gap in disseminating healthy behaviors in the community.

Chapter 28: #4 The Community Level of Influence on Behavior Change

An essential level of influence on changing behavior resides in the formal or informal social networks, norms, and standards that exist among individuals, groups, and organizations in a community. People frequently seek guidance from friends, social media, and support systems — guidance that at times is valued more than information from experts. There are innumerable opportunities to connect with community groups to provide leadership, utilizing their trusting relationships with their constituents to mobilize change.

Community norms may influence whether individuals perceive themselves as able to engage and may increase their capacity to participate in person-centered decision-making activities. Current social environment events can be used to trigger behavior change, and social marketing strategies can guide community messages.

Community Engagement Visibility:
Creating a Brand and Motivational Triggers

Community visibility includes social marketing strategies and opportunities that allow motivated individuals to act. An interesting model of behavioral modification asserts that motivation is not the only prerequisite for change. Rather, change requires the simultaneous convergence of three elements: motivation, ability, and triggers. The Fogg model recommends asking three questions when a desired behavior does not occur: 1) Is the person motivated? 2) Do they have ability? and 3) Are there triggers?[1]

Furthermore, the Fogg model asserts that if a person is motivated, and has ability, all that is needed are triggers. If a person is not motivated, all the triggers in the world will not make a difference. And, if a person is not motivated, it is important to make the change easier to perform by breaking it into small steps. Motivation, therefore, may not need to be the initial requirement for behavior change. I have frequently encountered varying levels of motivation when facilitating ACP conversations.

There are individuals who arrive at the meeting confident with a list of decisions they have already made. These individuals no longer need to be motivated; rather, they simply need the skills to accurately document and communicate their preferences so they will be honored. Conversely, some individuals are overwhelmed by the entire process of ACP, cannot participate in dialogue of their goals, values, or preferences, or express fears in completing a legal document. Despite the lack of motivation to complete the ACP process, these individuals may benefit from breaking the planning process into smaller, more manageable steps, such as choosing a health care agent.

Social marketing recommends the creation of a brand that is used to easily communicate the product, or service, being offered. For Respecting Choices, the community brand is "Making Choices," accompanied by a starfish logo. Both serve as triggers that may stimulate the individual to learn more, talk with a healthcare provider, or access other resources.[2] A trigger should be noticeable and actionable. You should know what to do when you see it. Today, through years of social marketing, the Making Choices brand is well recognized throughout the La Crosse community.

When a brand and image are created, they can be utilized throughout the community as familiar triggers — promoted in brochures, educational offerings, newspaper reports, clinic posters, health fairs, among other avenues. The Respecting Choices poster, for example, states: "We can't respect your choices for future medical care unless we know what they are." The poster's message is not about the completion of a document. Rather, the message is focused on the value of communication and personal control over healthcare decisions, communicating a commitment to honor individual choices when they are known.

The corollaries of motivational triggers to promote behavior change within a community can be significant. For example, a reporter from National Public Radio (NPR) visited La Crosse, Wisconsin to learn about the success of the RC program and to talk to community dwellers. The NPR reporter randomly knocked on the doors of several homes in one La Crosse city block to explore people's understanding of ACP.[3] She discovered that all but one family — all healthy individuals — had completed written advance directives and were well versed in the community dissemination of Respecting Choices.

Moreover, several of the families interviewed were concerned about one of their neighbors on the block whom they knew had not completed the planning process. Intrigued, the reporter decided to visit this family, who chuckled at the reporter's questions and acknowledged their neighbor's concerns and gentle nudging to continue the planning process. During the visit, the couple's 17-year-old-daughter joined the conversation, proclaiming that she knew what her parents would want if they became too sick to make their own decisions.

Additionally, she proudly announced that she had chosen "Terry's Song" by Bruce Springsteen in preparation for her father's funeral when that day should arrive. Though this couple had not completed a written advance directive, it was apparent that fruitful planning conversations were occurring within the family.

This story demonstrates community engagement outcomes that extend far beyond the increase in the prevalence of advance directives. An effective community engagement campaign can improve an individual's skills and confidence to navigate tough social problems, and create strong relationships among families and between neighbors. The impact of the diffusion of innovation can extend to future generations and equip our children with problem solving solutions to resolve social dilemmas.

For example, community engagement strategies have been created for young adults that include presentations in high schools, colleges, and community forums. One community was successful in distributing ACP brochures as a component of registration for a driver's license. Another community produced a video depicting the tragedy of teenage accidents that results in tough life-sustaining treatment decisions for parents. I fondly remember fulfilling a request for an ACP presentation for the La Crosse chapter of the United States Junior Chamber — the Jaycees — a civic organization to support community members, ages 18-40, in developing leadership skills in helping solve local problems.[4] These monthly meetings included education, conversation, and socialization. The chapter lead welcomed me by offering me a Pabst beer, a familiar brew of this Wisconsin community.

These community engagement activities are not intended for everyone to leave with a completed advance directive. To the contrary, they are intended to promote healthy decision-making behaviors.

Social Environment Triggers

A concept called "reciprocal causation" describes how the social environment influences individual behavior in simple and profound ways. People are influenced by those around them and current events.[5] The above NPR story illustrates the power of neighbors in influencing behavior change. National and local events also serve as triggers for community-wide motivation and activity.

For example, the local, state, and national events surrounding the widely publicized case of Terri Schiavo spurred community interest around the U.S. in having dialogue and resolving controversy about how life-sustaining decisions should be made for loved ones who are incapable of making their own healthcare decisions.

The Terri Schiavo saga began in 1990 when she suffered a cardiac arrest in her Florida home, and did not end until 15 years later.[6] Ms. Schiavo suffered a severe lack of oxygen from the cardiac arrest, eventually resulting in the diagnosis of persistent vegetative state (PVS), a condition that describes the loss of cerebral cortical function with partial brainstem activity. PVS creates a form of eyes-open unconsciousness and sleep-wake cycles, but afflicted individuals have no awareness of themselves or the environment. With good care, patients with PVS may survive indefinitely. Terri's husband, Michael, along with her legal guardian, provided oral evidence that Terri would not want to continue to receive artificial nutrition and hydration — the life-sustaining treatment keeping her alive — if there were no hope for recovery.

In 1998, after years of therapy and confidence in the PVS diagnosis, Michael petitioned a Florida court to have the feeding tube removed. Terri's parents disagreed and shepherded a series of court battles to have her life support continued. In 2001, however, Michael's request was honored, and the feeding tube was removed for the first time, only to be reinserted several days later. Local, state, and federal politicians were thrown into the debate, and after a series of court appeals, petitions, and motions at the local and state level, U.S. President George Bush moved the case to the federal court system, causing a seven-year delay before Terri's feeding tube was removed on March 31, 2005, and she died.

The Schiavo case spurred local and national dialogue on several fronts: the medical diagnosis of PVS, right-to-die and pro-life perspectives, and disability advocates. But despite the conflicting personal, moral, religious, medical, and political perspectives, one overarching principle guided the ultimate decision to allow Terri's feeding tube to be removed — the rights of surrogate decision makers to make life-sustaining treatment decisions based on clear and convincing evidence of an individual's goals and values.

The Schiavo case afforded the La Crosse community with an engagement activity to convert people's motivation to complete advance directives into an opportunity to understand the power of advance care planning. Community presentations were organized to highlight the value of conversations in conjunction with written documents — the impact of informing family of one's goals, values, and decisions. Partnerships with local media and broadcast organizations in the La Crosse community raised awareness of ACP by conducting interviews, publicizing presentations, and writing articles, reminding people of the Making Choices resources available to assist with ACP.

The Covid-19 pandemic of 2020 offered another example of reciprocal causation. Communities around the world were exposed to the uncertainty and sequelae of this unknown and lethal enemy. Interest in creating advance directives surged. Social distancing constraints raised multiple barriers to document completion, including compliance with statutory witnessing requirements in completing an advance directive, facilitating in-person ACP conversations, and communicating personal preferences to family, healthcare professionals, and organizations.

RC leaders, implementation teams, and national partners seized this opportunity to engage communities in ACP. Respecting Choices published Covid-19 specific open access resources which provided practical strategies to talk about ACP: how to facilitate telephonic ACP, choosing a healthcare agent, or revising an existing advance directive.[7] Consistent with the Schiavo case described above, the overarching principle of ensuring family understanding of goals and values is of paramount import.

Community Engagement Partnerships

Creating community partnerships — for example faith-based organizations and attorneys — has been a consistent and effective strategy to promote person-centered decision-making behaviors.

Faith-based organizations have been a cornerstone of most Respecting Choices ACP program implementations. ACP fits well within the mission of these organizations whose leaders are well-positioned to provide basic education for their respective communities and increase motivation to participate in planning activities. Several examples of faith-based program implementations are discussed later in this Part.

Creating partnerships with attorneys can yield positive outcomes for clients and the legal community. Many individuals become exposed to advance directives when constructing financial wills with their trusted attorneys. Attorneys view this activity as an essential component of their elder law services. My personal experience exemplifies a typical approach to an individual's initial exposure to advance directives. My objective in seeking legal advice was to produce a financial will and designate a power of attorney for finance.

During the final stages of this work, the attorney gave me a stack of papers to sign, including the statutory advance directive form he had partially completed. The attorney was unaware of my role with Respecting Choices or the fact that I had previously completed an advance directive and filed it with my physician and healthcare organization. I seized this as a "teachable moment," and after further conversation the attorney was intrigued. He eventually became certified as an ACP facilitator and forever changed his approach with his clients seeking legal advice on planning for the future. For several years, he invited me to speak to an elder law course he coordinated for novice attorneys on the importance of ACP conversations as a component of advance directive completion.

Partnerships with local attorneys can increase their awareness of ACP processes and assist in making referrals to local resources for clients needing more information on decisions specific to their medical condition and the importance of transferring completed documents to the patient's local physician and healthcare organization.

Lastly, a collaboration with Respecting Choices, the State Bar of Wisconsin, the State Medical Society of Wisconsin, and the Wisconsin Hospital Association resulted in a statewide public service campaign to promote future health care planning.[8] Respecting Choices faculty and elder law experts hosted a series of "town halls" across Wisconsin to increase awareness of the importance of planning ahead, talking, and completing a written plan. The creation of a written booklet, "A Gift to Your Family," accompanied the presentations. Produced by the collaborative parties, the booklet includes Wisconsin state forms and promotes the relevance of family conversations. This collaboration delivered an important message to the legal community.

During the town hall series, a well-known and respected elder law attorney (and program collaborator) began her presentations with the following introduction: "I have been doing advance directives for a long time; and I have been doing it wrong." This single message helped to promote collaboration between the legal community and the Respecting Choices ACP program mission.

There are innumerable community partnership opportunities, including home health agencies, hospices, long-term care facilities, and county health departments.

Community Volunteers

Community volunteers are an unexpected and effectual strategy for engaging individuals in person-centered decision-making behaviors. Volunteers are recruited from many walks of life: faith communities, retired health care professionals, the spouses of healthcare staff, educators, and others who are interested in helping people learn about and take control of their healthcare decisions.

In a study of the impact of community volunteers on ACP program outcomes, a specific group of community dwellers — those without healthcare experience — were certified in the skills of facilitating ACP conversations for adults with serious illnesses and at risk for complications. Once qualified patients were recruited for the study, volunteers scheduled time to meet with them and their selected caregivers to discuss the value of incorporating personal goals and values into their healthcare decisions and talking to their chosen healthcare agent(s). The following story, told through the eyes of a community volunteer facilitator, illustrates the impact when one member of a community interacts to change the behavior of another.

What if I Cannot Speak and Discuss My Decisions with My Healthcare Agent?

I [the community volunteer] met with Alexandra, a patient with advanced heart problems, who had been given information about advance directives from her insurance agent, her physician, and even from a speaker through her church's senior group. "I thought about it a lot," she told me, but had not taken the next step. Alexandra had personal experiences as a caretaker for both parents, a sister, and a cousin. She had chosen a friend to be her primary healthcare agent and was confident her friend "will carry out whatever I have written down." Alexandra wanted the following goal included in her advance directive: "I don't want to prolong life without quality of life." As a community volunteer, I have learned to explore these types of statements and so I probed a bit further into its meaning. I presented the following scenario to help Alexandra clarify her values about "quality of life."

If you have a complication from your heart condition and are being given treatment, but there is less than a five percent chance you will recover the ability to know who you are or who you are with…would you want life-sustaining treatment to continue?

Alexandra paused and said that she would talk it over with her friend at the time and come to a decision. Once I clarified that, in this situation, she would be unable to communicate, which is the reason why pre-crisis planning conversations are critically needed. With renewed insight, Alexandra announced, "Oh, if I cannot speak, then my friend must carry out my wishes? I am really glad you brought this up. I need to talk to my friend now so she can be the type of caregiver that I have been for my parents."

This type of peer-to-peer engagement strategy is an invaluable component of a community engagement campaign.

Targeted Community Engagement Activities

A community comprises populations that differ in age, gender, race, geography, readiness to learn, among other variables. All populations will not respond equally to a single engagement campaign to promote person-centered decision-making behaviors.

Targeted education involves an understanding of the characteristics of a population and integrating this information into a single engagement approach for that group. Customization of the engagement strategy will be unique to the target subgroup. For example, an ACP program within a Catholic community would ideally include a representative from the religious group — a priest or parish nurse — who actively participate in ACP presentations or awareness activities and remain active resources to integrate the traditions and beliefs of the Catholic faith as appropriate.

Moreover, it is impossible to meet the needs of an entire community simultaneously and decisions are made about priority populations, available human and financial resources, and time. Over the years, a variety of targeted engagement activities have been created and disseminated:

1) *Group Facilitation of Advance Care Planning*

Providing education to increase knowledge, awareness, and skill is effective when offered in a group setting, such as faith communities, senior centers, disease support groups, and health promotion programs. Group facilitation is an attractive strategy to increase dissemination of information and use existing resources widely. The content of group presentations, however, often needs to shift from providing information about advance directives to the importance of ACP conversations, choosing a healthcare agent, scheduling a facilitated conversation if needed, and specific steps and resources for completing a document.

2) *Topic-Specific Education to Build Skills of Person-Centered Decision-Making*

Rather than provide education on "everything you would ever want to know" about advance directives, or treatment decisions, selected topics can be presented that focus on a specific content or skill to motivate behavior change — such as how to choose and prepare a qualified healthcare agent, the CPR decision, the options for kidney dialysis, or the pros and cons of an implantable defibrillator. Focused education can assist with helping individuals understand and simplify the steps involved in person-centered decision-making in non-crisis situations.

One of the favorite focused programs I enjoyed facilitating was entitled: "How to Choose a Healthcare Agent" and was offered in community settings, to include long-term care settings, disease-specific support groups, and caregiver support meetings. It was typical for participants to be accompanied by an individual they assumed would be their chosen healthcare agent. The audience was asked to break into small groups and reveal their preferences in selected hypothetical situations requiring substitute decision-making. It was common for partners to be surprised by each other's preferences. This simple activity clearly demonstrated the importance of talking to a chosen healthcare agent and avoiding assumptions of goals and values. It was more valuable than any lecture or presentation.

3) *Care Management Educational Programs*

Person-centered decision-making behaviors can be effectively integrated into the routine management of patients with serious illness, such as heart failure or diabetes. Patients participating in care management programs typically receive group education on preventative health strategies as diet, medications, and lifestyle changes. Advance care planning topics can be readily added to this list of proactive healthcare behaviors. Beyond ACP content, patients who belong to disease-specific support groups, such as pulmonary rehabilitation, find it useful to discuss airway management options in non-crisis times and to prepare them and their families for a future role in making treatment decisions. These group settings allow engagement of several individuals who share a common healthcare experience, helping to normalize the conversation and address disease-specific questions and concerns.

Targeted community engagement activities are intended to provide information, increase awareness, and develop decision-making skills but are not intended to be stand-alone activities. For participants who are motivated to take the next step in their planning process, follow-up activities include access to additional resources, online tutorials, written instructions, and contact information for those who desire individualized assistance.

Social Media and Engagement Tools

Patient and family engagement strategies abound — resources that allow patients and families to learn about their illness, share stories, questions, and concerns with others, and use technology to improve their health outcomes. Many of these "patient and family" engagement resources include recommendations that can be extended, improved, and applied more intentionally to promote and improve person-centered decision-making behaviors.[9]

The Agency for Healthcare Research and Quality (AHRQ) published a "Guide to Patient and Family Engagement in Hospital Quality and Safety," an evidence-based resource for patient and family engagement strategies. This stellar resource is chock full of helpful tools to assist hospitals in partnering with their patients and families "to improve quality and safety,

respond to health care reform and accreditation standards, improve CAHPS®
Hospital Survey scores, improve financial performance, and enhance market
share and competitiveness."[10]

For example, the AHRQ guide recommends improving discharge planning
processes to help reduce preventable readmissions through better patient and
family engagement in the transition from the hospital to home or another
care facility. What a stellar opportunity to revisit advance care planning.
Patients who have recovered from a medical crisis and are feeling capable
of learning about advance care planning are typically more motivated to
learn and act. As a result, patients are more educated and understand what
is expected of them when they go home. Additionally, patients who have
experienced a complication from a serious illness and received aggressive
life-sustaining treatment may be motivated to discuss their preferences
upon discharge about future complications.

Another recommended patient engagement strategy is the "Patient-
Preference Passport," a patient-owned tool that provides a dynamic description of an individual's medical conditions, medications, care preferences,
and support systems.[11] This tool was created by a patient and family action
team convened by the National Quality Forum. The passport has the capacity to communicate valuable information as patients transition across the
healthcare continuum. For example, in reviewing the current passport
template, information on person-centered decision-making could be added
on the status of advance care planning, previous treatment decisions, and
preferences for shared decision-making activities.

Social media is becoming a principal avenue for individuals to absorb information about their illnesses. "Patients Like Me" is a personalized social
healthcare network that has produced amazing results.[12] It began with
one family's experience with amyotrophic lateral sclerosis (ALS). Stephen
Heywood, diagnosed with ALS in 1998, and his brothers were hungry for
information about disease progression and found a gap in information
about the real-world stories of patients living with the illness. They initiated

the Patients Like Me website to connect ALS patients, which has quickly expanded to other illnesses. Their mission and effectiveness are laudable: "Through continued advancements in our learning health network, and by connecting with a community of people like them, patients can discover new paths forward to improve their health today, and in the future."

A survey conducted on patients' perspectives of sharing information on this social networking site revealed that a majority (94%) are willing to provide personal data and information to help others with similar afflictions and assist doctors and researchers in providing better care.[13] I was excited to peruse this website and inspired by patient and family stories, insights, and suggestions. This network offers a wonderful avenue to encourage and promote person-centered decision-making, including advance care planning and related disease-specific treatment decisions.

The Center for Advancing Health has published a framework listing multiple actions an individual can take to improve their healthcare.[14] "Make Good Treatment Decisions" is one specific action that recommends that patients gather expert opinions and evidence-based information, evaluate treatment options, and negotiate a plan with a physician. While a laudable recommendation, more detailed person-centered decision-making behaviors also include identifying personal goals and values, talking to family, and considering do-not-treat options.

In summary, a plethora of patient and family engagement tools are available, and most could be improved by the addition of suggestions for helping individuals expand their capacity for person-centered decision-making behaviors.

Conversation Starters

There are a variety of scalable engagement strategies that are focused on promoting conversations about person-centered decision-making to include computer-based modules and websites, such as Prepare for Your Care and

The Conversation Project.[15] Additionally, digital technology — video and audio tools — provide rich information easily accessible to everyone. To increase the effectiveness of conversation starters, they should be designed to complement and enhance the local or organizational efforts to improve person-centered decision-making.

In 2003, I provided education and consultation on the Respecting Choices ACP program to the Coda Alliance, an organization in California that partners with families, health and religious professionals, communities, hospitals, universities, hospices, elder care facilities, and global partner organizations to improve advance care planning conversations as a standard of care.[16] The coalition's leaders created an impressive community engagement campaign that continues to exist and includes education, tools, and social media activities.

The coalition created the popular "Go Wish" cards that serve to promote conversations between individuals and their families to identify goals, values, and preferences for future healthcare decisions, and ensuring these decisions will be honored.[17] This engagement activity is enhanced by additional resources: in person assistance, news blogs, and written information.

Digital platforms are being developed to assist individuals, patients, and families in navigating challenging medical conditions, helping them become informed and better prepared to make healthcare decisions aligned with goals and values. For example, Naveon is a proactive Palliative Care digital solution that allows patients, families, and doctors to navigate serious illness together across the continuum of care.[18] Delivered through an application that can be installed on personal smartphones or unit-based laptops, information is presented to support a patient and family's ability to participant in difficult conversations necessary for better outcomes and experiences. Optimally, digital platforms are designed to complement organization-specific materials and professional practice. For example, Respecting Choices partnered with Naveon to create videos that present information that is aligned with RC implementation strategies, including written information, and facilitated person-centered decision-making conversations.

Community Involvement in Person-Centered Decision-Making Activities

National guidelines foster the involvement of patients' and family's engagement in the development of tools and strategies that directly impact their lives. During the creation of the RC CPR Decision Aid (DA), a focus group of patients with heart or lung disease was convened to provide feedback on an initial draft of the DA. Patients were asked for feedback on their understanding of the DA, language, amount of information, layout, the presence of bias, and suggestions for improvement. The feedback was valuable and improved the final product.

For example, patients had suggestions for the color scheme used in the tool for differentiating the options for CPR. The feedback also included affirmation on the content provided, such as "I was surprised by the information, but think it's important to have," and "Everybody should get this information. When I put my mom in a nursing home, no one ever told me this stuff."

Chapter 29: #5 The Policy Level of Influence on Behavior Change

Naturally, the local, state, and federal policies and laws that regulate or support person-centered decision-making behaviors have a critical impact on the ability for individuals, organizations, and the community to support healthy actions and practices. Policies can both hinder and help people engage in healthy behaviors. In the article, "Why is changing health-related behavior so difficult?" the authors state: The short answer...is that it is difficult because policy makers make it so.[1]

Advance Directive Statutes and Policy Barriers

The Patient Self-determination Act was designed to promote autonomy by allowing individuals to express their preferences for medical treatment in advance of an illness or injury. Yet, variability in state statutes on advance directives poses a host of problems, including required disclosures, mandatory phraseology for selected interventions, witnessing requirements, diagnostic requirements — the diagnosis of "terminal" — and limitations on withdrawal of nutrition and hydration.[2]

A robust discussion on the barriers to statutory advance directives is described earlier in this book.

Advance Care Planning Reimbursement

In January 2016, Medicare adopted and began reimbursement for Common Procedural Terminology (CPT) codes that describe advance care planning services.[3]

Physicians and other qualified healthcare professionals (advanced practice nurse, physician assistant, and licensed clinical social worker) may offer voluntary ACP services as an optional element of a patient's Annual Wellness Visit or as a separate Medicare Part B medically necessary service. These ACP services may include discussion about a patient's healthcare decisions, with or without the completion of a relevant legal form.

The Medicare reimbursement policy has created opportunities to financially support the investment in ACP resources and spurred interest from healthcare professionals to learn the skills of facilitating conversations and making referrals to existing organizational resources. The potential negative consequence of this policy, however, is the gap in ACP services for those not covered in this target population. An organization must decide if ACP is a right of all individuals, regardless of ability to pay or be reimbursed.

Local Policies Impacting Person-Centered Decision-Making Behaviors

Organizational policies or state statutes have presented many barriers to person-centered decision-making programs, such as advance care planning. These barriers make it difficult for motivated individuals to receive needed assistance, activate local resources, and ensure their preferences and decisions will be honored. Over the years, progress has been made in breaking through these barriers, yet several examples illustrate the conundrum that exists when policies thwart patient preferences.

A renal dialysis regional network requested RC consultation to improve ACP efforts for their patients and families. Their request was predicated on experiences with patients with advanced kidney disease who had — or were at risk of — complications from their illness. Staff caring for patients were challenged with uncertainty in emergency decision-making situations for those who suffered cardiac or respiratory distress during dialysis treatments.

In facilitating a problem-solving session on the opportunity for renal dialysis staff to initiate conversations with their patients on CPR preferences and document decisions, a shocking organizational barrier was discovered. While there was widespread support for facilitating conversations and honoring decisions, several renal dialysis centers had a policy to rescind a person's DNR (do not resuscitate) preference during dialysis because, since these were stand-alone clinics, they had no physical place to move a deceased individual.

An organization's policy for honoring an individual's DNR decision during surgery has been a topic of intense discussion and tension for years. For example, consider a patient with advanced dementia who suffers a hip fracture from a fall and requires reparative surgery. The patient has an existing advance directive that includes a request not to be resuscitated (DNR) in the event of a cardiac arrest. It is understandable that an organization would have a policy to suspend the DNR request during the hip fracture surgery due to the need to provide resuscitation efforts (vasopressors, mechanical ventilation) to counteract the effects of anesthesia and to improve surgical outcomes.

However, there are many consequences to this policy that are often left inadequately addressed and risk violating a person's healthcare decisions. Some surgeons and anesthesiologists believe the DNR order should be automatically suspended, without discussion with the patient and/or family, despite professional guidelines that recommend thoughtful conversation prior to surgery.[4] Others are unprepared to facilitate these conversations and individualize the final decision based on the patient's preferences, goals of care, and clinical situation.

Additionally, there exists a risk that the DNR order is not reinstituted postoperatively, as this requires professional vigilance and responsibility to determine the patient's medical stability and individual circumstances.

Over the years, I have been exposed to long-term care facilities that have policies that may be in direct opposition to an individual's preferences. For example, some long-term care facilities do not provide cardiopulmonary resuscitation (CPR) services within the walls of their organization. Internal policies to address a cardiac arrest include calling emergency services (911) and transferring residents to a local hospital. This policy naturally delays effective treatment and cardiac arrest outcomes.

The communication of such organizational policies should be a component of the admission assessment process to ensure residents' understanding and consequences of admission. Residents who prefer to attempt CPR would then choose a different healthcare facility. Other long-term care facilities are constrained by state statute in their abilities to honor specific informed treatment decisions. Consider the case of Susan Saran:

Susan Saran, an individual with frontotemporal dementia — a fatal brain disease — has encountered the gap that exists when organizational policies and regulations present roadblocks to the ability to honor healthcare decisions.[5] After suffering two cerebral hemorrhages, Saran was motivated to plan for future healthcare decisions. She worked with an attorney to complete an advance directive for dementia that included her decision to withhold hand feeding and fluids at the end of her life. She also financially secured her living arrangements at a New York retirement community. However, when she presented her dementia-specific advance directive, she was told that New York statutes do not allow for voluntary stopping and eating and drinking (VSED). Due to statute and practice, the facility representatives said they are required to offer food to all residents who are willing to eat, including hand feeding if needed. Susan's dilemma remains unresolved as of this publication.

Chapter 30: Global Experiences Engaging Diverse Communities in Person-Centered Decision-Making Activities

"The true test of a culture of engagement is that opportunities to engage and influence change extend to all participants, even those who traditionally are the most difficult to reach."[1]

Engaging whole communities in person-centered decision-making becomes more complex when the characteristics of all groups are incorporated. Individuals from groups such as non-dominant races, cultures, and religions, as well as the homeless and those with disabilities may become disenfranchised. They are less likely to participate in ACP or the completion of documents due to distrust of the medical system, differing values in relation to decision-making authority, and lack of individualized approaches for those with disabilities.[2]

The Respecting Choices ACP person-centered decision-making program has been implemented around the U.S. and in several countries, including Australia, Canada, Germany, Singapore, and Spain. It was a privilege to partner with and learn from diverse cultures throughout implementation. The overriding message I learned was that we are more alike than we are different.

Despite the obvious diversity of these communities, I witnessed a shared philosophy from around the globe focused on respect of an individual's goals, values, and beliefs and to the imperative to create improved systems that allow healthcare providers and families "to know and honor." A few of the teams I had the fortune to work with provide testimony to the generalizability of ACP program principles but also highlight important cultural differences that necessitated program customization. The research-related outcomes from implementation around the world are reported later in this book, but a few community engagement observations are described below.

The Australia Implementation Experience

This was the first country that requested consultation to improve ACP. Spurred by the experiences of an ICU intensivist and staff, the initiative garnered financial support from its ministry of health. First, there was little history of ACP or the completion of advance directives. This fact made it easier to begin implementation of an innovation. Contrary to experiences in the U.S., the Australian team and patients involved had no preconceived ideas about what would work — or what would not work. They had no history of advance directives being poorly completed and not useful to the treating healthcare team. They had a strong leadership team commissioned and supported for successful implementation and dissemination.

The healthcare clinicians that attended the first facilitator skills certification program were immediately open to learning new skills and putting them into action. The facilitator certification program occurred at the beginning of the week. A follow-up meeting was scheduled to field questions and concerns regarding their newfound skills at the end of the week. During this follow-up meeting, most clinicians had already tested their newfound skills by completing person-centered decision-making conversations with patients and families. They experienced the power of these conversations and were able to communicate their stories and experiences to motivate others in the organization to participate.

The Singapore Implementation Experience

The Agency for Integrated Care in Singapore invited us to assist in examining the impact of the RC approach to ACP within their healthcare system.

This invitation came in conjunction with a publication of the views and attitudes of physicians in Singapore towards end-of-life care. The report, "What Doctors Say About Care of the Dying," was the result of qualitative interviews of 78 physicians representing a wide range of disciplines. One goal of the study was to engage healthcare professionals, patients and families, and lawmakers in a dialogue about the issues surrounding the care of patients at the end of life.[3]

Many interesting perspectives and assumptions were discovered in this study that had an impact on how the RC program would be adapted for implementation. For example, physicians viewed themselves as having the responsibility for deciding when to shift the goals of care from treatment and cure to comfort. This viewpoint was most evident in deciding how to involve patients in decisions regarding CPR. Because physicians retain the authority to decide whether CPR should be attempted, information about CPR was removed from the ACP conversation.

A strong belief that patients and families would not be willing to participate in ACP conversations, or actively avoid them, was expressed based on distrust and suspicion of the healthcare system, fears that planning discussions would infer that physicians were giving up on the patient, or fear that relatives would be accused of wishing their loved one's dead in order to secure financial and property benefits. The taboo of speaking about death is reinforced in the teachings of Buddha, one of the traditional Chinese religious communities. ACP conversations, therefore, needed to focus on building trust, identifying fears, and understanding the impact of decisions on the distribution of wealth among the family.

Lastly, the Western concept of patient autonomy is not typically an operational value in clinical practice in Singapore. The Western value of autonomy assumes that individuals desire information, want to participate in medical decision-making, and are willing to talk about benefits and burdens of life-sustaining treatment. Although patient autonomy is incorporated into law in Singapore, healthcare decision-making is a family affair.

The report gave many examples of the physician's imperative to reveal a bad prognosis to the family before telling the patient. This lack of disclosure on the part of the family was well-intentioned, including relieving the burden of decision-making, lessening reaction to receiving bad news, and preserving hope of a recovery. From the patient's perspective, they often wanted to avoid decision-making and preserve harmony within the family. This family decision-making style was quite easy to adapt to the RC ACP facilitated conversation since the approach is intended to promote understanding among all family members.

A concern emerged about how healthcare providers would resolve a Chinese patient's request to have his elder son make all his healthcare decisions and not be included in decision-making conversations. Our response was a breakthrough moment for this implementation team. Patients have the right to waive their decision-making authority if that is their clear and informed decision — a decision that should be documented and integrated into the approach for current and future treatment decisions. A different challenge was encountered in the scheduling of ACP conversations since family decision-making was the norm. Since many families are large, scheduling a convenient time for everyone to gather was an implementation barrier.

With program adaptations, the planning strategies were well received by Singaporean healthcare providers, patients, and families.

The German Implementation Experience

Our experience in Germany was initiated through a research team interested in promoting decision-making for individuals living in residential (long-term) care facilities.

The implementation in Germany was the first location where the RC materials needed to be transferred to another language. The German team first came to La Crosse for education and certification in the RC program, facilitation courses, and systems, which allowed them to begin the translation process. Interestingly, there was no existing word for "advance care planning" in German, requiring the researchers to brand a new term for ACP, called "beizeiten begleiten."

During our first visit to Germany to assist in the delivery of the inaugural First Steps ACP facilitation course, we encountered an audience of nurses who would be conducting the ACP conversations in their respective residential facilities for the research study. The course was delivered in German by the research team, with translators available for RC to assess fidelity to the program and support the faculty. However, we needed no translation for the emotional reactions that oozed from several participants during the course.

During one emotional reaction from a nurse, we discovered that prior conversations about end of life simply were "off-limits" for these clinicians who were never given permission to initiate such topics or gain personal comfort with the content and its implications for patients and families. One participant revealed her remorse at her lack of skill and avoidance in talking about decisions that would be instrumental in the care of the residents she cared for and loved.

While we were conscious of the history of the Holocaust era, we were uncertain of its impact on ACP program implementation. During Hitler's reign, "healthcare" was focused on eliminating the disease factions, including Jews, homosexuals, and Jehovah's Witnesses, ridding the world of a "life unworthy of life." This history has left its mark on medical decision-making in Germany.

The research study team, nurses, and physicians were now being expected to facilitate conversations that involved withholding or withdrawing life-sustaining treatments. These clinicians needed time to resolve concerns about the consequences of ACP conversations, how their residents would perceive life-sustaining treatment decisions, and the clinician's personal and emotional reactions. Practice sessions were essential in order to become more confident and comfortable with person-centered decision-making skills and the completion of written plans.

Health Literacy

Health literacy will impact the ability of individuals to understand information and consequently become engaged in person-centered decision-making behaviors. In 2015, a health literacy assessment was completed on the First Steps ACP Conversation Guide by an outside expert who provided guidance to modify the language, phraseology, and format of the guide to conform to a 6th-grade reading comprehension level. In the process, the consultant noted several features of the guide that would support engagement of low-literacy individuals.

The conversation guide emphasizes the value of oral communication rather than relying on written or digital information, promotes learning by starting with an assessment of what the individual already knows, integrates cultural and spiritual beliefs, and offers several opportunities for clarification, such as "teach back" and summarizing themes. Lastly, the conversation guide promotes conversation, thus reducing the shame for individuals who do not understand written or digital information.

Faith-Based Initiatives

Naturally, a person's religious or spiritual values and beliefs will impact community engagement activities. For many who belong to faith-based communities, it would be unthinkable to make life-and-death decisions without the support of their advisors, mentors, and endorsement from the relevant theological and ethical perspectives.

Three stories of implementation in faith-based communities are provided that represent common engagement strategies: the use of ACP facilitators who are members of the community, the support of faith leaders in promoting a culture of person-centered decision-making, the teachings of the religious community, and the provision of support from community members to share their experiences with others.

1) *African American Baptist Church*

An early implementation experience occurred in a predominantly African American Baptist church. The leader of the church was passionate about integrating ACP as part of the ministry of his congregation. We recruited a dedicated member of his congregation, an African American parish nurse. She was a known and trusted community member, familiar with the values, norms, and traditions of its members and the teachings of the Baptist faith. These qualities allowed her to offer education and awareness sessions, organize ACP clinics for the members, and offer one-on-one facilitation.

2) *Catholic Healthcare System*

Implementation of ACP programs in the Catholic healthcare system requires sensitivity to community norms such as the integration of the Ethical and Religious Directives (ERDs). These guidelines, developed by leaders of the Catholic Church and other scientists, are published to communicate the Church's teaching on medical and moral issues related to the decision-making in the era of providing modern healthcare.[4]

For example, Ethical Directive #58 states: "In principle, there is an obligation to provide patients with food and water, including medically assisted nutrition and hydration for those who cannot take food orally."

This obligation extends to patients in chronic and presumably irreversible conditions (e.g., the "persistent vegetative state") who can reasonably be expected to live indefinitely if given such care. Medically assisted nutrition and hydration become morally optional when they cannot reasonably be expected to prolong life or when they would be "excessively burdensome for the patient or [would] cause significant physical discomfort, for example resulting from complications in the use of the means employed."[5]

ERD #58 served to assist with customization of RC implementation strategies in Catholic healthcare communities:

- First, the implications of this principle required extensive dialogue among the Catholic leaders and theologians involved in the ACP implementation. It was critical to reach consensus on definitions of "irreversible conditions," "excessive burden," and "significant physical discomfort" in order to provide guidance on how ACP conversations should be facilitated and how decisions about discontinuing assisted nutrition and hydration would be made.

- Second, the organization's medical ethics leaders and ethics committee members were intimately involved in designing and revising policies to guide medical decision-making, communicating, and interpreting these policies to healthcare professionals.

- Third, ACP materials were customized to reflect the Catholic teaching on assisted nutrition and hydration and providing resources for conflict resolution.

- Lastly, understanding of the ERDs were integrated as context-specific resources for those participating in the First Steps ACP facilitator course.

While customization of the ACP program occurred through respectful and thoughtful dialogue, the ultimate mission "to know and honor" resonated within this religious community. During implementation at one Catholic healthcare organization, each session began with a prayer by a Catholic nun, one of the program leaders. The following prayer was provided at the conclusion of our consultation:

> As we near the end of this journey and three days of training, we ask for your blessings as we move forward to change our culture and to keep our patients at the center of our decisions. The past three days have also given me an opportunity to reflect on the stories I hear weekly, sometimes daily that sadden my heart, and I know saddens yours, dear Lord. For example, this week a nurse relayed her frustration over a patient who was dying. She asked for a referral to hospice only to be told the patient was going to a nursing home for therapy and rehab. The patient died twelve hours later. The family was unprepared and lost their opportunity to say their goodbyes. We have many gaps and failures as we care for your dying people, dear Lord. I am sure your heart is heavy with sorrow as you see this, and I am sure both you and the Blessed Mother weep for your people. Please give us the courage, strength, and wisdom to be successful as we move forward. We all know what a privilege it is to birth someone into this world. Please help us to understand and remember what a privilege it is to birth someone into the next world to be with you. We ask this all in God's name. Amen.

3) *The Jewish "What Matters" Initiative*

"What Matters" is an ACP program initiated by the Jewish Community of New York.[6] Their mission is to "...engage New Yorkers in compassionate, value-driven conversations about advance care planning, so they may live with the comfort of knowing their choices will be honored by loved ones and health care professionals." The community serves thousands of individuals throughout five NY boroughs, with a broad spectrum of theological perspectives. Their communal approach reaches out to synagogues, academic settings, healthcare organizations, and other community settings.

The leaders of the "What Matters" initiative use a variety of engagement strategies. Volunteer facilitators, certified in the RC communication skills of person-centered conversations, are extensively disseminated to provide education, increase awareness, and provide personalized individual or group conversations. An educational booklet — "Understanding Advance Care Planning as a Jewish Process" — is distributed to impart knowledge and awareness of the connection between Judaism and ACP, including engaging messages on the value of ACP conversations, "Honest and caring conversations about healthcare decisions participate in the tradition of sacred dialogue."

To assist volunteer ACP facilitators in integrating Jewish perspectives into the conversations, an online curriculum was developed to complement their RC facilitator certification. The importance of diffusing this innovation into the Jewish community is supported by an engagement video, "Voices From the Field," that features the experiences and wisdom of community sages who have participated in ACP conversations and invite others to understand the consequences of this important work.

Implementation in a Safety Net Healthcare System

A substantial underserved population is those from lower socioeconomic groups. A safety net organization that implemented RC was interested in uncovering the barriers to ACP conversations and the creation of planning documents. Their healthcare "community" of patients and families included religious diversity, ethnic diversity (44% Hispanic, the majority were Spanish speaking), and a high percentage of members living in poverty (73% receiving Medicaid). Their initial attempts to create targeted engagement for ACP activities were not as successful as they had hoped; their rates of acceptance of ACP assistance fell well below the norm of 50%.

To understand this reality, they investigated the reasons people were unwilling to take advantage of a new, free ACP service. Their findings were instrumental in creating more effective engagement strategies. They discovered that many people had no working phone number, and a majority did not return for medical appointments, making follow-up meetings for ACP challenging. Many had no one to select as a healthcare agent. This specific population had a lower than average understanding of ACP, feared speaking about the future, and preferred to focus on the "here and now" as their basic needs for food and shelter were their healthcare priority. Armed with a new understanding of the barriers, the leaders of the ACP initiative regrouped. They created an engagement video in English and Spanish that provides information about the value of ACP delivered by Hispanic individuals who had experienced the process. This engagement video resulted in a two-fold increase in those who were willing to complete the ACP conversation.

To improve communication on the importance of ACP, the topic was embedded into the routines of care, introduced by physicians and advanced practitioners during scheduled appointments. When they discovered that patients use prepaid cell phones, which are discarded after several uses, the organization began collecting updated phone numbers with every clinical encounter to keep their contact database current.

ACP in Drug Addiction Recovery Program[7]

A medical student became engaged in ACP through an organization that was implementing several RC ACP programs. He became certified as a First Steps ACP facilitator and decided to put his newfound skills into action. Through his clinical rotations, he became exposed to "Recover Together," a community drug addiction support group focused on providing effective and affordable treatment to recover from opiate use. This program uses group interventions versus individual appointments with healthcare physicians. People at different stages of recovery come together to learn from each other, build collective wisdom, and hold each other accountable.

The medical student decided to test the effectiveness of increasing ACP knowledge and awareness in this group setting. After the group engagement activity, he surveyed the participants for their reactions to the information. Of approximately 60 surveys, 97% found the information "very useful," and most discovered ACP was "very important." Participants expressed motivation to continue to learn and 70% said they were "very likely" to complete an AD. Moreover, group discussions allowed participants to share experiences. Several members of the group were surprised to learn that, unless they proactively chose a healthcare decision-maker, based on state statute, medical decision-making would be deferred to their parents. Many were estranged from these relationships and became motivated to ensure this surrogacy standard would not affect them.

Chapter 31: Assisting Miss Sara in Making Healthcare Decisions Revisited

In a culture of person-centered decision-making, Miss Sara's story would look different:

Miss Sara was a 72-year-old woman with advanced heart failure who had experienced two hospitalizations in the preceding six months for increasing angina and shortness of breath, necessitating a few days of mechanical ventilatory support during the most recent episode. Miss Sara's cardiologist recommended that she meet with an ACP facilitator to review her goals and preferences regarding her illness complications and future treatment decisions, adding, "We will meet again to discuss any questions you have and assist you in creating a plan that will help us provide the care you want and one that your family understands."

During the ACP conversation, we explored Miss Sara's goals for living well, her hopes, and her fears. She was tired of managing her illness and uninterested in another stint on a breathing machine. Having little understanding of her treatment options in the event of future complications, I used a CPR decision aid to provide information and promote discussion. We also discussed her options for airway management other than mechanical ventilation. We developed a list of questions to review with her cardiologist, to include what specific outcomes he would predict — given his knowledge of her heart disease — if she attempted CPR. I documented the ACP conversation in the medical record and alerted the cardiologist of the questions Miss Sara intended to discuss at her next appointment.

Summary

This Part has provided many examples that are consistent with the African proverb — "Oran a azu nwa" — it takes a village working together for social change to occur. Designing community education and engagement campaigns to promote person-centered decision-making behaviors is a monumental task, mandating partnerships among the various influences — intrapersonal, interpersonal, organizational, community and public policy — that synergistically interact to impact behavior change. While this may be a monumental task, this Part has presented multiple examples of effective implementation around the globe. While cultural, religious, or socio-economic diversity is often used as a barrier to the implementation of PCDM programs, we are more alike than different. And we can replicate strategies that help deliver on a universal promise "to know and honor" an individual's goals, values, preferences, and decisions.

Personal Exercises

1) Describe the "community" in which you live. What barriers to ACP and SDMSI (Shared Decision-Making in Serious Illness) exist?

2) Make a list of assumptions you have about your community's values and norms. What surprises you?

3) Make a list of community education and engagement activities that exist to improve person-centered decision-making behaviors. What data exists that demonstrates successful outcomes?

4) What improvements would you recommend?

Part Six

Chapter 32: The Promise of Quality Improvement, Research, and Evidence-Based Practice in Building a Culture of Person-Centered Decision-Making

If We Only Knew

In the mid-1980s, Dr. Bud Hammes received three ethics consultations from the dialysis unit concerning treatment decisions for patients on hemodialysis who had suffered complications. In all cases, the patients had advanced renal failure, were receiving hemodialysis, had recently suffered severe strokes, were not able to make their own decisions, and were unlikely to regain cognitive function. The medical staff and family were faced with decision-making dilemmas: should life-sustaining treatments such as feeding tubes and dialysis be continued? How were these decisions to be made? In conversations with the families of these patients — unaware of their loved ones' preferences — they regrettably uttered the collective refrain, "If we only knew."

Overview

Although the opening story happened decades ago, the common refrain of "If we only knew" continues to be uttered among patients and families faced with the consequences of future and current healthcare decisions. In a 2016 commentary in the Journal of the American Medical Association, a daughter reflects on the angst she and her father experienced over not being offered a choice in changing the battery on her father's defibrillator. Without conversation, she was simply told, "He needs a new one."[1] As complications ensued, resulting in her father's death, she reflects on what it would have been like if a different choice had been contemplated.

Delivering and improving person-centered decision-making is an omnipresent challenge, deserving of our finest endeavors to provide person-centered care — care that centers on what matters most to patients and families. Although I began my nursing career as a clinician and educator, I swiftly discovered the power of analytical activities to produce varying levels of evidence — evidence valuable for healthcare professionals, patients, and families in making treatment decisions. I became an eager researcher. This Part is dedicated to the imperative to design, test, implement and continuously improve person-centered decision-making programs, strategies, interventions, and outcomes.

This Part begins by clarifying terminology: evidence-based programs, clinical practice guidelines, practice-based evidence, quality improvement, and implementation science. The commitment to these activities has been the lifeblood in the evolution of the Respecting Choices (RC) program. Ongoing improvement of the RC program has been guided by four fundamental principles described in Chapter 33: 1) gathering evidence of effectiveness; 2) the Five Promises framework; 3) creating, testing, and improving microsystems and; 4) quality improvement. Quality improvement stories from within the RC program and from external customers are illustrated that exemplify the strides that are gained from such endeavors (Chapter 34).

Evidence-based programs typically require adaptations that reflect local terminology, culture, policies, best practices, and resources — adaptations consistent with the RC "freedom within a framework" philosophy. Selected program adaptations are depicted from organizations and communities within the United States and from Australia, Singapore, Canada, Europe, Germany, and Spain (Chapters 35 and 36).

Measurement conundrums persist in documenting the effectiveness of ACP (advance care planning) interventions, conundrums illustrated in systematic review articles that have created skepticism on the value of ACP and influenced a challenging future research agenda (Chapter 37). The measurement conundrums are reflected in a summary of the lessons learned through decades of research partnerships, lessons that have informed RC's role in educating, advising, and mentoring research teams devoted to the collection of data to improve person-centered decision-making outcomes (Chapter 38). This Part concludes by revisiting the Opening Story and demonstrating the power of using evidence to guide clinical decision-making.

Terminology: Levels of Evidence to Guide and Improve Healthcare

Optimally, professionals utilize evidence in making treatment recommendations; evidence utilized by individuals, patients, and families to make healthcare decisions. Balancing the best evidence science has to offer with personal goals and values is the essence of person-centered decision-making.

Evidence is derived from different sources. The following terms and definitions are suitable to frame the stories, examples, and experiences illustrated throughout the remainder of this Part.

Evidence-Based Programs

"Evidence-based programs are programs that have been rigorously tested in controlled settings, proven effective, and translated into practical models that are widely available to community-based organizations."[2] Evidence-Based Programs (EBPS) are not synonymous with research-based evidence which refers to results discovered from research, but which have not been proven to be effective in practical settings. EBPs have undergone peer review by experts in the field who concur with the definable outcomes that can be realized if the program is implemented.

Organizations and communities search for EBPs that are a good fit to meet the needs of their target populations, implementation settings, resources, and desired outcomes. Once an EBP is selected, implementation involves attention to quality improvement and evaluation to ensure program fidelity — fidelity that increases the likelihood that the populations served will experience similar outcomes to those found in the original evaluation.

Clinical Practice Guidelines, Best Practices, Consensus Statements and Position Papers

Clinical practice guidelines (CPGs), best practices, consensus statements, and position papers offer supplementary levels of evidence to guide and optimize the healthcare of individuals and their families.

Clinical practice guidelines (CPGs) are created to aid healthcare providers and patients in making healthcare decisions in specific circumstances. "CPGs are statements that include recommendations intended to optimize patient care. These statements are informed by a systematic review of evidence and an assessment of the benefits and costs of alternative care options."[3]

Although not interchangeable, alternative terms may be used to describe CPGs, such as best practices, clinical pathways, protocols, and standards. For example, a best practice is "a technique or methodology that, through experience and research, has proven to reliably lead to a desired result. A commitment to using the best practices in any field is a commitment to using all the knowledge and technology at one's disposal to ensure success." Best practices are often guided by clinical wisdom or consensus rather than a systematic use of available evidence.[4]

Consensus statements and position papers provide recommendations on specific topics based on the opinions of experts in the field or professional societies.[5] These recommendations do not promise certain outcomes will be achieved but are intended to drive organizational policies.

Practice-Based Evidence

The real world of healthcare is complicated; patients are unique, and providing individualized care requires adaptations. Just as research informs practice, practice informs research. Practice-Based Evidence (PBE) emerges from shared experiences, clinical examples, and expertise during implementation. PBE compliments evidence-based practices and includes knowledge about local traditions, culture, and societal norms. "Interventions grounded in PBE range from those practices that are ultimately validated by randomized controlled trials to those that, while not yet subjected to rigorous empirical testing, appear to be effective based on the experience and observations of practitioners, family members, or entire communities."[6]

Quality Improvement

Quality improvement is a sine qua non tool used by organizations to enhance internal performance. No innovation is perfect; addressing issues and challenges during and after implementation is fundamental to discover the evidence required for wide-spread adoption and dissemination of practices to improve care.

Quality improvement (QI) programs are intended to improve health outcomes, improve the efficiency of the managerial and clinical processes of care, avoid waste and costs of program failures, proactively recognize and solve problems before they occur, and improve communication and partnerships among key stakeholders. "When an organization implements an effective QI program, the result can be a balance of quality, efficiency, and profitability in its achievement of organizational goals."[7]

Organizations are guided by several eminent quality improvement models to include the Institute for Healthcare Improvement (IHI), Six Sigma, and Lean. Each model integrates different improvement strategies, but all incorporate several common principles: leadership, clearly stated goals, a focus on systems and processes, the use of data and measurement tools, iteration, the involvement of stakeholders, monitoring and feedback during implementation, and a focus on patient/customer outcomes.[8] These quality improvement models begin with small-scale tests of change, finding evidence of what works and what does not, and building stakeholder support for more widespread dissemination.[9]

Implementation Science

Although EBPs have been critically reviewed and promoted to improve care, dissemination faces multiple barriers. EBPs take an average of 17 years to be fully implemented, and only about half reach the clinical setting.[10] Implementation science, "the scientific study of methods to promote the systematic uptake of research findings and other evidence-based practices into routine practice and, hence, to improve the quality and effectiveness of health services," has emerged to facilitate the spread of EBPs.[11]

The emergence of implementation science — stimulated by fixed budgets and federal funding resources — does not mean to imply that this field of research is new. It has a rich history beyond the scope of this publication that stems back to the 1970s and fortified by quality improvement agencies (National Academy of Medicine, Agency for Healthcare Quality and Research, Robert Wood Johnson Foundation, Patient Centered Outcomes Research Institute), conceptual frameworks (Roger's Diffusion of Innovation, PRECEDE, REAIM, and PRISM), publications (Cochrane Collaboration review groups, Agency for Healthcare Research and Quality), evidence-based practice centers, and journals, such as Quality and Safety in Healthcare, to name a few important influences in the field of implementation science.[12]

Implementation science often begins by identifying and resolving the reasons why an EBP is under-utilized by addressing gaps at the provider, clinic, or system level, typically centering on processes rather than outcomes. An implementation strategy is "an integrated set, bundle, or package of discreet implementation interventions ideally selected to address specific identified barriers to implementation success."[13]

Ultimately, implementation science seeks to disseminate interventions that can be applied to other systems, requiring the formation of unique and diverse trans-disciplinary research teams that include formal expertise from economists, sociologists, anthropologist and those on the front line — administrators, patients, families, clinicians — who deliver and experience the impact of the intervention.[14]

The commitment to ongoing improvement and evidence-based practices has been the lifeblood in the development and evolution of the Respecting Choices program. Conducting and participating in quality improvement projects, research studies, and garnering practice-based evidence experiences have enriched my personal and professional encounters.

Chapter 33: The Respecting Choices Principles for Quality Improvement, Evidence-Based Practice, and Research

For over thirty years, Gundersen Health System, its providers, and staff, and the La Crosse community provided a "living laboratory" for the testing of new ideas, program development, quality improvement, and research. With the dissemination of the national RC program in 2000, this "living laboratory" was extended to organizations and communities around the world, exponentially mounting improvement strategies and procuring a wealth of practice-based evidence and research data.

Four fundamental principles have guided the RC program improvement process.

Principle #1: A Commitment to Gathering Evidence of Effectiveness

Providing evidence of the program's impact on patient care has been and remains a strategic priority. With three decades of quality improvement and research, the RC ACP model is broadly acknowledged as an evidence-based program.[1] Aspects of the RC program have been evaluated in multiple peer-reviewed research publications, featured in white papers and QI reports. Additionally, RC faculty have partnered with multiple research projects and have assisted with implementation in organizations and communities throughout the country.[2]

In 2020, the RC ACP program was formally approved as an evidence-based program by the Administration for Community Living (ACL). ACL's stringent health promotion program approval criteria include evaluation of effectiveness in improving health and well-being or reducing disease and injury among older adults, the use of experimental or quasi-experimental design, peer-reviewed publications, full translation in other community settings, and publicly available disseminations products.[3]

In responding to the ACLs approval criteria, RC provided the following levels of evidence:

- **Improving health and well-being** - Research on the impact of the RC ACP program has revealed several outcomes: 1) increased congruence in treatment preferences, decreased decisional conflict, reduced survivor stress, anxiety, and depression,[4] 2) willingness of patients from diverse populations to engage in ACP, including the completion of written plans,[5] and 3) application of ACP in a variety of settings.[6]

- **The use of experimental or quasi-experimental design** - Current and past research studies involving the RC First, Next, and Advanced Steps ACP programs have consistently used experimental design (research conducted with a scientific approach, use of subject randomization to a control group compared to experimental group who are exposed to an intervention) or quasi-experimental designs (similar to experimental design without subject randomization).

- **Peer-reviewed publications** - Several research studies have resulted in 34 publications in peer-reviewed journals.[7]

- **Full translation** - Translation of the RC programs has (or is) occurring in 300+ U.S. medical centers, and testing has occurred in 12 countries.

- **Publicly available dissemination** - Dissemination strategies include the certification of RC Instructors to replicate the classroom and virtual ACP Facilitator skills-based programs, ACP and SDMSI Faculty fellowships, consumer education and engagement materials for purchase and customization, online educational programs for physicians, advanced practitioners, and others interested in improving ACP communication skills. National conferences are held biannually to expose individuals, teams, and organizations to the design elements in implementing an ACP program.

Principle #2: The Five Promises: A Framework for Program Assessment, Evaluation, and Quality Improvement

A promise is a pledge to do something; promises set expectations that certain behaviors will be performed. What are the promises needed to build a culture of person-centered decision-making? The commitment "to know and honor" an individual's healthcare preferences and decisions is multi-faceted and complex. Most organizations and communities assume they are performing better than they are. These assumptions are famously reflected in the "Lake Wobegon Effect," a fictional town featured in the radio series *A Prairie Home Companion* where "...all the women are strong, all the men good-looking, and all the children are above average."[8]

The Five Promises framework was initially designed to stimulate a thoughtful examination of the constituents of an ACP program but was expanded to include the SDMSI (Shared Decision-Making in Serious Illness) program more generally. The Five Promises framework integrates the five design elements in building a culture of person-centered decision-making illuminated in this book, outlines key quality indicators, and explores questions to examine the effectiveness of existing organizational or community services.

While the Five Promises framework can be used to expand an organization's perspectives on the meaning of person-centered decision-making or as a brainstorming activity to raise awareness of program gaps, it is also instrumental in identifying quality improvement activities, creating momentum for change, and articulating an organization's or community's mission and vision of person-centered care. Many organizations and communities have used the Five Promises framework to communicate the mission and vision of their ACP programs.

Each promise begins with "*We*," crystalizing an undeniable commitment to teamwork. No individual member of the healthcare team, profession, or community group can successfully work in a vacuum to provide person-centered care. Individuals benefit from the assistance of many resources when making health care decisions. Each promise requires an analysis of several questions — questions that assess the current environment and offer guidance for improvement. Specific microsystems to support each promise are discussed in Part Three.

Promise #1: We will initiate conversations.

This promise begs for operational definitions of "initiate" and "conversation." ACP conversations are intended to promote understanding, reflection, and discussion of an individual's goals, values, and preferences for *future* medical care. Initiating ACP conversations, therefore, involves more than the standard admission question, "Do you have an advance directive?" and "Would you like information?" While these standard questions may suffice in meeting regulatory requirements, they do little to commence a planning conversation. In fact, such questions are often "conversation stoppers" as they typically result in perfunctory "yes" or "no" responses.

This promise also examines where ACP conversations are occurring. Are they only occurring on admission to a healthcare organization? Or are they occurring proactively in care management programs, in the outpatient setting, in chronic disease management support groups, and in the community?

A multicenter prospective study of elderly patients who were at risk of dying in the next six months and their families revealed that although the majority of these individuals had discussed their preferences for life-sustaining treatments, there was inadequate communication with the healthcare team.[9]

Less than one-third of patients and families reported being asked about their preferences upon hospital admission. Moreover, in more than two-thirds of the cases, the documented treatment decisions were discordant with the patient's actual preferences.[10]

Written advance care plans — advance directives and POLST forms — cannot replace the value of ACP conversations. A nursing home study examining the reasons for discordance between ACP documentation and current resident preferences reported several gaps in communication: asking residents to complete the POLST without conversation or assistance, residents re-evaluating previous decisions, deferring to surrogates, or being unable to remember prior conversations.

Initiating conversations upon admission to a healthcare facility and using this information to create a medical plan of care is of paramount importance. "Investing in ACP is perhaps the single most important thing we can do as a society and as stewards of our health care system to improve the quality of care from the perspectives of patients and family members and to reduce healthcare costs at the EOL."[11]

Similarly, Shared Decision-Making in Serious Illness conversations are focused on the interaction between patients and their physicians and advanced practitioners to assist those with serious illness in making *current* treatment decisions and involve more than giving patients the typical "informed consent" presentation of risks, benefits, and alternatives. Initiating SDMSI conversations requires a commitment to gaining individuals' perspectives on what matters most, offering options that are aligned with their goals and values.

Promise #2: We will provide assistance with
person-centered decision-making.

This promise examines the meaning of "assistance," incorporating a shared decision-making approach between individuals, their loved ones, and the healthcare team. The goal of person-centered decision-making is to improve individuals' ability to make healthcare decisions consistent with their goals and values. This promise does not rest on helping people complete documents or obtain signatures on informed consent forms. Providing assistance requires an assessment of the level of assistance required, exploring such questions as, "What is the individual's stage of illness? What is the individual's readiness to participate? What is the urgency of the decision?" and "What is the impact of the individual's religious, spiritual, or cultural beliefs on the decision-making process?"

Providing assistance with person-centered decision-making also compels a commitment to acquire the requisite communication skills, holding oneself and the entire team accountable to provide a consistent and reliable service. What standardized, competency-based programs are available to the team? Can these programs be tailored specific to the role of each team member? Are members of the team required to achieve competency in the skills of person-centered decision-making, or are these skills merely optional? Does a referral system exist that allows team members to utilize the most appropriate member to provide the level of PCDM (patient-centered decision-making) assistance required?

Lastly, this promise requires evaluation of the effectiveness of the team approach to providing person-centered decision-making assistance. Are patients and families satisfied with the level of assistance provided? Do they feel better prepared to make future and current healthcare decisions? Do staff feel they have adequate time and resources to provide assistance? Is this assistance available to all individuals?

Promise #3: We will make sure plans are clear.

The promise to ensure plans are "clear" is multidimensional. First, do plans created truly reflect the individual's goals, values, preferences, and decisions? Are medical orders concordant with information obtained from advance directive documents, POLST (portable medical order) forms, and shared decision-making conversations?

For example, the POLST program has been demonstrated to provide care consistent with POLST form medical orders.[12] Most POLST studies, however, have not asked the question, "Are the medical orders concordant with the individual's *current* treatment preferences?" Concerns over the quality and accuracy of POLST forms and advance directives in protecting patient rights and safety have consistently emerged from skeptics concerned that patient autonomy will be threatened. For example, a pilot study examining the quality of POLST decisions found discordance with one or more of the POLST orders in 64% of nursing home residents. Half of these discordances necessitated further discussion resulting in participant agreement with the existing orders.[13]

A recent study assessing the degree of concordance between medical orders and preferences of nursing home residents in 40 Indiana nursing homes (20 using POLST; 11 not using POLST) reveals an ongoing challenge "to know and honor" treatment preferences.[14] Concordance was measured by comparing existing medical orders (resuscitation, mechanical ventilation, hospitalization) with current treatment preferences, assessed by facilitated conversations by certified research interventionists using the RC Advanced Steps ACP conversation guide.

While concordance was higher for residents with POLST than without POLST (59.3% versus 34.9%), there remained a disturbing number (41%) of medical orders that were discordant with current treatment preferences. Further investigations into the causative variables of this discordance is planned.

Second, are plans accurately completed and documented? Advance directive documents, for example, have legal requirements for completion and may be complicated by the inclusion of ambiguous statements that contribute to decision-making uncertainty. For example, "I don't want to be hooked up to machines" is fraught with varying interpretations. Similarly, POLST forms have guidelines for accuracy and completion. Selected team members must be taught and assigned to review planning documents for accuracy and completion prior to entry into the medical record.

Lastly, this promise asks if plans are understood by surrogates, family, and healthcare providers. Is the designated surrogate included in planning conversations? Are these individuals prepared to make substitute decisions that are aligned with patient preferences? How is the written plan communicated to surrogates and other family not present during planning conversations? What strategies are in place to involve the patient's physician or other healthcare providers in the creation of the plan, answering patient-specific questions, or providing other resources as needed? Do SDMSI conversations result in documentation of an individual's rationale for making a current healthcare decision — rationale that provides transparency of the individual's goals and values that may form the basis for other healthcare decisions?

Promise #4: We will store, update, and use plans.

This promise involves the implementation of appropriate organizational and community policies and practices that ensure plans are entered into a medical record, are available when needed, revised as appropriate, and used to design a person-centered care plan. This promise necessitates a culture that is committed to continuity of patient care throughout the community.

An effective storage system entails an analysis of several questions. What is the system for entering plans into the patient's medical record? Are plans entered in a timely manner regardless of where they are created (e.g., attorney's offices, outpatient, or community settings)? Are physicians and other healthcare providers notified of the entry of advance directives? Is there an electronic platform that highlights an individual's goals and values — goals and values used to assist with person-centered decision-making? Are plans available when needed to make decisions, and upon transfer to another healthcare facility?

This promise also includes a commitment to update plans over time and at regular intervals, for example, upon admission and transfer to healthcare facility, as serious illness progresses, when life circumstances change, or whenever individuals verbalize changing goals and values.

Lastly, this promise pledges that health professionals and others will search for and review previously developed plans — advance directives, POLST forms — and shared decision-making conversations, use this information to guide clinical decision-making conversations with individuals and surrogates, and apply this information to design a customized plan of care.

Promise #5: We will honor preferences and decisions.

This promise demonstrates a commitment to monitor the ultimate impact of person-centered decision-making efforts: the provision of person-centered care.

Ultimately, all other promises lead to this sentinel goal and require quality improvement systems in place that routinely gathers evidence of care concordance and makes recommendations for improvement in policies, practices, and behaviors.

Although the measurement of goal concordant care is challenging, efforts to analyze this outcome include retrospective and concurrent chart audits, post-death surrogate surveys and interviews. When evidence of discordant care exists, what actions are taken? Are Serious Safety events due to discordant care eliminated? Do morbidity and mortality rounds consistently examine advance care plans as part of the review process? Do the number and kind of ethics consultation change as a result of more proactive assistance with person-centered decision-making? Are healthcare agents and families of those who have died satisfied that their loved one's goals, values, preferences, and decisions were followed?

Moreover, the "we" in this promise includes the ability for healthcare agents to make decisions that honor an individual's dynamic preferences and decisions. A well-prepared healthcare agent is perhaps the most important variable in decision-making for individuals who have lost their decision-making abilities. The role of a healthcare agent does not end with a single conversation or a designation of authority on an advance directive document. Rather, healthcare agents who stay actively engaged in their loved ones' ongoing illness experience, understand the dynamic nature of goals and values, and participate in ongoing conversations will result in improved confidence in making substitute treatment decisions if needed.

Respecting Choices has often referred to the "enduring power" of person-centered decision-making conversations — initial conversations that build a foundation for ongoing communication between a healthcare agent and a patient and increased congruence in treatment decisions.

The measurement of the enduring power of conversations is best reflected in a recent evaluation of longitudinal congruence in a randomized controlled trial of the FACE (FAmily CEntered) intervention for adults with HIV.[15]

The intervention dyads (a patient with HIV and a selected healthcare agent) received the Respecting Choices Next Steps ACP conversation compared to the control group. The intervention dyads had eight times the odds over the controls to have an excellent understanding of the patient's treatment preferences at 12-months post-intervention, even when the patient's preferences changed over time. This data reflects the impact of a single communication strategy over time, allowing a healthcare agent to continue to remain engaged and informed.

The demographics of the study population are also significant. Of the 155 dyads randomized to the intervention group, 86% were African American ranging from age 22-77 years, 42% had a high school education or less, and 39% had incomes below the Federal poverty level.

In summary, the Five Promises framework assists in a comprehensive assessment of person-centered decision-making programs and the development of microsystems to support behavior change.

Principle #3: Creating, Testing, and Improving Microsystems

An indispensable focal point in building a person-centered decision-making program centers on creating, testing, and improving microsystems — systems more fully described in Part Three of this book. "Clinical microsystems are the small, functional front-line units that provide most health care to most people. They are the essential building blocks of larger organizations and of the health system. They are the place where patients and providers meet. The quality and value of care produced by a large health system can be no better than the services generated by the small systems of which it is composed."[16]

Microsystems shape behavior, satisfaction of care, effectiveness, safety, and costs of healthcare. They function to accomplish the work of patient care and evolve over time. A person-centered decision-making microsystem may be clinical staff working as a team to promote person-centered decision-making and competently facilitating person-centered decision-making conversations, or information on ACP conversations that is readily available to clinicians to use in transferring preferences to medical orders, or an advance directive document that is user-friendly and able to accurately communicate individual preferences for future medical care, or an EMR that quickly identifies the legally appointed surrogate decision-maker. Microsystems can result in the delivery of high-quality, personalized, and efficient care, or result in care that is harmful, wasteful, and costly.

In partnership with implementation teams, quality improvement, and research studies, RC shares its experience in creating, customizing, and testing microsystem strategies.

Principle #4: Quality Improvement: Test, Improve, and Disseminate

Typically, the initial microsystems-materials, workflows, processes-designed are not perfect. Time-limited, rapid-cycle waves of implementation provide a mechanism to test and improve microsystems that can be more confidently hardwired into the routines of care prior to widespread dissemination.

Although the preferred organizational QI model — IHI, Six Sigma, Lean — is used during implementation, RC consultants typically use the familiar "Plan-Do-Study-Act" (PDSA) rapid-cycle improvement model to test and improve key microsystems that have been created by the implementation team.

"Underlying the concept of PDSA is the idea that microsystems and systems are made up of interdependent, interacting elements that are unpredictable and nonlinear in operation. Therefore, small changes can have large effects on the system."[17]

The following RC PDSA implementation strategy illustrates the process used to test and improve newly created microsystems, identify barriers to change, and create momentum for dissemination and sustainability.

The Planning Phase

The planning phase, typically lasting six to eight months, sets the stage for successful initial "waves" of implementation and includes the following objectives:

Identify, educate, and mentor the executive and implementation team and faculty fellows. The executive team is responsible for aligning the implementation as an organizational improvement strategy from the outset — rather than an afterthought — and providing the human and financial resources for success. The implementation team is organized to lead the design of the improvement projects, creating and customizing the microsystems used during testing, and providing ongoing mentorship and support.

Project and quality improvement experts are assigned to the implementation team to lend their expertise in analytics and are responsible for the tools and strategies instrumental in studying the achievement of project outcomes.

The identification and mentoring of faculty fellows are an essential element of successful implementation, dissemination, and sustainability of the RC programs. These qualified individuals have key responsibilities for initial and ongoing leadership engagement, system changes, implementation success, measure and monitor performance, and long-term sustainability. Faculty fellows provide leadership for program development and system-wide implementation of person-centered decision-making programs across health systems to meet clinical and strategic objectives.

Create microsystems to be tested during implementation (described in Part Three). Several key microsystems — planning documents, community engagement materials, medical storage and retrieval — are typically designed by small workgroups comprised of local experts and technical advisors. Sample materials are revised or created for customization or adoption during the testing phase.

Develop and communicate a program metrics plan. RC acknowledges the desire to document and achieve long-term goals that will impact the delivery of person-centered care, such as care concordance, resource utilization, ICU lengths of stay, and cost savings. However, long-term impact outcomes cannot be achieved overnight; they require continuous development, monitoring, and improvement of systems and practices that become hardwired into behaviors of all healthcare professionals.

The program implementation leadership team is responsible for selecting the initial (process) and impact (long term) metrics, identifying how the data will be collected, reported, and analyzed, establishing baseline data, and identifying comparative benchmarks that may exist within and outside of the organization.

Initially, the success of implementation is focused on *process* measures — measures that evaluate the effectiveness of the microsystems developed, microsystems necessary to meet each of the Five Promises described above. Process measures assess adherence to the workflows, policies, and procedures developed to improve the delivery of a consistent PCDM service and include an evaluation of:

- the new workflows developed to initiate conversations (For example, are individuals routinely invited to participate in ACP conversations? Are the recruitment strategies effective?)

- the number of PCDM conversations, with and without a healthcare agent or family member present, scheduled and completed

- fidelity to the quality of the conversation

- the frequency and quality of documentation of PCDM conversations

- the quality of the plan created, such as an advance directive, POLST form, or person-centered care plan

- selected patient-reported outcomes, such as patient and healthcare agent satisfaction with the ACP conversation

When new ACP and SDMSI microsystems are hardwired into the culture of person-centered decision-making norms, the long-term impact outcomes can be realized. Care concordance is the ultimate outcome of a person-centered decision-making program, but it is not the only one. More insight into standardization of ACP outcomes in described in Chapter 37.

Collect baseline data. When a program metric plan is created, baseline data is collected that identifies the "starting" point and is used to demonstrate gradual improvement. Gathering baseline data also serves to raise awareness of the current situation, to counter the Lake Wobegon effect and to motivate participation in the program's goals.

Prepare a written implementation or action plan. RC provides action plan templates for customization that include recommended process metrics for each of the Five Promises.

The "Do" Phase

For three to six months, the constructed plan is implemented in short-cycle, small tests of change, monitoring signs of success, and identifying problems for resolution. Revisions are expected throughout this timeframe; new strategies developed as needed and ineffective strategies abandoned. Implementation teams collect standardized metrics, share data and lessons learned, and hold each other accountable to reach the identified data points.

At the conclusion of the implementation cycles, teams congregate in a half or full-day *Share the Experience* workshop where successes, challenges, and stories are revealed. New implementation teams and organizational leaders participate to prepare for their respective implementations.

The "Study" Phase

This phase involves an analysis of the collated data from the implementation teams to identify the final revisions required for more widespread dissemination. Did the intervention succeed in achieving its anticipated goals? Is more testing and adaptation required? What lessons can the initial implementation teams share with others? Typically, a written report of recommendations is created and submitted to the leadership executive team for consideration.

The "Act" Phase

This is where many implementations lose momentum. Implementation teams work intensely to complete their projects and then ease up when they are completed. Many factors can lead to a loss of momentum, including a lack of accountability to continue to implement the innovation, lack of data to demonstrate improvement, and inability to create broad buy-in for the change.

The final stage of the PSDA improvement cycle involves designing a plan for dissemination and sustainability. What protocols, policies, and standards will be expected across all aspects of the organization or community? What resources will be required? What parts of the program will be maintained, supported, and sustained? If the initial program is abandoned or adapted, what will the new program look like?

There is no simple pathway to achieve the long-term impact of program implementation. However, with a sustained and organized improvement process, incremental progress can be measured. As this progress is recognized, improved person-centered decision-making processes and materials become hardwired into the routines of care, resulting in a culture of person-centered decision-making.

Chapter 34: Quality Improvement Experiences in Person-Centered Decision-Making

Quality improvement projects yield countless rewards and opportunities, allowing the testing of new ideas in the real world, engaging people to participate in the innovation, building momentum for change, and discovering program adaptations. In some situations, quality improvement projects can lead to more formalized studies, contributing to evidence-based research.

The following stories elucidate a few examples of the rewards and opportunities that emerge from quality improvement activities.

Quality Improvement Story # 1: The Results and Impact of a Death Chart Audit in an Academic Health Care System[9]

A "death chart" audit of 80 randomly selected deceased patients at Dartmouth Hitchcock Medical Center in New Hampshire was completed by 4th-year medical students. The chart audit gathered information on the patient's decision-making capacity, presence of an advance directive, decisions made by a legally documented decision-maker, and presence of DNR orders and POLST documents. The audit tool included an assessment of whether care provided was concordant with patient preferences.

The results were eye-opening for the medical students. Forty-six patients (57%) did not have an advance directive in the medical record. Sixty-nine (86%) of patients were unable to make their own healthcare decisions, but only 9% had explicit documentation. Loss of capacity was largely inferred due to patients being intubated, sedated, or having altered mental status. In 30% of the cases, it was unclear if the patient's preferences were honored as there was no AD in the medical record or prior conversations with family documented.

For the students, these results provided a personal engagement opportunity on the importance of ACP. Moreover, the results prompted the need for several system-wide policy changes to "help busy professional do the right thing," including: the documentation of ACP conversations in the "Advance Care Notes" section of the EMR (electronic medical records), identification of the legal surrogate decision-maker in the EMR banner, templates for documenting assessment of decision-making capacity, and the use of smart phrases for activating the advance directive.

Quality Improvement Story #2: Telephonic Advance Care Planning (TACP) in a Health Plan Environment

Insurance plan case managers at Priority Health in Grand Rapids Michigan provide telephonic services for frail individuals with complex needs. In collaboration with local implementation of the Respecting Choices ACP programs within the community and in a regional healthcare system, leaders of the initiative wondered how the skills of ACP facilitation could be transferred to the telephonic case managers at the health plan, who admittedly lacked facilitation skills and desired new strategies to engage their members in planning ahead. I assisted this team in designing the necessary adaptations of the RC conversation to the telephonic environment.

First, the needs of this vulnerable patient population required both a First Steps (FS) introduction to ACP with the specific decisions explored in the Advanced Steps (AS) ACP conversation. Therefore, we created a combined — FS and AS — conversation guide that was integrated into the case managers' electronic assessment protocols.

Second, we created a POLST-like form to allow for documentation of a patient's decisions for life-sustaining care, called "Patient Orders for Scope of Treatment." This POLST-like form was necessary because at the time of implementation, Michigan did not have a statewide POLST program.

Third, the ACP facilitator certification skills-based program was adapted to include the combined FS and AS content, telephonic strategies, and role-play scenarios. Lastly, fidelity monitoring of the certified case managers occurred through role play certification, monthly support meetings, self-assessment surveys, and ongoing consultation with the medical director, a Respecting Choices Instructor.

In a 12-month evaluation of the newly designed TACP service, 576 health plan members were offered FS conversations, with 198 of those interested in further ACP assistance. Using established criteria for AS conversations, 56 members were provided additional AS assistance, resulting in 55 new or updated FS advance directive documents and four AS documents.[10] The TACP service was disseminated to the entire Medicare case management team.

Quality Improvement Story # 3: Advance Care Planning in a Tertiary Care Cancer Center: Start Small and Spread.[10]

In an examination of existing ACP practice at the Moffitt Cancer Center, the rate of completion of advance directives was 32 % and were viewed as applicable to only those who were dying. The quality improvement team established the following goals: to enhance communication of patient's understanding of their diagnosis, prognosis, and treatment options, clarify goals of care, decrease decision-making conflicts at end of life, and improve staff morale.

Using the RC ACP facilitation model, key nurse and physician champions, employee health nurses, and all cancer center social workers and chaplains became certified as ACP facilitators to integrate ACP conversations as a standard of care.

The Blood and Marrow Transplant (BMT) program elected to conduct and test the first wave of implementation with the following results: the percentage of Ads completed gradually rose to over 80 %. In a review of the care received by BMT patients who died, 100% had an advance directive versus 88% baseline. Median length of stay in the hospital decreased from 27 to 22 days, and the number of ethics consults decreased from 8% to 0%. The results of this project supported expansion of the model across the cancer center.

Quality Improvement Story #4: Measuring the Effectiveness of the Building Physicians Skills in Basic Advance Care Planning Online Course

In August 2017, Respecting Choices received a grant from the Gordon and Betty Moore Foundation to create, disseminate and evaluate a three-module, online curriculum for physicians and advanced practitioners in integrating basic advance care planning into practice.

Given my experience in online curriculum development, I was privileged to lead this project, accompanied by a team of content experts, an external ad hoc committee representing the online development vendor and an RC attorney, and a national advisory group of physicians, nurses, and other content experts in ACP and curriculum development. The final product, "Building Physician Skills in Basic ACP," was created and disseminated.[11]

In developing a plan for evaluation, extensive alpha and beta testing were completed that was focused on the functionality and quality of the content. However, the entire team was committed to creating an evaluation methodology that would focus on the impact of the online curriculum on clinical practice. The team wanted to measure more than satisfaction with the content.

An "impact survey" for each module was created to measure the extent to which the curriculum changed participants attitudes in three domains: 1) self-perceived competence (attitudes, knowledge, and skill) in providing ACP services; 2) commitment to change their practice to provide ACP services; and 3) self-reported actual change in practice three months after completion of the curriculum.

Between July 2019 and June 2020, an analysis of 4604 impact surveys was completed, representing advanced practice nurses (31.1%), physicians (23.6 %), social workers and nurses (29.2%) resulting in the following responses from participants:[12]

- 65% reported significantly or moderately improved competence in introducing, motivating, guiding, and documenting basic ACP conversations.

- 85% reported being extremely likely or likely to invite and motivate patients to participate in ACP, guide and document more ACP conversations, and seek out ACP resources.

- 85% reported being extremely likely or likely to work with their team to design a consistent way of offering ACP to more patients, design strategies to store, update and use advance directives, and document ACP to support ACP billing and coding guidelines.

This ongoing quality improvement study provides evidence that the online curriculum is effective at changing practice. Notably, these results reflect self-reports that may not be representative of actual practice.

Quality Improvement Story #5: The Evolution of the Next Steps ACP Program

Shortly after joining the Respecting Choices program in 1999, activities were designed that gave me opportunities to become involved in the operations of the ACP program at Gundersen Lutheran Hospital, now called Gundersen

Health System (GHS), learn from the ACP team, and create an avenue for quality improvement activities.

These activities helped me glean insight from front-line clinicians, interact with patients and families, and assist in the development and improvement of the local and national ACP program. Moreover, I learned first-hand what it means to facilitate person-centered decision-making conversations, gaining practice-based evidence for application to new environments.

In 1999, we convened a multidisciplinary group to assess the status of the ACP program — now fully operational for four years — to identify opportunities for improvement. For 90 minutes, the group reviewed the Five Promises framework, reflected on the quality indicators, listened to others' perspectives on what was — and what was not — working, and created an impressive "wish list" of future improvements to include online education, a more effective electronic documentation platform, and a request for additional ACP facilitator resources.

Among the more pressing issues identified was interest in providing proactive and timely ACP assistance for patients with serious illness in the outpatient setting and prior to hospitalization. We designed a quality improvement project, "ACP in Special Patient Populations," that launched an unpredictable chain of events that included clinical experience, research, and the development and dissemination of the Next Steps (NS) ACP program.

ACP in Special Patient Populations: A Quality Improvement Project

The Planning Phase: Step One

First, baseline data was gathered on the status of ACP in two patient populations, those with advanced heart failure (HF) and chronic obstructive pulmonary disease (COPD):

- The outpatient medical records of 111 patients with COPD or HF were examined for evidence of advance care planning, revealing that 48 percent of patients had executed an advance directive, 94 percent of these were in the medical record but only 15 percent of the records had evidence of documentation of an ACP conversation.

- Standardized interviews were conducted with 20 primary care physicians to explore their views regarding the ACP needs of patients with serious illness. While most physicians reported the importance of and comfort with initiating ACP conversations, they admitted to reserving these conversations for patients most seriously ill or older, citing lack of time and inadequate pool of resources as the main barriers to consistently providing ACP assistance.

- Phone interviews were conducted with 20 patients whose medical records indicated they had completed an AD. Only 31 percent of patients had discussed their preferences for future healthcare decisions with their physicians, 36 percent had a discussion with their chosen healthcare agent, and 33 percent with other family members.

This baseline data was effective in raising awareness and engaging professionals in the need to improve ACP strategies in the clinic setting. Approval was gained to increase the number of ACP facilitators in the clinic environment and clarify ACP services in the outpatient setting.

To enhance communication between the patient, chosen healthcare agent, and physician, an "Information Card for Healthcare Agents" was designed that outlines the healthcare agent's decision-making responsibilities and suggests strategies to promote increased understanding of patient preferences. In addition, Respecting Choices faculty incorporated strategies for strengthening the role of the healthcare agent into the facilitator manual and certification program.

The Planning Phase: Step Two

Next, a review of three ethics case consultations involving decision-making uncertainty for patients who had undergone cardiac surgery prompted further investigation. In all cases, it was estimated that these patients had a small chance of survival, would require ongoing aggressive medical support for an unknown period, were at high risk for further complications, and were likely to experience a decline in functional and cognitive abilities.

Without written or oral evidence of the patient's goals and values, physicians, the healthcare team, and family struggled with treatment decisions. We wondered if such ethics consultations could be eliminated or reduced if ACP was integrated into the routine preoperative preparation of cardiac surgical patients and their families.

Interviews conducted with the cardiovascular team — two surgeons and two advanced practice nurses — involved in these ethics cases resulted in consensus that preoperative ACP would be beneficial for patients facing cardiovascular surgery, their families, and the healthcare team. While the surgeons expressed conflict in personally facilitating these preoperative conversations, they were supportive in delegating this role to the advanced practice nurses.

Armed with new information from these investigations, a group of patients were identified who would benefit from a different ACP facilitation approach than what had originally been created. Initially, these "special patient populations" were categorized as follows: 1) individuals with advancing chronic illness where complications in the next two years could be expected; 2) individual facing high-risk surgery or procedures; 3) individuals who have ACP needs beyond the more familiar decisions to withhold or withdraw life-sustaining treatment, such as those with early dementia or mental illness; and 4) individuals who lack decision-making capacity (developmental disabilities) or authority (minors), and must rely on guardians or parents to make substitute decisions and plan for the inevitable.

The Planning Phase: Step 3: The Design of a New ACP
Intervention for Patients with Serious Illness

To begin to answer the question, "What are the ACP needs of patients with serious illness," we explored existing research. Terri Fried's study of 23 patients 60 years of age with serious illness who participated in an in-depth focus group interview to discover the process they used to make health-care decisions and what they would prefer for future decision making was enlightening.[1] Transcript analysis revealed three factors important to decision making: treatment burden, outcome, and the likelihood of outcome.

The interrelationship to these factors revealed that some treatment burden was acceptable if the outcome was desirable, marginal outcomes were less acceptable, and some outcomes were unbearable regardless of the burden. The authors concluded, "A patient-centered approach to advance care planning needs to incorporate a consideration of both treatment burdens and treatment outcomes, including the likelihood of these outcomes. Patients' valuations of these outcomes may change over time."

Fried's perspective and ongoing investigations provided a strong foundation for the creation of a decision-making tool, the Statement of Treatment Preference form, to assist patients in reflecting on their goals and values in future, hypothetical — yet realistic — situations, situations of high burden, low functional outcomes, and low cognitive outcomes. This first draft was reviewed by a small number of patients for feedback on comprehension and readability.

Next, we examined our existing guidelines in facilitating ACP conversations. How would the ACP needs of patients with serious illness be incorporated? How would the newly created Statement of Treatment Preference form be woven into the conversation? A new ACP conversation guide was created that combined existing RC interview questions with additional strategies uncovered from the "Representational Approach to Patient Education" — originally used in the management of pain — which provided a strong theoretical foundation for designing a novel intervention for patient with serious illness.[2]

Based on Leventhal's Common-Sense Model of Illness Representation, a person's thoughts about an illness has five dimensions: identity, cause, timeline, consequences, and cure/control.[3] Exploring a person's understanding of their illness using these five dimensions sets the stage for a highly effective interview. Using this framework, the new ACP conversation guide (now called Next Steps ACP) had five stages.

Stage 1 is Representational Assessment, which explores the individual's understanding (representation) of their illness, its cause, and potential complications. Stage 2 is Exploring Misconceptions, which investigates the individual's previous experiences with illness complications and with decision making for family or friends. This exploration helps the patient identify the importance of planning ahead and motivates them to take additional steps to continue the process. Stage 3 is Creating Conditions for Change, which is a transition stage that offers people the opportunity to explore future medical complications and prepare the surrogate for a future decision-making role. Stage 4 is Introducing Replacement Information, which uses the disease-specific Statement of Treatment Preference form to provide an opportunity to express goals and values regarding future medical care and treatment, and Stage 5 is Summary and Next Steps, which provides recommendations for further conversation, information, and completion and documentation of written plans, such as the Statement of Treatment Preference form, POLST form, and/or advance directives.

This novel approach to address the ACP needs of patients with serious illness resulted in a research partnership with the University of Wisconsin led by Dr. Karin Kirchhoff, who recommended the collection of pilot data to provide evidence in support of an application for federal funding for a randomized controlled trial.

The "Do" Phase: Testing New Materials and Processes

A pilot study of the newly designed ACP facilitation approach for patients with serious illness was conducted in 2001 called "Patient-Centered ACP in Special Populations."[4]

The heart failure (HF) clinic, renal dialysis (RD) unit, and open-heart (OH) surgical department agreed to participate in the recruitment of patients and their surrogates for this pilot study. Twenty-seven patient/surrogate pairs were recruited, meeting the eligibility criteria of advanced illness (those we would not be surprised died in the next 1-2 years) and patients facing high-risk surgery. Thirteen patient/surrogate pairs were randomly assigned to receive the intervention, and 14 were assigned to the control group.

The intervention included a semi-structured interview with the patient and surrogate and use of the Statement of Treatment Preference form to assist with "disease-specific" healthcare decisions. Those in the intervention group experienced significantly better congruence in the understanding of the patient's treatment preferences than those in the control group, satisfaction with the decision-making process, and less decisional conflict.

For consistency, I personally facilitated all 13 patient/surrogate interviews during this pilot study. It was an invaluable experience that fortified my confidence in this new intervention and informed the development of the skills-based educational program that would be needed for future research and program disseminations. I learned the importance of ACP conversations in building and strengthening relationships between patients, families, and the healthcare team, among other lessons.[5]

First, I discovered that facilitating tough conversations is not only hard work for patients and their families, but also for the facilitator. After facilitating three conversations in one day, I was exhausted and wondered if I was effective and helpful. This new work would require attention to the needs of the facilitator.

Second, creating an environment of intimacy among strangers was possible. I was introduced as "the lady doing the study," but trust was quickly created. I entered their lives as a researcher but left knowing I had established a therapeutic relationship. Third, I learned that patients are often concerned about expressing their treatment preferences with their family and valued the assistance of a neutral person in bridging communication and understanding of when, for example, life-sustaining interventions would no longer be wanted.

Lastly, I learned the power of listening — the power of using communication techniques to promote dialogue, helping patients self-discover their goals and values, coined as the "ah-ha" moment of self-discovery.

The "Study" Phase

The research partnership with the UW School of Nursing resulted in funding from the Agency for Healthcare Research and Quality (AHRQ) to conduct a multisite randomized controlled trial of this novel ACP intervention (called "Disease-Specific ACP") across six outpatient Wisconsin-based clinics between January 1, 2004 and July 31, 2007.

The aim of the study was to determine whether this ACP process would improve surrogates' understanding of goals for future medical treatment of patients with life-limiting illness, patient and surrogate knowledge of ACP, and quality of communication of the ACP conversation. Three hundred thirteen patient-surrogate pairs with advanced heart or kidney failure completed the study and were randomized to receive the ACP intervention (described above) or usual care. Intervention group surrogates demonstrated a significantly higher degree of understanding of patient goals than control group surrogates. Although not an intended outcome, we discovered that intervention patients withdrew from dialysis at twice the rate of the control group.[6]

Concurrently, a graduate student member of the UW nursing research team was interested in conducting a specific pilot study of this newly designed ACP facilitation approach for patients undergoing cardiac surgery. The cardiovascular surgical team had become engaged in ACP and welcomed the opportunity to participate in the study.

To support the student's research interest, a NS Statement of Treatment Preference form for cardiac surgery was designed, customizing the hypothetical scenarios to this patient population. Dr. Hammes served as the student's advisor, and the ACP team at GHS provided clinical access and mentoring for this investigation. Thirty-two cardiovascular surgical patients and their surrogates were randomly assigned to receive usual care or the "Disease-Specific Patient Centered ACP (DS-ACP) Intervention." Compared to the control group, DS-ACP improved patient surrogate congruence and reduced decisional conflict. There were no reported changes in anxiety levels pre and post ACP.[7]

The graduate student pursued her research interest in this ACP approach, creating an adapted intervention, called SPIRIT (Sharing Patients Illness Representations to Increase Trust), producing evidence of its effectiveness to improve communication of end-of-life treatment decisions between African American patients on dialysis and their designated healthcare agents.[8]

The "Act" Phase

To facilitate the integration of this research-based evidence into the clinical setting, a NS ACP program was created to complement the existing First and Advanced Steps ACP programs. The NS ACP program incorporates and customizes the related program implementation strategies, including leadership, systems redesign, ACP education and certification, community engagement materials (decision aids), and quality improvement.

Most quality improvement studies do not result in randomized controlled trials; rather, they are designed to inform local initiatives, program adaptations, and dissemination goals

These selected quality improvement stories reflect the power of evaluation to test new ideas, make revisions, engage key stakeholders, inform dissemination, and design research investigations. Quality improvement projects also lead to program adaptations and customized programs — programs that require further evidence of their effectiveness.

Chapter 35: Adaptations of the Respecting Choices Evidence-Based ACP Program

Adaptations to an evidence-based program are often required to ensure it is compatible with a specific population, setting, policies, best practices, and organization or community infrastructures. Adaptations can include changes to program content, delivery, or core components of the EBP — adaptations consistent with the Respecting Choices "freedom within a framework" implementation philosophy.

For example, redesigned advance directive documents must be consistent with state statutes, community engagement materials must reflect local terminology, cultural diversity, and available resources, information regarding cultural or religious beliefs must be integrated into facilitator certification programs, role-play scenarios must be customized to a target audience, and documentation guidelines must be compatible with electronic record applications and technical resources.

At what point, however, does an adaptation compromise fidelity and weaken the outcomes of the program? Ideally, adaptations to an EBP should be discussed, analyzed, and negotiated prior to implementation. This will require the EBP to identify the core components that must remain intact to ensure fidelity to the original program.

The decision to make adaptations should also be driven by acceptable motives. For example, updating an EBP's factual information and/or adjusting activity scenarios to make them more suitable to the population being served are typically seen as acceptable motives for adaptations... However, adaptations are not encouraged when the purpose is to make it easier or more convenient to implement the program; to stick to what is familiar or fun; to drop controversial topics; or because educators lack appropriate training or preparation. - Welcome To ACF[1]

For example, during implementation of the NS ACP program at a large medical center, the legal department refused to allow the entry of the Statement of Treatment Preference form — a planning tool to document treatment goals following the NS ACP conversation — into the patient's medical record.

Despite our attempts at understanding and resolving the concerns of the legal department, they did not relent. The documentation and communication of the outcomes from the NS ACP conversation is essential to an organization's ability to meet Promise #5, "We will honor preferences and decisions." It was one of the rare RC program implementations that was aborted prior to completion.

More commonly, RC has provided consultation and education to many high-profile organizations and programs throughout the world who integrated the core design elements of the program in creating customized adaptations — adaptations that in some cases have produced program-specific evidence of effectiveness.

Adaptations of the RC Program: United States Examples

Honoring Choices Minnesota

Honoring Choices Minnesota (HCM) is a statewide ACP public health initiative of the Twin Cities Medical Society (TCMS). In 2007, in consultation with RC, the leadership of the TCMS organized exploratory meetings with community members and senior leaders of hospital systems and health plans in the Minneapolis-St. Paul area. Dr. Hammes presented the RC program and described the ongoing education and consultation that could be provided to assist with geographic implementation.[2]

The exploratory meetings resulted in unanimous support to 1) not compete; 2) provide resources to support an initiative; and 3) advocate with respective organizations to support the initiative. Subsequently, Dr. Hammes and I provided consultation to assist in the development of the leadership infrastructure (the creation of an advisory group), the "Honoring Choices" brand, a new Minnesota specific advance directive and community engagement materials, and provided RC education and pilot site implementation guidance.

HCM represents the first "convener" experiment facilitated by RC to promote a coordinated implementation of ACP in a large geographic area.

In a qualitative description of the origins of HCM, the goal of the initiative was stated as follows: "Honoring Choices Minnesota (HCM) was organized with the goal of recruiting all Minneapolis–St. Paul metropolitan area healthcare systems to adopt the RC model of ACP to increase, to the La Crosse level, the proportion of individuals with healthcare directives (HCDs) in their electronic medical record (EMR)."[3]

The report further described three outcomes achieved with the convener model. The initiative was successful in building a healthcare infrastructure for ACP among key organizations, building community partnerships to support engagement activities — web-based information, documentaries on end-of-life decisions, public service announcements — and five healthcare organizations reported an increase in the documentation of advance directives from pre-program levels.

Today, HCM shares its experiences and strategies nationally. Those interested in using the trademark "Honoring Choices" must receive permission. "Joining the Honoring Choices National Network allows states to support one another as advance care planning programs are developed. Members of the network have access to resources and take part in regular communication opportunities to give updates and describe growth and development, ask questions, and share ideas and materials in mutually beneficial ways."[4]

Life Care Planning Program, Kaiser Permanente Northern California

Kaiser Permanente is one of the nation's largest not-for-profit health plans and includes several medical groups throughout the country, including Northern California, whose leaders made a decision to invest in the RC program after investigating the evidence, conducting a system-wide assessment of ACP practices, and scheduling two RC leadership engagement workshops to learn about the program, gain understanding, and garner support.[5] In March 2012, we began our consultation with the Northern California ACP team, the first organization to implement all three stages of planning (FS, NS, AS) concurrently. Over the ensuing years, this well-equipped and supported ACP program conducted many quality improvement studies which informed their adaptations and ability to effectively disseminate ACP practices throughout its multiple medical groups. The ACP program at Kaiser is called *Life Care Planning* and offers written, video, and online resources, group facilitation classes, an updated advance directive document, among its program accomplishments. Over time, this program created adapted ACP facilitator courses.[6]

Chapter 36: Adaptations of the Respecting Choices ACP Program: International Examples

Interest in ACP outside of the U.S. resulted in several partnerships with organizations, research teams, and individuals. Extensive variability in implementing ACP in European countries continues. In a report of the investigation of the prevalence of advance directives among deceased individuals in 322 long-term care facilities in six European countries revealed wide variability, with only 32.5% of the 1384 residents having a written plan.[1]

The Australian Adaptation

Australia has a rich history of ACP program development, adaptation, and research. The RC connection with this history began in 2001, when Dr. William Sylvester, an ICU intensivist in Melbourne, Australia began a search for solutions to common clinical dilemmas he had witnessed involving seriously ill patients whose preferences were not known, and whose family were uninformed, resulting in uncertainty in how treatment decisions should be made.[2]

I vividly remember sitting in a conference room with Dr. Hammes in 2002 when he received a page from the operator informing him of a call waiting from an Australian physician. This phone call resulted in continued conversations, a materials license agreement, and consulting contract to bring the RC program to Australia. Subsequent to a week-long consultation and educational program provided in August, 2002, the Australian team "...formed a reference group; gained executive support, prepared policy and advance care planning documents; worked with key stakeholders within hospitals, such as the medical records department, on how these new documents would be filed; and, most importantly, gained the interest and support of the doctors and nurses in the clinical areas where the advance care planning model was to be trialed."[3]

Financial support was garnered from the Australian Department of Health and Ageing to the tune of $1million to disseminate the program in aged care homes, community palliative care services, and in several Australian territories. The RC program was adapted to reflect Australia laws, terminology, and culture — and was named Respecting Patient Choices (RPC).

The dissemination of the RPC program progressed throughout the country, allowing the continued customization and refinement of its materials, strategies, and research. To gather evidence of the RPC adapted program, researchers conducted a randomized controlled trial between August 2007-March 2008 in a Melbourne hospital, enrolling 309 patients age 80 years and older.[4] Patients were randomized to receive usual care or the intervention, which was usual care plus facilitated ACP, based on the RC program, and described as "... a coordinated approach to advance care planning whereby trained non-medical facilitators, in collaboration with treating doctors, assist patients and their families to reflect on the patient's goals, values, and beliefs, and to discuss and document their future healthcare choices."

Of the 154 patients randomized to receive the intervention, 81% accepted the facilitated ACP, and 84% expressed their preferences for future medical care, appointed a surrogate, or did both. Of the fifty-six intervention patients who died during the study period, 86% were significantly more likely to have their end of wishes known and honored than the control group (30%). Family members of patients who died in the intervention group experienced significantly less stress, anxiety, and depression than those in the control group.

The ACP program in Australia continues to evolve. A National Framework for Advance Directives was disseminated in September, 2011,[5] and in June 2019, staff from the Office of the Royal Commission into Aged Care Quality and Safety — a department established by the Governor-General of the Commonwealth of Australia — published an extensive overview of the practice of ACP in Australia.[6]

The Canadian Adaptation

In January 2020, spearheaded by the Canadian Hospice Palliative Care Association (CHPCA), a National Framework for ACP was created, updated, and disseminated that describes the ongoing collaboration and partnerships in Canada to disseminate ACP best practices. The development of this framework was funded by Health Canada as part of a $1.9 million project to assist Canadians in preparing for future healthcare decisions.[7]

In a podcast, the "History of Advance Care Planning: Part I," the speakers identify two health authorities — Frasier Health in British Columbia and Calgary Health in Alberta — that stimulated attention to ACP and their relationship with RC consultation and education services.[8]

In October 2004, the four-day RC Organization and Community ACP course was offered to Fraser Health, an organization comprised of 12 Acute Care Hospitals including three regional hospitals and nine community hospitals. The Fraser Health Authority (FHA) is one of six publicly funded health care authorities within the Canadian province of British Columbia.[9]

The four-day program — accompanied by pre and post-consultation and mentoring — stimulated several successful outcomes by the Fraser ACP team:[10]

- A planning document, called "My Voice: Expressing My Preferences for Future Healthcare Treatment," was created — modeled after the La Crosses Power of Attorney document — to assist in the documentation of people's preferences following ACP facilitation.

- Educational materials were produced to include online education for facilitating ACP conversations and ACP videos for patients, translated into Chinese, French, and Punjabi.

- A "green sleeve" documentation system for document portability was implemented. Originally invented in the La Crosse AD program, the green sleeve is a plastic pocket to house ACP information. It is used as a medical storage system and patient-specific "passport."[11]

- A quality improvement project from the organization's renal dialysis unit was published.[12] A diverse population of thirty-five patients from Punjabi, First Nations, Hindu, Muslima, as well as Greek, Cantonese, South Asia, and Vietnamese communities were willing to participate in facilitated ACP conversations. All expressed a sense of relief and gratitude for the opportunity.

In October 2005, the RC consultation and educational programs were provided to the Calgary Health Authority, resulting in a contract to deliver the four-day Organization and Community ACP program to Calgary leadership and implementation in March 2006. The Calgary leadership team elected to create their own program, and in May 2007, the Canadian leaders hosted the "Inaugural Canadian Symposium on Advance Care Planning" with speakers from Respecting Choices, the Australian RPC program, the Canadian Hospice and Palliative Care Association (CHPCA) and both the Fraser and Calgary health authorities.

The experiences of the Frasier and Calgary ACP program initiatives are described in a written report, "Implementation Guide to Advance Care Planning in Canada: A Case Study of Two Health Authorities."[13] Informed by the RC ACP program, the report describes the four building blocks of ACP as Engagement, Education, System Infrastructure and Continuous Quality Improvement.

Canada's national ACP campaign, "Speak Up," is currently organized and led by the Canadian Palliative Care Organization, promoting a four-pillar ACP program infrastructure of engagement, education, system infrastructure, and continuous quality improvement.[14]

The Singaporean Adaptation

In a 2020 description of ACP in Singapore called "Living Matters," the program stresses the importance of having conversations and talking to loved ones. "Advance Care Planning is a facilitated process that helps you and your loved ones to plan for future healthcare needs together. Making decisions about your healthcare is not always just a simple 'yes' or 'no.' This process gets harder should your loved one be unable to understand or communicate their choices."[15]

These were not the ACP messages, tools, or strategies being delivered a decade earlier. The Agency for Integrated Care (AIC) was given a charge to investigate the development of an ACP program for Singaporeans and subsequently contracted with RC for consultation and education over several years to adapt and implement the FS, NS, and AS ACP programs. Dr. Hammes and I began our partnership with the AIC team traveling to Singapore for an initial ten-day education and consultation program in 2009, which included a licensing agreement to replicate and adapt all three ACP programs.

We returned in 2010 for an extended consultation to include observation and mentoring of the certified FS, AS, and NS Instructors. Our partnership continued in 2012 with the design of an onsite consultation for the Singapore team to continue their education, meet with local community and healthcare leaders, and observe ACP systems in action.

The "Living Matters" program includes patient educational materials, certified ACP facilitators, and a storage and retrieval system for written plans. To study the impact of the adapted RC ACP program components, a retrospective cohort study was conducted between January 2011 and December 2015 across participating organizations. The study evaluated patient responses to end-of-life preferences as documented in three different forms that correspond to a person's stage of illness (general, disease-specific, and preferred plan of care form).[16] Over 3000 documents were completed, and 53% were deceased at the time of the data collection.

The study supported the ongoing development of ACP programs to assist in understanding patient's end-of-life preferences to better inform the need to create programs and resource allocation. For example, 40% of patients preferred to be cared for at home, prompting the need to provide home services for end-of-life care.

The "Living Matters" program continues to promote its aims "to systematize the elicitation and documentation of medical and care preferences, with a long-term goal of normalizing death and dying conversations in the community."[17]

The German Adaptation

In 2007, Dr. Hammes was contacted by a German research team interested in studying the impact of the RC ACP program in long-term nursing homes in Germany. A research partnership was formed that provided education on the RC ACP program, a one-week training in La Crosse, WI., to expose the team to the design and implementation strategies, facilitator and instructor certification, and the opportunity to meet with local healthcare leaders, professionals, and patients.

In addition, the partnership included permission to translate the educational materials into German to be utilized to certify social workers, the research interventionists, in the skills of ACP facilitation, and to educate others in preparation for the study implementation. Dr. Hammes and I provided consultation by phone and email to assist with the research design and ACP implementation strategies. This consultation included a 5-day visit to Germany in 2008 to guide the German team in teaching their first facilitator certification program and providing additional research recommendations.

Armed with this education and consultation, the German research team designed a study to evaluate the feasibility of implementing an RC adapted ACP program — "beizeiten begleiten® — through a prospective, regional, non-randomized controlled research methodology that compared four intervention nursing homes in one town with a control region of five nursing homes in two German towns.[18]

Several RC ACP program design adaptations were integrated into the research methodology: 1) The creation of standardized advance directives for capable patients, proxy documents, and a "POLST-like form" for documenting physician orders for life-sustaining treatment; 2) a customized ACP Facilitator Certification for the research site interventionists; and 3) ACP education and engagement of the primary care physicians and nursing staff from the participating nursing homes on the merits of ACP and use of non-physicians facilitators, the creation of written plans and the importance of organizational design elements.

The main research intervention was the provision of ACP facilitation using the RC adapted conversation. Outcomes from 136 residents from three intervention nursing homes who accepted the ACP invitation were compared with 439 residents in 10 control nursing homes. The primary outcome of the study, an increased completion of advance directives, was achieved. Residents in the intervention group had twice as many completed advance directives than those in the control group (52% vs 25%). Moreover, the completed documents were of high quality, including the designation of a proxy (90% vs 35%), signed by a physician (69% vs 14%), and included clear instructions regarding resuscitation (72% vs 11%). The median total ACP facilitation time was 100 minutes and included a median of 2.5 conversations.

The ACTION Trial: A European Adaptation

The ACTION Trial was a multicenter cluster-randomized clinical trial in multiple hospitals in six European countries (Belgium, Denmark, Italy, the Netherlands, Slovenia, and the United Kingdom) to study the impact of an adapted Respecting Choices ACP approach on quality of life with patients with advanced lung or colorectal cancer.[19] Patients in the intervention group received assistance from an ACP facilitator compared to care as usual.

As members of the research team, Dr. Hammes and I provided consultation on the definition of "adapted RC approach," resulting in a combined First Steps (FS) and Advanced Steps (AS) facilitated conversation intervention. Other adaptations were required to support this intervention's delivery, including a customized ACP facilitator certification course, patient educational materials (for example, a CPR pamphlet), and a POLST-like form for documentation of a patient's goals and values and relevant FS and AS conversation guides.

Our research partnership with this team included the provision of education, consultation on the research methodology, instructor certification, fidelity monitoring recommendations, and ongoing support throughout the study. Representatives from the six European countries, who would become the ACP facilitator course Instructors for the future research interventionists, and the project coordinator traveled to La Crosse, WI, to participate in education on the five design elements of an ACP program, and facilitator and Instructor certification courses.

Education was challenging due to language barriers (some were not fluent in the English language and RC was only fluent in English), lack of previous experience with ACP in Denmark, Slovenia, and Italy (ACP was an unknown concept), and there being no legal status for advance directives in Italy.

Once the program adaptations were approved, translation into the respective languages progressed. To support fidelity-and prior to patient recruitment-to the adapted FS and AS ACP facilitator curriculum, I provided onsite mentorship and certification of the Instructors from all six countries as they demonstrated their knowledge and teaching techniques in a mock course in the Netherlands.

This was a challenge for those who were not fluent in English — a challenge they met with grace and expertise. These individuals would serve as Instructors in their respective countries and use the adapted course to certify future research interventionists. Fidelity monitoring recommendations were provided to assist the research team in evaluating the ongoing competency of the research interventionists.

From 2015-2018, the ACTION trial recruited 1,117 patients with advanced cancer; 442 received the intervention and 675 remained in the control group. The main outcome — quality of life — was no different between the intervention and control groups, a finding that deserves further examination.[20] It is commendable that the ACTION researchers commenced and persevered to implement this multi-site and multi-cultural study that from the beginning faced many barriers and challenges. Several lessons can be gleaned from this study — lessons that may inform other ACP research studies.

First, the ACTION trial demonstrated several positive outcomes of ACP facilitation, even in diverse cultures with little experience in ACP and for patients with advanced illness. Sixty-seven percent of patients reported the ACP conversation was 'quite or very helpful', while 16% reported they were 'quite or very stressful'. These are impressive findings given the reality that most of the study's facilitators had little experience facilitating ACP conversations or working within a culture that was used to supporting the facilitator's work as a component of quality cancer care.

In a qualitative sub-study of the ACTION trial, the experiences of the study's facilitators was examined.[21] While they appreciated the opportunity to facilitate challenging conversations, they struggled with using a conversation guide, and identified the importance of ongoing training in advanced communication skills. Moreover, the facilitators recognized that most patients were positive with the outcome of the conversation that helped them identify preferences and share them with others.

The ACP intervention was successful at increasing the number of completed planning documents. Thirty-seven percent of patients in the intervention group presented a copy of a completed My Preferences form. No information is known about how many other patients may have completed a written plan.

Second, the quality-of-life outcome selected for this study was not optimum as it does not measure the impact of ACP activities. As discussed in the following chapter, the ideal outcomes to measure ACP have not been standardized, but recommended metrics include goal concordant care and behavior change, such as ability to have family conversations. In addition, "quality of life" in a population of advanced cancer patients is appropriately limited by multiple variables not likely to be improved by an ACP intervention delivered within three months of death.

It is common for researchers to strive to find avenues to move the impact of their studies into clinical practice. Researchers involved in the ACTION trial created an online ACP tool embedded in a website created by general practitioners for the community, called "Thuisarts" (doctor at home).[22] The website intends to provide clear patient information on health topics, is visited by millions of people monthly, and has received international awards. According to the ACTION trial project coordinator, Ida Korfage:

> We are happy with this opportunity since it ensures the ongoing availability of the ACP tool. It also ensures the support of general practitioners, who will most likely refer their patients to this tool.[23]

The Spanish Adaptation

In 2004, Javier Júdez, a bioethics and healthcare services physician and researcher interested in the U.S. phenomenon of advance care planning, attended the First Steps ACP Facilitator and Instructor courses in La Crosse, Wisconsin, in conjunction with a nursing research network on aging and elder care in Madrid, Murcia, and Andalucia. Dr. Júdez eventually moved to Murcia, Spain, adapting the ACP model and gaining new funding to create a Spanish validated version of the Next Steps program with research application for individuals with chronic disease, including those with cognitive dysfunction.

To support this goal, a personalized, week-long education and consultation program was designed. In January of 2007, Dr. Júdez was to travel to La Crosse, WI, become certified as a Next Steps ACP Instructor, receive permission to translate the materials into Spanish, and contemplate how to customize the program into his culture and healthcare environment.

I fondly remember Dr. Júdez's visit to Wisconsin when he first came to Madison for a tourist weekend. He was surprised when my husband offered to be his guide on his first snowmobile adventure during a snowy Wisconsin winter. Although he had never been on a snowmobile, worn a hefty helmet or a winter coat, he was thrilled with the opportunity. This adventurous spirit, I think, also guided his ACP improvement journey.

In 2008, armed with additional funding, Dr. Júdez invited me to Murcia for additional Next Steps educational workshops with his research team. This invitation coincided with a vacation I had scheduled to visit my son in Madrid, where he was attending college. Fluent in the Spanish language, my son accompanied me as my interpreter when meeting with the research team.

Dr. Júdez provided the English to Spanish translation of my presentation and visual aids. In roundtable discussion, the group raised questions and concerns about the application of the NS intervention within their dementia population. Although I do not speak Spanish, my responses to their questions seemed to break through our language barriers. During one emotional interchange, my son leaned over and said, "They understand what you are saying. They get it."

Dr. Júdez represents the experiences of lone physicians, nurses, community advocates, and others who encountered the challenge of engaging their colleagues and healthcare professionals in the importance of ACP and figuring out how to disseminate its advantages. Dr. Júdez describes two of his research studies of the adapted ACP program, KAYRÓS-Helping Conversations, with patients with early Alzheimer's Disease and Amyotrophic Lateral Sclerosis (ALS) at the Advance Care Planning and End of Life (ACPEL) conference in 2011.[24]

In a 2020 personal communication, Dr. Júdez provides an update on the progress of ACP in Spain:

> Shared Care Planning, the twist that could save the unfilled potential of advance care planning in Spain.

> The 'right to grant and register an advance directive' has spread within Spain's health care legislation. The current reality is that documents are completed by less than 1% of the population. This reality does not sympathize with the way we human beings suffer, endure, and face illness.

> While this "administrative or contractual" approach remains stuck, a few but significant number of healthcare professionals from different regions of Spain have shared an intellectual journey and created a rationale and roadmap for a new twist in Spain's theoretical, ethical and policy development, promoting ACP implementation into public health care systems.

In 2017, the "Spanish Working Group on Shared Care Planning" (GET-PCA in Spanish) was established to discuss how to use our National Health System strengths and merge the concept of shared decision-making (SDM) for current care decisions with the pursuit of ACP for future care, We named this approach "shared care planning"(SCP) and in 2020 the working group evolved into the "Spanish Association of Shared Care Planning" (AEPCA).

AEPCA defines SCP as "a deliberative, relational, and structured process that facilitates reflection and understanding of illness' and care's experiences, among all involved, focusing on each person facing a disease trajectory, to identify and express their preferences and expectations within their context of care. Its goal is to promote SDM in relation to current context and ACP to future care challenges, such as when the person might not be competent to decide for herself."

The journey resembles the evolution of Respecting Choices® from an ACP program to a person-centered care approach. SCP may save the day for Spain.

The challenges in conducting quality improvement and research studies is reflected in the national dialogue on the value of ACP and the importance of standardization in measuring the effectiveness of ACP interventions.

Chapter 37: ACP Research: Measurement Conundrums and Future Directions

Overwhelming interest in ACP has continued long past the Patient Self-Determination Act of 1991 and related court battles over the rights of individuals to influence healthcare decisions, even when they have lost decision-making capacity. However, mixed results from ACP research studies have stimulated conversations over future directions. The following discussion will briefly review the design and measurement conundrums that have percolated over ACP studies, describe the emerging consensus on the standardization of ACP outcomes, and a proposed agenda for future research, including the author's perspective on missing research topics.

ACP Studies: Design and Measurement Conundrums

Studies attempting to evaluate the effectiveness of ACP interventions have been plagued with design and measurement conundrums to include the existence of diverse interventions and definitions, and lack of consistent metrics — conundrums that have cast skepticism on the value of ACP and created a challenging research agenda.

For example, ACP interventions investigated in research studies have ranged widely from the provision of information, the use of decision aids and communication strategies, efforts to increase the prevalence of written plans, "complex" interventions, and efforts to integrate ACP into existing palliative care services.[1] Studies that have used face to face conversations facilitated by a "trained" individual often do not define the "training" process.[2]

In addition, research studies have not consistently ascribed to a common definition of ACP. A systematic analysis of 69 ACP randomized controlled trials (RCTS) reported that while 16% of the studies gave no definition of ACP, 41% described ACP as a "process," 28% as making end of life treatment decisions, 7% as communicating goals of care, and 4% as completing Ads.[3]

ACP outcomes selected to measure the effectiveness of ACP interventions have been heterogenous, ranging from the completion of Ads, documentation of Ads, congruence, levels of survivor stress, anxiety and depression, knowledge, quality of communication, resource utilization, care concordance, and hospitalizations.[4]

The variability in the design and chosen metrics of ACP studies have made it difficult to compare interventions. Even studies that have demonstrated positive outcomes from ACP interventions conclude that more investigation is needed to standardize the outcomes and intervention for clinical implementation.[5]

The Evolution in the Design of Standardized ACP Outcomes

Making recommendations on how to measure the effectiveness of ACP interventions is demanding, especially given the lack of standardized outcomes and validated tools. Some of my experiences with ACP outcome measurement stems from consulting with organizations and teams during implementation of the First, Next, or Advanced Steps ACP program. For example, it was common for many organizations and communities implementing the First Steps ACP program to select the completion of Ads as a main outcome for the initiative. This inclination required negotiation and identification of other outcomes that more realistically represented the First Steps ACP program focus on patient engagement outcomes, such as the number of individuals "ready" to schedule an ACP facilitated conversation, the number of ACP conversations that included the chosen healthcare agent and documentation of ACP conversations — all critical milestones in an individual's readiness to participate in future planning.

In an effort to understand the ACP behaviors that reflect an "engaged" individual, Sudore and colleagues have reported on the design and evaluation of an ACP Engagement Survey to assess various "process measures" (knowledge, contemplation) and "action measures" (selection of surrogate decision-maker and exploration of goals and values) involved in an individual's capacity to participate in ACP. Once identified, these variables can be used to design specific interventions to improve ACP participation.[6]

Sudore and colleagues conclude, "Based on our findings, prior advance care planning interventions studies may have grossly underestimated their impact by solely focusing on advance directive completion and not on the processes of behavior change and multiple advance care planning behaviors."[7]

I am reminded of the power of ACP conversations to move people forward in their decision-making process — to move them from precontemplation to contemplation. During an ACP conversation with a patient with advanced renal disease who expressed frustration with his self-perceived declining quality of life and physical restrictions and was contemplating withdrawing from hemodialysis, we uncovered his fears: What would happen if he decided to stop hemodialysis? What symptoms would he experience? Who would take care of him? Would his family be supportive?

This single ACP conversation resulted in the identification of specific questions for his physician, a consultation with the palliative care team, and the creation of strategies to talk to his family. These outcomes were never measured as a consequence of our ACP conversation, yet demonstrated critical behavior changes that eventually led to his decision to withdraw from hemodialysis.

Current efforts to reach consensus on standardized ACP outcomes to measure the success of ACP interventions are commendable, necessary, and a work in progress. Achieving consensus will improve the validity of future research endeavors and confidence in the value of ACP interventions.

Through the work of a large, multidisciplinary Delphi panel, an Organizing Framework of ACP outcome construct was created that identifies different outcomes categories: Process (e.g., attitudes), Actions (e.g., having conversations), Quality of Care (e.g., satisfaction), and Healthcare (e.g., utilization).

The top five outcomes ranked by the panel were: 1) goal concordant care; 2) surrogate designation; 3) surrogate documentation; 4) discussions with surrogates; and 5) accessible documents of recorded preferences and decisions. Interestingly, advance directive documentation was ranked 10th.[8]

An updated version of the ACP Outcomes Framework was utilized in an analysis of eligible ACP randomized controlled trials (RCTs) aimed to identify promising ACP interventions and outcomes. Of 1464 studies, 69 met the eligibility criteria and 94% were perceived as high-quality using updated ACP Outcomes Framework categories: Process (readiness), Action (communication), Quality of Care (satisfaction), Health Status (anxiety) and Health Utilization. The varied ACP interventions described in the RCTs resulted in positive Process and Action outcomes, but mixed results in the other categories.[9] For example, they found positive outcomes in the area of patient/surrogate congruence and satisfaction with communication, but not in goal concordant care.

ACP Outcomes Research: Future Directions

In light of the mixed outcomes from ACP studies, McMahon and colleagues make several recommendations for future ACP research:

> In consideration for outcomes research, further work may be needed to refine the ACP Outcomes Framework (e.g., goal concordant may need its own category). Furthermore, decisions about which ACP stakeholder/pillar to focus on, which populations to include, which intervention to use, and which outcomes to assess will require a tailored approach based on the needs of the local environment.

That said, given the current heterogeneity of ACP outcomes, future research should consider using some standardized outcomes so that trial findings can be compared, as some studies are attempting. Finally, pragmatic trials measuring implementation strategies in real-world settings are needed, and several are underway. For effective ACP interventions, an impartial repository, as used in other fields, may help disseminate the interventions to clinical champions.[10]

The need for tailored interventions is instructive. However, not every intervention will impact all outcomes. For example, how would providing written information on ACP or Ads be the single intervention that would lead to goal concordant care? The Outcomes Framework provides a construct to select tailored interventions to achieve specific outcomes.

Additionally, Process and Action outcomes would be effective for studies aiming to improve ACP engagement, as in the First Steps ACP program, whereas goal concordant care would be an expected outcome of the Advanced Steps ACP program. Moreover, the lack of standardized and validated tools for all ACP outcomes complicates the interpretation of study results. McMahon and colleagues report that only 10% of studies achieved evidence of goal concordant, measured by retrospective chart review and post death surrogate or family input, strategies that cast doubt on the reliability of the data.

The concept of tailored interventions was a frequent topic of discussion in my RC consultation offered to implementation and research teams alike. For example, it was typical for leaders to envision that a First Steps ACP implementation would result in decreased hospitalizations for patients with serious illness, shortened ICU length of stays, or an increase in hospice or palliative care resources. However, First Steps ACP targets healthy individuals or those who have never engaged in ACP and is aimed at creating a system infrastructure to build a culture of person-centered decision-making.

In addition, teams interested in implementing the NS ACP facilitated conversation for patients with serious illness required the design of a combined intervention to first expose the target population to FS ACP behaviors, such as how to select a healthcare agent. Without this combined intervention, patients recruited for a NS ACP conversation with no previous exposure to basic ACP might resist participation or be overwhelmed by the NS ACP intervention. The FS ACP activities helped prepare the patient for a more specific planning conversation with his/her chosen healthcare agent.

Progress on creating a standardized ACP Outcomes framework may be enhanced by considering other elements of effective ACP.

ACP Outcomes Research: Two Missing Elements?

From my perspective, the robust research agenda proposed by McMahon and colleagues is missing two elements inextricably linked to achieving ACP outcomes: 1) reaching consensus on the definition of an *ACP program* and 2) identifying the *leadership outcomes* that make dissemination and sustainability possible.

Investigators have cautioned against the misinterpretation of a single ACP intervention as an ACP program: "…conceptualizing ACP as a whole process (instead of as a collection of individual, disjointed steps), composed of many interconnected elements and stakeholders, may provide insight on how to evaluate it better and produce higher quality evidence to improve its implementation and potential."[11]

Recognizing the complexities in achieving and measuring ACP outcomes, McMahon and colleagues elevate the concept of "pillars" to describe six ACP stakeholders — patients, surrogates, community, clinicians, health systems, and policy — and recommend the creation of strategies to measure the interaction between each pillar.[12]

The mixed results on the effectiveness of ACP interventions, for some, have resulted in a desire to abandon current ACP terminology and create new labels and tools. "So, if the term ACP is not helpful to the key stakeholders that are meant to be using it, maybe it's time for a change?... I would like to propose we rally around the concept of "Advance Serious Illness Preparation and Planning (ASIPP)."[13]

Pardon my frustration, but the perpetual inclination to reinvent the wheel rather than perfect the wheel remains puzzling and has thwarted our collective ability to make systematic change. Suppose we are always searching for new tools, strategies, communication skills training, among others. Is it possible we will perpetually avoid doing the hard work of implementing standards of behavior — ways of working that are embedded in the essence of how to provide person-centered care? If we are going to redefine ACP, why not redefine it as a "person-centered decision-making" program — a program to improve the delivery of person-centered care?

I am reminded of the vision of ACP that attracted me to this work, recanted in the history of the RC program in Part Two. ACP is more than preserving self-determination. It's even more than honoring a person's informed healthcare decisions. As Bud always said, "ACP is about how we care for those we love."

ACP has the ability to enhance and strengthen relationships, to open doors of communications, to help people be comfortable with their healthcare decisions (helping them sleep better at night), and to identify the qualities that make life worth living. ACP has the power to improve the way we provide person-centered decision-making assistance, working as an interprofessional team throughout the community, using systems to help busy people do the right thing, and building a culture capable of delivering person-centered care. The measurement of cultural transformation eluded me and the RC program.

I realize that not everyone will appreciate or agree with this vision of ACP but can agree that gaps currently exist in operationalizing ACP to achieve improved outcomes. Minimally, defining the components of an ACP program will assist in delineating ACP interventions as part of a whole, rather than the Holy Grail. Moreover, the responsibility, accountability, and impact of leadership behaviors must be acknowledged as ingredients for dissemination and sustainability of even one ACP intervention.

Envisioning ACP as a person-centered decision-making program paves a pathway for aligning measurement outcomes with patient-reported outcomes (PROs), defined as "any report of the status of a patient's health condition that comes directly from the patient, without interpretation of the patient's response by a clinician or anyone else." PROs have emerged as a vital component in measuring the effectiveness of person-centered decision-making programs. Examples of PROs include quality of life, symptoms, satisfaction with care, adherence to a prescribed treatment regimen, or perceived value of the treatment.[14] When PRO data is accurately collected and accessible in real-time, it can be effectively used to guide the delivery of person-centered care and clinical decision-making.[15]

PRO data is the hallmark of comparative effectiveness research promoted by the nonprofit organization, the Patient-Centered Outcomes Research Institute (PCORI). Funding hundreds of comparative effectiveness studies, PCORI aims to increase and promote research that improves the quality of evidence to assist patients, clinicians, policymakers in making healthcare decisions and impact PRO's included in other research studies. PCORI has published standards to assist with the identification and collection of PROs, admittedly more difficult to measure than counting advance directive documents or the number of hospitalizations.

While PROs are requisite for clinical trials, they can effectively be used in clinical practice as well, especially when collecting this data is automated and regularly assessed. A systematic study of 27 cancer setting studies reports that PROs improve patient-provider communication and satisfaction scores mainly since clinicians were required to talk to patients about their feelings, symptoms, and concerns, promoting better understanding of treatment goals and needs.[16]

In summary, envisioning ACP as a person-centered decision-making program rather than a series of ACP interventions opens the door to more widespread measurement opportunities-measurement that provides evidence of person-centered care.

Chapter 38: Respecting Choices Research Partnerships: What Lessons Have Been Learned?

The cacophony and debate over the effectiveness of ACP continues and ideally will lead to standardization in definitions, interventions, outcomes, and research priorities. I will admit that when I started my work with RC in 1999, I naively believed that by 2020 there would be substantial progress in the implementation of a standardized approach to ACP. I did not appreciate the multi-faceted complexities involved in producing evidence of effectiveness — evidence that would propel program dissemination and sustainability.

I did appreciate the value of gathering evidence and became a curious research partner. The Respecting Choices long-standing legacy of creating partnerships with research teams interested in evaluating a novel component of RC remains a program priority. Research partnerships with RC occur through negotiated roles as a co-investigator, consultant, or advisor, depending on the extent of consultation requested or required and reimbursement terms.

As a co-investigator, RC faculty offer widespread consultation to the research team on study design, methodology, metrics, facilitator skills certification, fidelity monitoring, interpretation of data, and publication. A consultant role is less formal, and services are negotiated based on the needs of the study, but typically includes providing email and phone recommendations, fidelity monitoring, and publication review and assistance. The advisor role is appropriate for research that is not new or typical and does not need ongoing RC involvement or oversight.

Research partnerships have enriched my professional experience in ineffable ways. I owe a debt of gratitude to the research teams who have been passionate investigators, committed to gathering evidence to improve person-centered decision-making. These partnerships revealed a wealth of practice-based evidence that expanded our collective expertise in consulting with ongoing research studies.

The remainder of this Part summarizes the lessons that I learned through multiple research partnerships — lessons that resonate with the mixed outcomes from ACP research described in the previous chapter. Reflecting on these lessons today, I understand why the research was challenging, why some studies never produced positive outcomes, while some highly effective interventions were never disseminated into clinical practice. Furthermore, I have some clarity on what I may have done differently to enhance my participation on the research team. It would be my aspiration that these lessons may inform others interested in contributing to the evidence on the effectiveness of ACP programs.

Definitions Matter

A consistent definition of ACP remains elusive and its potential influence unappreciated. The Delphi consensus panel description of ACP as "a process that supports adults at any age or stage of health in understanding and sharing their personal values, life goals, and preferences regarding future medical care" marked a significant step toward standardization of definitions and movement away from a focus on advance directive completion[1] Yet, the *process* of ACP remains undefined and often misinterpreted.

For example, the literature continues to equate the ACP *process* with *advance directives*, exemplified in the title of an editorial "Advance Directives/Care Planning: Clear, Simple, and Wrong," or in publications that simply want to reframe Ads by calling them "advance care plans."[2]

In addition, ACP continues to be narrowly equated with "end-of-life" decisions or "goals of care" conversations for patients with serious illness, reducing ACP interventions to an important but narrow population. This perspective leads some critics to propagate the danger in completing Ads early in the course of an illness or asking healthy patients to make "hypothetical" decisions when they are incapable of understanding an unknown illness trajectory. ACP critics note: "The key point is that planning for death under conditions of certainty (like when you have end-stage cancer) is not the same as planning for your serious illness (like COVID-19 pneumonia) where it is uncertain how you will turn out"[3] and "...conducting good serious illness conversations is not simple. Like learning a surgical procedure, it requires specialized knowledge and skills, training with feedback from experts, and ongoing practice."[4]

I agree with these criticisms, but the premise of these statements is inconsistent with the RC definition of ACP and its categorization as a person-centered decision-making program described throughout this book. ACP is not a "one-size-fits-all" conversation only appropriate for individuals with serious illness, nor should ACP conversations be facilitated by unqualified individuals. Rather, ACP is a dynamic process that requires different approaches, different skills, and different content for target populations. The Staged approach to ACP — described in Part Two — gives testimony to the need to customize ACP strategies based on an individual's stage of illness, becoming more specific as illness progresses, complications ensue (and the hypothetical becomes the reality), and goals and values change.

Of course, it makes no sense to ask a healthy individual to make decisions about what goals they would have if they had a hypothetical illness, such as heart disease. Rather, in a culture of person-centered decision-making, ACP (and SDMSI) conversations are integrated as a component of routine, quality healthcare — conversations that become more specific when illness progresses. ACP conversations for healthy adults, or those who have never planned, builds decision-making behaviors that will strengthen their capacity for making future, complex, and "real-time" person-centered decisions in times of declining health, complications, changing goals and values, and crisis events.

The power of consistent and ongoing ACP conversations are described by Kate Detwiller, a parent of a child with medical complexities, who participated in a pediatric ACP study described in the next Part:

> These conversations are individual building blocks that when put together, create something beautiful and strong; the peace of knowing that I cared for my child throughout his life and those cumulative moments will bring me peace at the end. The weaker moments and conversations during times of crisis are supported by the stronger conversations defined by the clarity of our lives and values outside of that traumatic moment. The more conversations you have, the more building blocks you have as a parent and the better picture you have of that final something.[5]

An ACP Intervention is NOT an ACP Program

An ACP intervention does not constitute an ACP *program*, yet research studies and some systematic reviews have disseminated this inaccuracy. A single ACP intervention will not be adequate to allow us to meet our promise "to know and honor" an individual's goal, values, preferences, and decisions.

The inconsistency in understanding these two concepts has led to questionable conclusions on the value of an RC program. For example, a systematic review of the level of evidence of the RC model using criteria developed by the Cochrane Collaborative identified an impressive list of 18 articles from 16 studies (nine RCTs, six observational, and one pre/post test). The authors concede the high level of evidence that the RC program and its derivatives lead to increased patient-surrogate congruence on treatment preferences and increased completion of written plans, such as advance directives and POLST forms.[6]

However, the authors opine that "The evidence is mixed, inconclusive, and too poor in quality to determine whether RC and derivative models change the consistency of treatment with wishes and overall healthcare utilization in the end of life."

The majority of the studies cited by MacKenzie and colleagues only investigated one aspect of the RC program, such as facilitated ACP conversations, therefore misrepresenting the impact of the RC "program" or "model." This theme is common within multiple research teams who have been interested in evaluating the effectiveness of one component of the RC program, most commonly the First, Next, or Advanced Steps facilitated ACP conversation. While we were eager to partner with research teams, it was imperative that the "ACP intervention" be accurately described as one component of a more comprehensive program.

For example, in consultation with the ACTION trial research team, the following description of the adapted RC intervention was crafted to distinguish it from the more comprehensive RC program:

> We developed and evaluated the ACTION RC ACP intervention. This was an adapted and integrated version of 2 of the 3 stages of the RC facilitated ACP conversations (First Steps and Advanced Steps). The ACTION RC ACP intervention includes 3 components (see S2 Text): (1) facilitated structured ACP conversations, (2) the My Preferences form, and (3) information leaflets.[7]

ACP Outcomes are Hindered by Inadequate Clinical Infrastructure

Many RC research collaborations have been hampered by a lack of basic infrastructure to support the ACP intervention, including lack of tools, community engagement materials, or an effective EHR (electronic health records) documentation system. As a result, our research roles typically provided extensive consultation on a study's design to identify and include infrastructure elements that would support the intervention.

For example, the type of advance directive used in the clinical arena will impact the ability of the facilitator to assist in the transfer of patient goals and values to the written plan. In one multi-site study, there were five different advance directive documents used in the clinical arena, making it challenging to teach facilitators consistency in documentation. In addition, studies aimed at evaluating the effectiveness of the NS ACP facilitated conversation require organizational support and approval to allow the Statement of Treatment Preference form be entered into the patient's medical record.

Multi-site research studies may have existing ACP education materials that are confusing or contradict the ACP intervention being tested. In some cases, there are no educational materials that exist to support the ACP process, such as Information Cards for Healthcare Agents or CPR fact sheets. Research teams often create their own materials or use standardized materials available for purchase. Regardless, the objective is that patients recruited for the ACP study receive standardized and accurate information that supports the ACP intervention.

Lastly, recruited study subjects receive care by an entire healthcare team — physicians, nurses, social workers, and others — who will need to be informed of the aim of the research study and ACP intervention; prepared to provide adequate team support and follow-up resources. According to the ACTION authors, "We could not ensure that ACP documents were routinely completed, included in the medical notes, and acted upon by physicians. Also, the intervention was delivered in a research context, which required standardisation. As a result, the programme was not integrated with routine services, nor adapted to local circumstances and needs, which may have reduced its effect."[8]

Fidelity Monitoring: An Essential and Complex Research Component

Fidelity is the state of being faithful. Monitoring fidelity is essential to ensure an intervention is replicated as intended. In the clinical arena and research setting, it can be easy for individuals — inadvertently or intentionally — to drift away from the treatment or intervention protocols. When this happens, the reported outcomes may vary from the expected outcomes, and it will be impossible to report on whether the program was implemented as intended.

Fidelity monitoring sets expectations for performance, enables documentation of an intervention, provides opportunities for feedback on individual performance, program improvement, and needed adaptations. Essentially, fidelity monitoring is quality improvement.

"Reporting documentation of fidelity to the implementation strategy will facilitate selection of optimal implementation strategies, more accurate replication, and ultimately more successful transfer of evidence into practice."[9]

When a research study intends to evaluate the impact of the RC approach to facilitating ACP conversations, attention to fidelity entails establishing the criteria for competency evaluation. What are the expectations of performance? How is fidelity to the intervention monitored? The RC fidelity monitoring plan includes (but is not limited to) the following guidelines:

- Demonstration of ACP facilitation skills via face-to-face or video demonstration of standardized facilitation competency criteria
- Practice of role-play situations of common problems, questions, and strategies
- Preparation of site mentors to support the competency of the research interventionists, provide practice and feedback sessions, and validate initial and ongoing competency achievement
- Creation of individualized improvement plans for competency certification as needed
- Creation of inter-rater reliability guidelines for mentors and instructors to improve consistency in evaluating competence and providing feedback for improvement
- Review of audio or videotape ACP conversations, providing individualized feedback and identification program concerns and themes for group learning
- Regular conference calls with interventionists to review lessons learned, identify themes for group learning, provide support and ongoing mentoring

These fidelity monitoring strategies were instrumental in ensuring the intervention remained stable and provided support as facilitators learned and practiced new communication skills and encountered real-life conversations.

Lack of Knowledge, Skills, and Resources of Frontline Providers: Misalignment of Research Evidence with Operational Priorities

Undoubtedly, the RC program is complex, requiring attention to the Five Promises framework. Research teams require education to understand the

ACP intervention, its evidence, content, materials, and implementation strategies. A lack of knowledge of these components can lead to poorly designed research studies. For example, many research teams have wanted to modify the Conversation Guides for facilitating ACP conversations even before the study begins.

Minor adaptations to the guides are understandable, such as providing a research introduction or providing disease-specific information within the context of the guide. However, changing or eliminating conversation questions and strategies risks changing the evidence-base of the intervention. Most often, we have found that, with education and experience, the research team's concerns and interest in making significant changes are resolved.

In addition, the patient's healthcare team can be instrumental in supporting an ACP intervention — or not. Professionals play a central role in the delivery of healthcare, and ACP interventions may conflict with this role. "Traditional norms of professionalism favor individual professional judgment...over standardized, codified policies and procedures."

Physicians and other healthcare providers caring for patients in the study population require an understanding of the ACP intervention and the potential follow-up questions and concerns elicited from the conversation.[10] Recruitment of patients willing to participate in a research study is impacted by the beliefs and actions of the healthcare providers. The authors of the ACTION trial identified this "gatekeeping" phenomenon from healthcare professionals as one explanation for the lack of positive study results. Gatekeeping behaviors from healthcare professionals stem from a variety of beliefs: fear of burdening vulnerable patients or their families, difficulty disclosing prognosis, doubts about the value of the intervention, and lack of skills to recruit patients.[11]

Last, many ACP interventions result in follow-up communication and assistance. Physicians and others will need to be prepared for questions that patients have identified or assistance with making specific treatment decisions. Patient goals may conflict with physician recommendations. Additionally, patients may require the assistance of palliative care resources, social services, ethics committees, or chaplains to provide support to meet the patient's identified goals of care.

Lack of Sustainability Once the Research Ends

Research-supported resources seldom remain at local study sites to support continued use of even successful interventions. The ACP service may be eliminated once the research funding and resources are gone. We did not effectively address this challenge, which left unresolved questions and loss of quality interventions.

For example, it would be helpful to develop strategies to engage the executive leadership teams at the study sites in understanding the intervention and keeping them abreast of research findings throughout the study, and offering strategies for dissemination of the intervention. RC offers a variety of services to assist organizations and communities to continue to replicate the intervention, including online and onsite education, facilitator and instructor certifications, and attendance at national programs.

Chapter 39: If I Only Knew Revisited

In a culture of person-centered decision-making, the opening story of this Part stimulated an organizational response to gather information and create an improvement plan which sparked the design of the original RC ACP program, "If I Only Knew."

A multidisciplinary team from the renal dialysis unit — including a patient receiving hemodialysis — was convened to study the problem presented by the ethics consultations and create a strategy to help patients understand how to participate in ACP.

Baseline data revealed that only four patients (2%) with kidney failure and on hemodialysis had completed an advance directive available in the medical record. An educational program was designed with three goals: 1) to encourage patients and families to understand the importance of making decisions prior to a medical crisis, 2) to assist patients to identify their goals for future medical care and define quality of life, and 3) to provide education on documentation of their preferences and decisions.[1]

The intent of this program was to promote conversation and not merely the completion of advance directives. The program included an ACP video introduction — with stories from hemodialysis patients — a workbook to encourage reflection on goals and values, and a follow-up appointment to answer questions and assist with decision making and documentation if appropriate. The immediate impact of this program resulted in 46% of patients having completed an advance directive and the design of a "green sleeve" to store the document in the medical record for quick identification by treating physicians in an emergency.

Qualitatively, the nephrologists reported a much easier time deciding to forgo dialysis when the patient was incapable of making decisions, and staff reported that even when patients remained capable, they were given support and information in helping them decide whether to continue with dialysis. In the words of one nephrologist, "When I have to make difficult decisions to forgo dialysis, I now know what my patients want, and I can sleep better at night."

Armed with information, data, and resources, a First Steps ACP intervention was designed to provide planning information and assistance for all patients within three months of initiation of hemodialysis, and a Next Steps ACP intervention for patients with serious illness at risk for complications requiring life-sustaining treatment decisions. Hemodialysis clinicians and a patient and family advisory group participated in the evaluation of these services, providing feedback on the importance of continuing to invest in the provision of ACP services throughout the illness trajectory.

Moreover, this small renal dialysis pilot program outcomes provided a best practice model that was used to create the community wide program in 1993, entitled "Respecting Your Choices" which led to the publication of the La Crosse Advance Directive Study (LADS) in 1998, detailing the results of the community-wide program after two years of implementation.[2]

Summary

This Part has emphasized the imperative to use and gather evidence to guide the creation and improvement of person-centered decision-making programs. The underlying principles and utility of the Five Promises framework, microsystems creation, quality improvement, and research have been demonstrated in a description of RC program adaptations around the globe.

Mixed outcomes from multiple ACP systematic reviews have cast doubt about the ongoing value of ACP and stimulated exciting work on a standardized

ACP Outcomes framework and future research agenda. What I fear is missing in this discussion is a vision of the universal impact of comprehensive ACP programs on the delivery of person-centered care.

The entire content of this book is dedicated to creating a vision for ACP that extends far beyond an ACP intervention to promote patient engagement, surrogate understanding, accessibility of documented preferences and decisions, and even goal concordant care. When will it be time to do the hard work of cultural transformation? Yes, we need standardization of the ACP Outcomes framework, but we also need standardization on the core elements of an ACP program and leadership outcomes that impact dissemination and sustainability.

While it is perfectly understandable to question the value of an isolated ACP intervention, it is unacceptable to abandon efforts to integrate ACP as a vehicle to improve person-centered decision-making, the pathway to the provision of person-centered care.

Personal Exercises

1) Describe the outcomes you have observed through person-centered decision-making quality improvement and/or research activities. What lessons have you learned?

2) What ACP "interventions" exist in your current practice? What interventions are missing?

3) What is your vision for ACP?

Part Seven

Chapter 40:
The Promise of Pediatric Advance Care Planning

Honoring a Child's Decision

My nephew was born with cystic fibrosis, a genetic disease causing the production of extra thick mucus in the lungs and digestive organs that results in cycles of lung infections and failure. He was a warrior, determined to live life to the fullest. In the process, he periodically resisted compliance with his arduous medical regime, which included antibiotics to treat lung infections, anti-inflammatory meds to decrease swelling, mucus thinning drugs, bronchodilators, pancreatic enzymes, and daily chest physical therapy and breathing exercises.

At 17 years of age, when his fragile lungs gradually succumbed to the unrelenting assault of the illness and the burdens of treatment outweighed the benefits, he made a decision to stop fighting the disease — a decision supported by his parents, who arranged for home hospice care. His hospital bed was artfully arranged in an open bedroom facing the woods, intravenous morphine and sedatives were on the bedside stand with administration guidelines provided by the hospice team, and there were short, frequent family visits.

My sister was a resilient woman, having tended to two sons with this fatal disease for over two decades, but after a few days of caring for her dying son, she reached out to me and my nursing background for help. I welcomed her request and was privileged to witness the last few days in the life of this brave young man, determined to live (and die) on his own terms. The intravenous morphine and sedatives helped to manage his secretions, shortness of breath, rapid breathing and heart rate, and anxiety.

The cycle of injections were interspersed with lucid periods that allowed him to be awake, talkative, and interact with family. At one point, however, the cycles of lucidity became grueling. Near the end, during a private conversation with my sister and me, he pleaded: "I am sick of being forced to stay awake for all of you. I am tired. It hurts to talk. It hurts to breathe." My sister heard his plea and asked me to give adequate medication to allow her son to remain comfortable and sedated until his death.

Overview

The past decade has seen an increase in the prevalence of chronic and life-threatening illnesses for infants, children, and adolescents and young adults (AYAs) while mortality from these illnesses has decreased.[1] The pediatric population ranges in age from prenatal to young adults, including some over the age of 21 who remain in the care of pediatric specialists or have healthcare needs that are best delivered by pediatricians.

As a result of medical, scientific, and technological advances, some children with complex chronic and life-threatening conditions who would have died from their illnesses years ago can be cured and live a long life; some are not cured but live well with their illnesses for many years. But others battle their illness every day, tolerating significant treatment burdens in their struggle to continue to live.

This Part is dedicated to the parents and competent AYAs who grapple with complex healthcare decisions that underscore the delicate balance between survival and the burdens of life-sustaining treatments. A brief history of pediatric advance care planning (pACP) explores childhood illness trajectories, acknowledges national support for end-of-life counseling as a standard of care for the pediatric population, and outlines the barriers to, and value of, pACP.

While my initial experience with pACP was personal, my role at Respecting Choices exposed me to robust opportunities to design a pACP program and produce evidence of its effectiveness. The early experience in pACP and quality improvement experiences are described in Chapter 41.

To support the development of a quality pACP program, parents' and physician perspectives were explored and are reported in Chapter 42. Research on the effectiveness of this pACP approach is described in Chapter 43 for two pediatric populations: parents of children with life-threatening illnesses unable to participate in decision-making and AYAs with serious illness.

The Part concludes with my perspectives on how the pACP strategies described herein effectively respond to the long-standing barriers to planning conversations, supporting the integration of pACP programs as a routine standard of care for children and AYAs with life-threatening illness. (Chapter 44)

A Brief History of Pediatric Advance Care Planning (pACP)

Unfortunately, when ACP conversations for the pediatric patients occur, they are typically stimulated by the anticipation of a looming death, in a time of crisis, and in the intensive care unit. For parents, these seemingly abrupt conversations occur when the healthcare team believes further treatment is non-beneficial or harmful. Ethics consultations and palliative care (PC) resources are employed to resolve decision-making dilemmas and assist in the care of this vulnerable population.

Pediatric palliative care specialists ascribe to four common pathways, or trajectories, for how children die that influence the type of PC services delivered. The first pathway comprise children who die suddenly from trauma, homicide, or premature birth, while the second pathway includes previously healthy children who contract a malignancy or degenerative disease that steadily declines to poor health and altered quality of life.[2] A third pathway emerges of children whose chronic illness trajectory — malignancies, cystic fibrosis, metabolic disorders — varies significantly, with alternating episodes of exacerbation and recovery that may include additional decompensation.

A fourth pathway for how children die include those whose chronic medical conditions are fragile, who experience repeated healthcare crises, and remain vulnerable to long-standing insults for months to years. The diverse illnesses in this pathway include children with congenital or acquired multi-system disease, severe neurologic conditions with functional impairment, or those with cancer and ongoing disabilities. "…the pattern of fragile health comes to define the way of life for these children and their families, as they often live waiting for the next crises and setback. As a clinician or family member, determining when the child is dying can be difficult. Deciding when to redefine the goals of care from life-extending to comfort-seeking can be divisive within families, between families and clinicians, and among clinicians."[3]

More recently, the fourth pathway is aptly described as "children with medical complexity (CMC)" to highlight "person-first" terminology and the requirement of multiple levels of expert resources to manage optimal outcomes.[4] These children require hospital and community-based services, rely on technology, pharmacology, and intensive home care for basic survival, experience frequent and prolonged hospitalizations, and require a high level of care coordination.

These distinct pathways for childhood illnesses are well-served by early and proactive PC services but in addition, ACP resources that are integrated as a standard of care from initial diagnosis throughout the unpredictable illness trajectory. The American Academy of Pediatrics and the World Health Organization recommend that ACP conversations begin at diagnosis of a life-threatening illness, include the patient (AYA) when capable, family, and primary healthcare provider, be individualized and become a routine and structured part of standard of care rather than be reserved until a medical crisis.[5]

Despite national recommendations for pACP and published guidelines from supportive organizations, programmatic implementation into clinical practice remains sluggish amidst an array of barriers.[6]

Barriers to Pediatric Advance Care Planning

Certain barriers to pACP are remarkably similar to those faced in adult populations, such as fears of causing distress or taking away hope, dealing with emotional responses, inadequate clinician skill and education, time constraints, lack of readiness to participate in ACP, and cultural, ethnic, or racial norms.[7]

There are distinct differences. First, there may be disparities in understanding prognosis between healthcare providers and the parent or child, complicated by prognostic uncertainty of the child's illness trajectory. My nephew with cystic fibrosis endured several illness complications throughout his 17 years that required mechanical ventilation and long hospitalizations — events that allowed him to recover and return to his life and activities, albeit at reduced levels. Through many of these hospitalizations, there was no prognostic certainty that he would get better, or if he might die.

Second, the parents' and AYAs cognitive and emotional development must be evaluated to assess their capability of understanding information, ability, and willingness to participate in three-way shared decision-making conversations. The decision-making capacity for pediatric patients range from those who are incapable of participation or providing consent to those who are developing capacity for consent and finally, to those who are fully capable of providing consent.

The mature minor, such as my nephew — not legally an adult — may possess the ability to weigh the benefits and burdens of treatment choices. For those minors who have evolving capacity, respect for autonomy requires they be informed of their choices, so they are either allowed to make their own healthcare decisions or provide assent through conversation that informs their parents or legal guardians of their goals, values, and preferences.

Third, parents and healthcare providers may ardently wish to protect children — to shield them from having to talk about their illness and the possibility of death. The consequence of this well-intentioned desire to protect children from painful conversations may result in the loss of the child's voice — especially those AYAs with capacity to participate — from the decision-making process and the potential of providing healthcare treatment decisions that may not be aligned with the AYAs goals and values.

This consequence rings especially true when a child turns 18 years of age, when they are legally afforded the right to choose the person who will make healthcare decisions if they become unable to do so. Parents who have held a decision-making role for the prior 17 years may find this transition to legal decision-making authority novel, frightening, and risks accepting an outcome and path of treatment that may be contrary to their own.

Fourth, pACP conversations are demanding, complicated by the lack of professional experience and competence in facilitating goals of care conversations for a child. Healthcare inexperience with pACP conversations results in inaction. Even for children with predictable prognoses, such as terminal cancer, professionals are hesitant to initiate ACP conversations. An international study of pediatric oncologists revealed that 45% do not initiate ACP conversations with their cancer patients, even though the trajectory of the illness is clear. For patients with serious illnesses, when the timing of death is challenging to predict (e.g., severe cerebral palsy, neurodegenerative disorders, short gut syndrome), conversations are even less common.[8]

Lastly, there are legal and ethical barriers that create uncertainty in honoring advance care plans for children and AYAs. For example, pACP may involve the drafting of written plans, such as advance directives, the POLST (portable medical order) form, or instructional letters (drafted by parents, or physicians) that indicate the actions that should be taken when a health crisis occurs. Written plans may not be respected, perhaps due to their lack of legal status or lack of education among appropriate parties. One U.S. study found that 80% of public schools did not have policies for implementing student DNR (do not resuscitate) decisions, and 76% reported unwillingness to honor the decision or uncertainty if it was legal to do so.[9]

Moreover, for parents of children with life-threatening illness, federal and state statutory and case law may restrict decision-making rights. Most states have adopted the federal Child Abuse Prevention Act of 1996 (CAPTA) that aims to prevent medical neglect, ensuring that appropriate care is provided to children to prevent or remedy conditions that may cause harm to include oversight by child protective services and authorized to initiate legal action if necessary.[10]

Under CAPTA, failing to provide appropriate nutrition, hydration, and medication to any infant with a life-threatening condition always constitutes "withholding of medically indicated treatment."[11] The notable exceptions to this standard of providing life-sustaining interventions include the presence of chronic and irreversible coma, or if the proposed intervention would only prolong the dying process, be ineffective in correcting the life-threatening condition, or be inhumane.

The decision-making rights of AYAs, age 14-18 years, bears other legal and ethical concerns. By law, only competent adults age 18 years and older can execute an advance directive.[12] While most authorities recognize that adolescents, beginning around the age of 14, possess capacity to make informed healthcare decisions, controversy over the autonomous rights of minors has received national attention.[13] The case of Abraham Cherrix raised ethical and legal questions regarding the rights of young adults to *refuse* life-sustaining treatment.[14] In an analysis of this case, the prominent ethicist Arthur Caplan asks the following questions: "What should a physician do when a young teenager refuses life-saving medical care?" and "How should society react if the teenager insists on not undergoing such care?"

In 2006, Abraham was a 16-year-old teenager diagnosed with Hodgkin's disease and had completed one round of chemotherapy resulting in typical treatment complications of baldness, weakness, and inability to walk. When his cancer returned two months later, he and his parents rejected a second round of recommended chemotherapy in lieu of an alternative condemned by the FDA (Food and Drug Administration), but available in Mexico.

Upon learning of the family's actions, Abraham's treating physicians reported them to the Department of Social Services, who determined that he was not receiving appropriate care. After court charges of medical neglect were levied, the family, court, and physicians reached an agreement to allow them to proceed with nonconventional treatment under supervision of a qualified oncology physician.

The Cherrix case exemplifies the rights of teenagers to self-determination while upholding society's obligations to ensure life-saving medical treatment is provided to children. However, the case also highlights the impact of effective communication between all stakeholders that eventually resulted in improved understanding of the treatment options and Abraham's and his parent's goals and values.

These variables were represented in the resulting Abraham's law that outlined the conditions under which a minor may refuse life-sustaining treatment: 1) the decision is made jointly by the parents or legal guardians and the child; 2) the child is 14 and capable of understanding information; 3) the parties have considered appropriate alternative treatment options; and 4) the parties are making decisions based on the best interests of the child.[15]

In May 2020, Callasandra Callendar, a 17-year-old with Hodgkin's lymphoma whose refusal of chemotherapy — a decision supported by her mother — resulted in the Connecticut Department of Children and Families' action to take legal custody of Callasandra. A legal battle ruled she did not meet the state's statutory requirements as a mature minor. Callasandra was forced to undergo chemotherapy for five months, held in the hospital against her wishes.[16]

The goal of improved communication between parents, children, and the healthcare team in times of conflicting opinions and values could decrease the need for court involvement and erosion of physician and parent relationships. In the face of long-standing barriers, the value of pACP for parents, patients and healthcare professionals is indisputable.

The Value of Pediatric Advance Care Planning

Most parents want physicians to discuss ACP options and assist in making shared decisions.[17] Parents who have participated in ACP conversations and creating written plans express satisfaction with the planning process, believing this results in providing good care for their child, preserving quality of life, and avoiding unnecessary suffering.[18]

A survey of 114 bereaved parents of children and AYAs with complex medical conditions at a large children's hospital was conducted to assess the impact of ACP on parent-reported end-of-life experiences and outcomes. Sixty-five percent of the recruited parents reported having had ACP conversations — conversations that helped them be more prepared for the end-of-life, allowed them to rate the quality of their child's end-of-life as excellent, and plan the location of their child's death.

Notably, ACP conversations that included a specific assessment of family goals were associated with a decrease in child suffering and parental regret. Seventy percent (70%) of the parents believed such conversations should start early during a child's illness.[19]

The content and quality of ACP conversations matters. The parents of children with medical complexity identified these factors to be most helpful as part of ACP conversations: a holistic approach, exploration of beliefs, goals, and quality of life, communication strategies that include shared decision-making, ongoing conversations, family readiness, and provider facilitation expertise.[20]

For AYAs able to participate in shared decision-making conversations, evidence of the value of pACP extends beyond improved end-of-life outcomes; evidence stemming largely from randomized controlled trials of the FACE (FAmily-CEntered) ACP intervention, described in Chapter 43. The FACE ACP intervention has demonstrated improved parental understanding of their adolescents' treatment preferences in the setting of cancer and HIV diagnoses, the delivery of earlier palliative care, and improvement in symptoms related to HIV.[21]

Pediatric ACP for AYAs can uncover and address the gaps that may exist between a parent and AYA's understanding of goals, values, and preferences for medical care and treatment. As a component of a larger FACE ACP study, researchers examined the end-of-life values of adolescents with cancer, and their families' understanding — revealing several areas of incongruence. A majority of adolescents preferred that ACP conversations occur early in the course of an illness (before getting sick, when first diagnosed), but less than half of the families were aware. While there was a high level of congruence between adolescents and their parents on the desire for honest communication and understanding treatment options, there was low congruence on the adolescent's views of a natural death and being off machines.[22]

Normal adolescent growth and development includes the desire to gain autonomy, yet AYAs with complex life-threatening illnesses must rely on their parents or legal guardians for making healthcare decisions. AYAs living with chronic illness battle physical and emotional changes, loss of school and social interactions, adding stress and psychological complications.[23] Being allowed to participate in healthcare decision-making, and providing appropriate support, can help fill their need for purpose and self-determination.

Many AYAs living with a life-threatening illness have clear views of what they want included in a written advance care plan. These individuals desire opportunities to make and record their choices in the kind of medical treatment they do and do not want, how they wish to be cared for, what they want their families to know, and how they wish to be remembered.[24]

Lastly, creating a shared decision-making process for parents and AYAs with life-threatening illnesses can resolve the stress, grief, and guilt that accompanies the role of surrogate decision-makers. Once a decision is made to withhold or withdraw life-sustaining treatment, such as CPR, even the process of signing a Do-Not-Resuscitate (DNR) order can raise negative emotions among family members.[25]

Chapter 41: Pediatric Advance Care Planning: The Early Evidence and Respecting Choices Experience

As the opening story depicts, my initial experience with pediatric planning was personal. Over time, I came to appreciate the courage required for my sister and her husband to respect my nephew's autonomous decision to stop fighting his cystic fibrosis, arrange for home hospice care, and face the realities of providing comfort throughout the dying process and eventually, to let him go. I came to realize why my sister never wanted to be the person to give her son the medication that would keep him comfortable, but also sedated. I do not think I fully appreciated the grief or guilt she may have felt in honoring her child's dying request.

My interest and experience with pACP quickly evolved through research partnerships and in personally facilitating pediatric conversations with parents of children with life-threatening conditions. These experiences produced evidence of the effectiveness of the RC approach to pACP and instilled in me a commitment to meet the needs of the pediatric populations, although this personal commitment remained an unfulfilled hope in the widespread programmatic expansions of pACP as a standard of care for the pediatric population.

Nonetheless, Dr. Hammes and I welcomed the opportunity to apply the ACP program principles and strategies developed for adults to two specific pediatric populations: parents of children with life-threatening illness and AYAs with complex chronic illness. The impact of these ACP principles were described in a 2013 systematic literature review that analyzed pACP practices from 13 studies. Only three programs met the studies' criteria for an ACP program; all three programs — FACE ACP, Footprints, and the pACP program at Gundersen Health System — are based on Respecting Choices.[1]

ACP for Parents of Children with Life-Threatening Illness

The Early Evidence

Although the RC ACP program was focused on consenting adults, the principles of person-centered decision-making were instinctively applied to pediatric ethics consultations facilitated by Dr. Hammes at Gundersen Health System, stemming as far back as the late 1980s.[2] This "pediatric ACP service" included two to three meetings of variable time limits with parents to explore their understanding of disease progression, prognosis, and the related medical treatment decisions that would be likely over time.

The length and frequency of the meetings were customized to meet the needs of the parents, and included the child's physician and other members of the healthcare team, such as chaplains or ministers, as appropriate. The ACP conversations included the documentation of the parent's treatment decisions in a letter format, signed by all parties, and entered into the medical record. In 1998 when the POLST system was operationalized in the organization, it was used to document DNR orders.

A medical chart review revealed that of the seventeen children in the study, 11 (65%) had an advance directive letter from their parents in the medical record, and four had completed POLST forms. For eight of the nine children who died, the parent's plan for treatment decisions was honored. Thirteen parent interviews were qualitatively analyzed to assess the ACP process in which they participated.

The parents reported the ACP process was valuable to assure the "best care" — defined as providing care to prolong life that had clear benefit and avoiding treatments with little or no chance for prolonging life — for their child, provide information and time for decision-making, present options to communicate treatment decisions, and provide peace of mind. Dr. Hammes believed there were additional benefits:

> Before pACP, I was involved in many cases where decision-making resulted in deep conflicts between mom and dad. In some cases, parents lost a child and their marriage at the same time. I wanted to help parents develop a shared decision so that in the crisis, they could be together, supporting each other through a terrible loss.[3]

As the RC program evolved and research produced evidence of the value and need for pACP, Dr. Hammes and I aspired to expand this approach to a broader population — one that would be integrated as a routine standard of care for children with complex medical conditions. Although the pediatric ACP service implemented by Dr. Hammes as a component of his ethics consultations was valuable, it was dependent on one person and was stimulated by an ethics consultation referral.

The development and research outcomes of the RC Next Steps (NS) ACP program — aimed at the decision-making process for adults with serious illness — provided a framework to apply these planning strategies, principles, and tools to the pediatric population. The research outcomes from the FACE studies for AYAs with HIV/AIDS (acquired immunodeficiency syndrome) and cancer provided evidence of successful application in this pediatric subgroup.

We embarked on a quality improvement (QI) process to gain interest in implementing a formal pACP program at Gundersen Healthcare System.

Pediatric ACP for Parents of Children with Life-threatening Illness: A Quality Improvement Approach

The QI planning process began by making adaptations to the adult and AYA version of the Next Steps ACP conversation guide, planning document, and ACP Facilitator certification curriculum. The questions and content in the Pediatric NS Conversation Guide was adapted to reflect the target population: parents of children with life-threatening conditions.

In lieu of the Statement of Treatment Preference form used for adult and AYA populations, a new planning new document was created — the Pediatric Advance Care Plan for Children who are Unable to Participate in Healthcare Decision-Making — that helps the parent(s) express how they want their seriously ill child to be treated in the event of a future medical crisis, including a description of the specific medical treatment the parent(s) want or do not want, what they want healthcare providers to know about their child, and their preferred place of death. A Pediatric ACP Facilitator Certification program was adapted to integrate appropriate pediatric information, legal and ethical issues, and video and role-play examples.

In September of 2012, I met with a small team of pediatric physicians, nurse care coordinators, social workers, and the program manager at Gundersen Health System — the team who coordinated the care of children with complex needs. The goal of this first meeting was to engage them in learning about our adapted pediatric ACP approach, Next Steps ACP research and publications in the AYA population, and create interest in expanding this approach for parents who struggle with making decisions for their children with life-threatening illnesses — children unable to participate in the decision-making process.

The team was curious, tentative, and recommended gathering input from a parent advisory group who would be interested in participating and providing feedback on a pACP program. Even though the team was cautious, they instantly described several current cases where pACP could be helpful.

- **An 18-year-old girl with Batten's disease, a progressive neuro-degenerative illness** - The care team had witnessed a physical decline in her symptoms and were worried that her mother "had not come to grips" with her daughter's decline. The team believed the daughter would minimally be able to participate in an ACP conversation. They sensed she was scared.

- **A 9-year-old male with a progressive neuro-degenerative disorder who struggles with constant seizures, is home-bound requiring a feeding tube** - He has a supportive family but has not developed a plan to address end-of-life situations.

- **A 17-year-old female with a progressive neuro-degenerative disease who is non-communicative** - Her parents have expressed interest in helping other families caring for children with complex medical conditions.

In order to create a pACP approach, we proceeded to gather more information from parents and physicians.

Chapter 42: Lessons from Pediatric ACP Conversations: Parent and Physician Perspectives

To gather more information on the development of our pediatric ACP (pACP) program, we wanted to learn from parents and physicians who had real-life experiences with children living with serious illness. It was a privilege to meet with several parents of children with complex medical conditions who agreed to participate as an advisory group to evaluate the proposed pACP program.

The following excerpts from three parent conversations provided valuable feedback and suggestions for programmatic revisions and personal insight into how ACP conversations would look and feel different from the adult conversations I had become familiar with.

What We Would Have Wanted for Our Child

Parents who had recently lost their daughter to the consequences of a life-threatening illness agreed to meet with me and one of the pediatric physicians who had cared for their daughter. The goals of the meeting were to: 1) solicit their experiences with communication surrounding treatment decisions for their daughter in the last year of her life; 2) provide feedback on the adapted pACP Conversation Guide for Parents; and 3) provide suggestions for integrating a pACP service as a standard of care for children with medical complexities. Their perspectives were invaluable.

First, while these parents received open and honest information about their daughter's medical conditions from the healthcare team throughout her illness, they admitted to the benefit of receiving added support from a neighbor — a pediatric physician — who helped them interpret complicated disease trajectory information and understand the benefits and burdens of treatment decisions, such as CPR (cardiopulmonary resuscitation).

Second, despite a few wording suggestions, all questions in the Pediatric ACP Conversation Guide were viewed as worthy topics to prepare for future healthcare decisions. Several questions spurred a recollection of past experiences with their daughter's progressive complications and hospitalizations in the last year of her life that included destructive seizures and respiratory difficulties, but since she recovered, they never fully appreciated the slow and steady decline she was experiencing: "We thought she would live into her early twenties."

Third, in reviewing the Pediatric Advance Care Plan document, the parents appreciated the opportunity to discuss the hypothetical clinical scenarios as an avenue to reflect on future treatment decisions. They would have welcomed the creation of a written plan — a plan that was periodically discussed but never completed. The father commented, "I would have had a different answer for my daughter two years before she died than I would have had in the last six months before she died," highlighting the importance of ongoing conversations and revisions to the goals of care over time.

Last, the parents supported the proposed pACP service as a standard of care for all parents of children with medical complexities.

Jessica is a Tough Little Bird: Carl's Story

As a single parent, Carl has been caring for his 18-year-old daughter, Jessica, since birth. Jessica has multiple chronic conditions which make her vulnerable to serious and progressive complications. Our pACP conversation followed a recent hospitalization where Jessica narrowly survived.

Initially, Carl was cautious, perhaps a bit suspicious, and warmed up slowly to the conversation. To help break the ice, I called attention to the logo

"Hooked on Fishing" inscribed on his blue tee-shirt. He smiled proudly as he revealed Jessica's love of their frequent fishing expeditions — an activity that gives her life meaning.

Despite her complex medical conditions, Jessica is a happy child, and although she is unable to communicate, they understand each other. "When she starts hollering, I can usually figure it out." Jessica goes to school, loves animals, listening to nature and music, fishing, and going for nightly walks.

In describing his hopes for her current and ongoing plan of care, Carl shifts uneasily in his chair. "There are a lot of things I'd like, but I know they are not in the cards." When encouraged to elaborate, he does. Carl hopes Jessica stays healthy, avoids more complications and infections. He hopes she does not have to "struggle" and that one day she might talk.

While he resists talking about other hopes, especially when asked to describe what he means by "struggle" he admits that he worries every day and does not sleep much at night. "I try not to think about the reality of life, but if it ever comes to it, I hope it is easy for her, that she does not suffer. I wouldn't want her lying around for weeks not getting better." He worries about the possibility of Jessica dying, but tries to block it out. "I don't like to talk to anyone about this."

As a side note: this theme of "not wanting to talk; yet being able to talk" continues to amaze me as a facilitator. Carl agreed to come to this meeting that lasted approximately two hours, talk to a complete stranger, give his permission to be videotaped, and allow us to share the conversation with others who might learn from his perspectives. Although informed he could stop the meeting whenever he wanted, he stayed engaged until the end. The conversations are hard, yet indispensable.

In discussing Jessica's recent hospitalization from complications from her illness, Carl admits he "had no clue what was going on" as he was told that "no one with her condition has lived past their early twenties." He was nervous, but he learned that Jessica "...is a tough little bird. She must struggle to live. She's a lot tougher than me." He learned that he wants to be present if Jessica dies, to be there for her, yet not be there. He had always hoped he would die before Jessica. I could sense the anticipatory grief and loss in his verbal and non-verbal expressions.

Understanding that this conversation was hard for Carl, I offered him the option of taking a break or ending the conversation. He simply shook his head "no." We continued to explore his goals and values for Jessica if faced with a future serious complication where she was hospitalized, and in which he was told that selected treatments would likely only prolong her life for a short time, and certain treatments may cause more suffering.

Carl vividly remembered her last hospitalization when the surgeon told him she only had a 10% chance of surviving the proposed surgery and offered him the option of keeping her "peaceful" and not doing the surgery. "I am not God. She survived the surgery because she is a fighter. I won't give up on her."

Carl welcomed the opportunity to have his goals and values for Jessica recorded on the Pediatric Advance Care Plan. He wanted his decision to continue all treatments so Jessica could live as long as possible — even if there was only a 1% chance of success — to be documented. He also wanted to communicate to healthcare providers that Jessica is "...a tough little bird and she has a will to live." Carl readily signed the document.

When the videotaped conversation ended after two hours, I saw the relief in Carl's face as he understood that I was not there to sway his views toward a specific direction or to judge his decisions. He agreed the conversation was helpful, giving him a sense of assurance that Jessica would receive the care she needed when serious complications occur.

As a facilitator and researcher, I was again confronted with internal dissonance of what had just happened. How would Carl continue to process this information? How would he deal with his own emotions, and where would he get support? How would the healthcare team integrate Carl's goals and values into an ongoing care and treatment plan?

This dissonance for me had occurred in the past, and to address these concerns, we invited the nurse care coordinator for Jessica and Carl to be present during the conversation, providing assurance that his goals, decisions, and concerns would be integrated into Jessica's ongoing care management.

After the conversation, I recorded the following reflections:

> Listen to the lived experience; respect what he had learned. Show respect, compassion, and understanding. Give him space to think about the questions; to reflect on his daughter's life. Slow down, acknowledge his strength and love.

We Have to Be Prepared: Heather and Greg's Story

Heather and Greg are the parents of Jamie, a 9-year-old son who suffered a severe anoxic brain injury at birth and is cared for at home, receiving multiple interventions and medications for his serious and progressive medical complications.

From the beginning of the conversation, Heather eloquently exposed her healthcare expertise. She had become a well-informed and competent caregiver with an amazing command of healthcare terminology, technology, and skill in managing the multiple interventions he receives at home, including suctioning, tracheostomy care, gastrostomy feedings, and a ketogenic diet. Despite his extensive care needs, the parents describe Jamie as a "strong little boy" who goes to school two days per week, participates in physical therapy every four hours, and with every complication, "he pulls through... he is meant to be with us."

In exploring their hopes for Jamie's current medical plan of care, Greg answers first. He hopes for continuous improvement, which he defines as "continuing to grow and do all the little things he does, fewer hospitalizations and medications, and less machines." Heather hopes for improved communication with Jamie, "I want to hear his voice," and "I want to keep him home with us." Heather and Greg love to travel with Jamie and their other children and hope to take them to Alaska, allowing Jamie to go whale watching. They smile at each other as they describe these hopes, affirming their commitment to Jamie's quality of life.

In probing a bit further, they discuss other hopes, especially if their expressed hopes do not come true. "That would be the hard part," Heather says as she looks to Greg for a response. "It's hard to think about. We are positive people. We would pick up and move on." But Heather elaborates, having time to think about "hoping for the best, but planning for the worse."

She hopes she does not react with her emotions so she can communicate effectively and remain strong. "I am Jamie's mom, his advocate. When I get too emotional, they think I am difficult to deal with, or that I have not come to terms with the realities of Jamie's diagnosis. If I get emotional, people will not listen to me, and Jamie will not get the care he needs." They agree with the value of this type of hope exploration. "We have to be prepared. It's not a happy thing to think about, but we need to acknowledge the reality."

If Jamie were to suffer another serious complication in which he was "not likely to survive," they openly debate their options. While they would not want Jamie to be dependent on a ventilator for the rest of his life, they would want a trial on the ventilator because "the doctors have been wrong in the past." They are resolved about not attempting CPR if his heart stopped. They are interested in continuing to review the Pediatric Advance Care Plan document and agree to discuss it further with their nurse care coordinator. They believe any plan created should be revisited on a regular basis, perhaps every six months, as goals and decisions may change.

After two hours, Greg expresses his feedback on the importance and appropriateness of the conversation we had just completed: "This is about education. It can open channels of communication and build relationships between parents and the healthcare team."

I could not have hoped for any better outcome for these parents.

The Influence of Physician Champions

The videotaped conversations with parents of children with medical complexities was effective in engaging most of the pediatric care management team, including the lead pediatrician who distributed the following email to the team after his review of feedback from the parent advisory group and his analysis of the evidence:

> I have had a chance to come to a better appreciation of the Respecting Choices Program and the Next Steps process. I think that having a chance to view the video recordings of actual patients and their family members has helped me to move my perception of the program from theory to an appreciation of practice. I see an alignment between what Linda represented to us and something that I learned about at the Montreal Conference that is called "Dignity Therapy" that has been developed and researched by Harvey Max Chochinov, MD, a psychiatrist at the University of Manitoba in Winnipeg, Canada.

> But the Respecting Choices Program does more than the process of Dignity Therapy, or storytelling, because I heard Linda describe a desire to move the patient's story from narrative to a description of practical decisions that can help the whole care team to provide the kinds of care that are consistent with the patient's perception of his/her own story.

I would like for us to be able to learn more about how we can make the benefits of the Respecting Choices Program available to our pediatric patients and their families. We are all familiar with the dictum regarding pediatrics that children are not little adults. But we must also recognize that a lot of pediatric practice has been adapted from practice that first was shown to be beneficial for adults.

This quality improvement approach resulted in revisions to the Pediatric Next Steps ACP Conversation Guide, adaptations to the Pediatric Advance Care Plan document, refinement of a pediatric facilitator certification program, certification of two pediatric healthcare providers, and medical record documentation guidelines.

Chapter 43: The Respecting Choices Research Partnerships in Pediatric Advance Care Planning

A long-term research partnership with Dr. Maureen Lyon and Respecting Choices began in 2004 with the creation and evaluation of an adapted approach to pACP for adolescents and young adults with HIV/AIDS called FACE (FAmily CEntered) ACP.

This research partnership expanded in 2015 when Dr. Lyon received interest in the submission of a grant to evaluate an adapted FACE ACP intervention specifically for parents of children with rare diseases, a population previously underrepresented in research studies and with few evidence-based interventions to support these families through the twists and turns of caring for a fragile child.

A description of both pACP research partnerships, outcomes, and publications is described below.

Pediatric Advance Care Planning with Adolescents: The Emergence of FACE for Adolescents and Young Adults with HIV/AIDS and Cancer

As thousands of adolescents and young adults (AYAs) battle life-threatening illnesses each year, the obligation to integrate end of life conversations into their care is supported by the American Academy of Pediatrics, the Institute of Medicine, and the World Health Organization, acknowledging their capacity to participate in treatment decisions developmentally and emotionally.[5]

The obligation to address the planning needs of AYAs with chronic illnesses has been a longstanding goal of Dr. Maureen Lyon, a Clinical Health Psychologist and Professor of Pediatrics at the Children's National Research Institute. Early in her investigation into the end-of-life decision-making attitudes of adolescents, Dr. Lyon used a convenience sample of 25 adolescents with chronic illness compared to 25 healthy adolescents and reported that the majority of both patient groups (96% and 88% respectively) desire to participate in shared decision-making if serious illness occurs, although adolescents with chronic illness are less likely to want to discuss EOL issues early in their illness trajectory.[6]

Intrigued with these initial research results, Dr. Lyon contacted Respecting Choices to explore our interest in the application of the Next Steps ACP intervention to AYAs with chronic, progressive illness. A long-term research partnership was formed that resulted in the creation and evaluation of FACE (FAmily-CEntered) ACP, a novel approach to the end-of-life planning needs of AYAs living with serious illness. Dr. Lyon's commitment to garnering research funding was phenomenal, securing support from the National Institute of Nursing Research, NIH National Center for Advancing Translational Sciences, and the American Cancer Society.

As principal investigator in randomized controlled trials, she orchestrated multi-site collaboration with Children's National Health System, Washington, D.C, Children's Diagnostic and Treatment Center, Fort Lauderdale, Florida, Johns Hopkins University, Baltimore, Maryland, St. Jude Children's Research Hospital in Memphis, Tennessee, University of Miami Miller School of Medicine, Miami, Florida, and Akron Children's in Ohio. And last, but not least, Dr. Lyon authored multiple publications that allowed the widespread dissemination of the outcomes and value of ACP for the pediatric population.

An Adapted Respecting Choices ACP Intervention: The FACE (FAmily-CEntered) ACP

As co-investigator of the FACE ACP studies, my responsibilities have included consultation on study design and methodology, creating program material adaptations (for example, creating a Next Steps Conversation Guide for AYAs and pACP Facilitator Certification course), providing facilitator certification for research interventionists and ongoing fidelity monitoring, and assisting with interpretation and publication of study results.

The effectiveness of the adapted FACE ACP intervention was initially evaluated in AYAs living with HIV and their families for increasing congruence and quality of communication and decreasing decisional conflict.[7] The FACE ACP intervention included three sessions:

1) The Lyon Family-Centered Advance Care Planning Survey, administered through an interview to assess the AYA's interest in a decision-making role in end-of-life care

2) The Respecting Choices NS Conversation, adapted for AYAs with HIV which included the completion of a Statement of Treatment Preference form that reflected the goals and preferences for treatment in hypothetical situations of high burden and low survival and altered functional and cognitive outcomes

3) The option to complete the Five Wishes document, which served as a legal directive of the AYAs goals, values, and preferences for treatment in the event they lost decision-making capacity

One hundred and five dyads (AYAs aged 14-21 years and their surrogates, aged 18 years and older) were randomized to intervention or control groups.

It is significant that 92% (50) of the intervention patients were black, and 53% (29) had no high school diploma.

Several predetermined benchmarks for enrollment and retention were met or exceeded, for example, 99% of those who started Session 1 attended all three sessions; retention was 85% once participants were enrolled, and there were no adverse events reported.[8] A majority of the adolescents and their families felt the intervention was helpful and worthwhile.

The first FACE ACP study concluded: "Family-centered advance care planning by trained facilitators increased congruence in adolescent/surrogate preferences for end-of-life care, decreased decisional conflict, and enhanced communication quality. Families acknowledged a life-threatening condition and were willing to initiate end-of-life conversations when their adolescents were medically stable."[9]

Similar results of increased congruence in treatment preferences, feelings that the sessions were worthwhile, and decreased anxiety were found in a replication study of the FACE ACP intervention for AYAs with cancer (FACE-TC).[10]

In addition, FACE-TC reported that intervention dyads were more likely to limit treatments than the control counterparts. Moreover, FACE-TC has demonstrated the long-term impact of pACP conversations. As compared to those in the control group, FACE-TC families reported significantly increased positive caregiving appraisals for their teen with cancer at three months post-intervention. The intervention did not result in undue distress or strain.[11]

Given the success of the FACE ACP studies for AYAs, Dr. Lyon spearheaded a research study evaluating the impact of an adapted FACE intervention for adults living with HIV on immediate and long-term congruence.[12] The Statement of Treatment Preference form — discussed during Session 2 of the FACE ACP intervention — was used to assess treatment preferences for each patient-surrogate dyad.

Congruence across all scenarios was significantly higher among the intervention dyads compared to the controls immediately post-intervention and 12 months post-intervention. The surrogates in the intervention group accurately reported on changes in patient preferences throughout this time period. This first-of-its-kind study demonstrates the enduring power of ACP conversations to maintain open communication between patients and their healthcare agents as goals, values, and preferences are apt to change over time.

The success of FACE (FAmily-CEntered) pediatric ACP for Teens with Cancer (FACE-TC) was recognized by the National Institutes of Health as a Research Intervention Tested Program (R-TIPS).[13] The R-TIPS website offers a database of evidence-based cancer programs that have been tested in a research study, results disseminated through publications, and offer program materials and products to assist with implementation.[14]

Experiences With FACE ACP Intervention Facilitators

As a component of my fidelity monitoring responsibilities for the FACE ACP studies, I collaborated with Dr. Lyon and the research team to review recorded Respecting Choices NS conversations for consistency with the published competency criteria and to provide feedback to facilitators for ongoing learning and communication skills improvement. Monthly facilitator conference calls provided a forum for group learning to discuss identified themes and explore suggested strategies that promote a consistent and robust pACP conversation. A few examples of the themes that emerged from a review of recorded conversations are described as follows:

- **Adolescents who are quiet and unable or unwilling to answer all questions** - Naturally, being quiet may be a personality trait, an adolescent developmental phase, an attribute of the subject matter, or all of the above. Remaining silent and providing additional space and time to respond to questions may be needed. At times, parents may be able to provide information or observations to assist the teen in expressing him/herself.

In addition, using reflection, such as "Do you agree or disagree with your mom's statement?" may provide an opportunity to engage in mutual dialogue. Continuing with the conversation may stimulate more dialogue over time; be prepared to revisit questions or explore new comments. There are times when dialogue remains limited despite communication strategies. For some, the dialogue may come well after the scheduled conversation.

- **Parents/guardians who believe they are unable or unwilling to honor their teen's expressed preferences** - It was common for parents to express uneasiness upon hearing their teens goals and values — goals and values they perhaps had never expressed and were contrary to the parent's viewpoints. It is important to recognize that congruence in understanding differing points of view may take time.

A few strategies to attempt to promote the parent's understanding include asking the teen to repeat the reason behind their goals, values, or decisions, paraphrasing your understanding of the teen's preferences. Acknowledging the parent's perspective ("It must be hard to think about these decisions.") by verbalizing empathy may also be helpful. For parents that remain resistant, facilitators can recommend follow-up support from an ethics consultation, the healthcare team, or a trusted chaplain or social worker.

- **Facilitator assumptions that the conversation "won't go well"** - When reviewing background information on the patient's clinical condition or reflecting on prior experiences may create personal biases prior to the conversation. Identifying concerns and barriers and discussing these with another team member prior to the conversation can present new suggestions and insights for how to resolve these.

Periodically reaffirming the purpose of the conversation can set the stage to address the patient's barriers or concerns. During one conversation in which the adolescent refused to answer many of the questions, the facilitator acknowledged her frustration and anxiety, but she kept the conversation going. Midway through the conversation, the teen "came to life" as he encountered a topic in which he was passionate.

Pediatric Advance Care Planning for Parents of Children with Rare Diseases (FACE-Rare)

A new partnership with Dr. Lyon created an adapted pACP intervention for this pediatric population that would integrate the previously described programmatic strategies for parents of children with life-threatening illness developed by Respecting Choices with Dr. Lyon's research outcomes from the FACE ACP intervention for AYAs. The newly created intervention, FACE-Rare (Family-Centered pediatric ACP for parents of children with rare diseases), consists of four sessions.[1]

- **Session 1**: The Carer Support Needs Assessment Tool (CSNAT), adapted for parents of children with rare diseases.[2] This evidence-based, practitioner-facilitated tool is used to assess the level of parental support needed to care for a child with medical complexities, and to continue to take care of their own personal health.

- **Session 2**: Review of the action plan to address the prioritized support identified in Session 1.

- **Session 3**: The facilitated Respecting Choices Next Steps pACP conversation for parents of children with life-threatening conditions who cannot communicate. This conversation, delivered by a certified RC facilitator to support shared decision-making, explores fears, values, hopes, and goals for future medical care and prepares the parent or guardian for a future decision in the event of a medical crisis.

- **Session 4**: Follow-up discussion and completion (if desired) of a written plan. Given time to reflect on the exploration of goals and values in Session 3, this session provides a forum for remaining questions, concerns, and the need for additional resources, such as the identification of questions for the child's pediatrician, or referrals to appropriate services. The opportunity to complete the Pediatric Advance Care Plan for Children with Life-limiting Illness who are not able to participate in healthcare decision-making is offered, but optional.

Initial Evaluation of FACE-Rare

The initial evaluation of this intervention was conducted with six families, meeting all expected benchmark measures for feasibility and acceptability. All parents found FACE-Rare helpful, including the quality of facilitator communication, and completed the RC Pediatric Advance Care Plan document, along with suggested modifications that were integrated into the document. Support for a larger, randomized controlled trial of FACE-Rare was awarded to Children's National Research Institute in 2020 with Dr. Lyon as the Principal Investigator.

My research role in the initial evaluation of FACE-Rare was to provide input into the study design and methodology, provide the pediatric ACP tools (pACP conversation guide and Pediatric Advance Care Plan), and assist with program revisions as appropriate.

In addition to these roles, I actively participated in the collection of data by facilitating pACP conversations with two recruited parents, using the adapted Pediatric NS Conversation Guide. This is when I met Kate Detwiller and her son Nolan. Telemedicine was used with four families, including with Kate and Nolan, and although I had prior experience using video conferencing to facilitate ACP conversations, it was not my preferred modality, especially given the novel pACP intervention we were evaluating.

Nevertheless, this modality worked best for a busy mom who was balancing work and care of a child with medical complexities. Although I had never met Kate, the conversation flowed easily. Not because the subject matter was "easy," or that I was a good facilitator, rather, it was "easy" because of Kate's experiences, ability, and willingness to communicate what was most important to her in caring for her son. It was emotional to listen to her describe her multiple encounters with the healthcare system and how she learned to navigate Nolan's ongoing needs and healthcare decisions.

Kate reviewed the Pediatric Advance Care Plan document and was interested in recording important messages about how to care for Nolan, and also how to make healthcare treatment decisions. At the end of the conversation, Kate asked if I would like to "meet" Nolan, who proceeded to waddle into view of the camera displaying a toddler's smile and enthusiasm for life.

I wanted all children with life-limiting illnesses to be cared for by someone like Kate, her husband Brian, and a supportive family care system. This family had already begun to process how they would make decisions for Nolan as his illness progressed; I am unsure if they even needed the pACP facilitation that day. But I do know that many families are not like Kate's family. I was ever convinced of the importance of providing a pACP service for all parents of children with complex medical conditions.

Kate provided invaluable feedback on the facilitation approach, wording suggestions for the pACP conversation guide, and the Pediatric Advance Care Plan. I remain grateful for her honesty, openness, and commitment to support pACP for all parents:

> These conversations are individual building blocks that when put together, create something beautiful and strong; the peace of knowing that I cared for my child throughout his life and those cumulative moments will bring me peace at the end. The weaker moments and conversations during times of crisis are supported by the stronger conversations defined by the clarity of our lives and values outside of that traumatic moment. The more conversations you have, the more building blocks you have as a parent and the better picture you have of that final something.[3]

Experiences Facilitating FACE-Rare pACP Conversations

As a component of fidelity monitoring of pACP interventions, research facilitators review recorded conversations to identify and discuss themes that emerge — themes that set the stage for future program revisions and implementation plans. I have chosen the following personal themes and reflections to demonstrate the commitment to ongoing learning for pACP facilitators.

- **Parents are the experts in the care of their child.** It is important to affirm this role during pACP conversations. Parents of children with medical complexities are often required to teach medical students and nursing staff how to care for their child; teaching that, at times, is minimized or disregarded. Fathers can often feel excluded from conversations, and their role as caregiver minimized.

For example, in my pACP conversation with Heather and Greg, while both were invited to respond to questions, I was impressed with the added information and feelings offered by Greg. The effectiveness of the two-way conversation was evident in their constant interaction, nodding heads, smiling, and sharing personal insights that perhaps they had not previously done.

The concept of "expertise" often pits parents against the healthcare team at critical points when they need to be on the same side, the child's side. The reality of being a parent with a child with a complex medical condition is illustrated in an editorial by a pediatrician who, when confronted with the challenges of caring for her son with a rare skeletal dysphagia, apologizes to other parents and their children with medical complexities for not better understanding what they were experiencing.[4] "I can remember sitting in care conferences and wondering, "Why is this family being so difficult?" or "Why can't they just accept the expert advice and do the right thing?"

The pediatrician proceeds to describe why she is now "that parent" — the demanding, obnoxious, and crazy parent who questions the experts, fires them, and seeks for answers to new questions. "We are no longer looking for the right answers. We are looking for the right partner; someone willing to stand shoulder to shoulder in solidarity with, to discover all the things we still don't know about my son, about parenting, about medicine, and about ourselves as finite human beings."

- **Specific disease trajectory knowledge is not required in order to facilitate pACP conversations.** In fact, possessing in-depth knowledge may interfere with one's ability to listen to the parent's description — to allow them to tell their story. Professionals often have a tendency to be the "expert" on the child's medical condition, and ACP facilitators have expressed this concern to be knowledgeable in the myriad of complex medical conditions. This was not my experience. Rather, listening to the parent's description is revealing and poignant. My lack of knowledge in the disease trajectory did not inhibit dialogue; perhaps it encouraged dialogue. This theme also supports the use of a facilitator who is not a direct caregiver — not responsible for ongoing case management.

- **Parents' experience of grief and loss is unending.** As one parent expressed, "I deal with perpetual grief" and "live on the precipice." These parents have extraordinary experience with uncertainty, of navigating through serious, life-threatening events, of dealing with healthcare provider bias. During the admission process for her child, one parent recanted the following comment from a healthcare provider, "Why do you keep bringing [child's name] back to the hospital?" Naturally, these comments are insensitive and value-laden, but I believe contribute to the perpetual grief experienced by these parents.

- **There is complexity in every medical decision.** A common condition that is easily treated for most children becomes an overwhelming situation for a fragile child. There is "unchartered territory with each step." Any prognostic proclamation can be proven false. Recall Carl's experience with a surgeon who predicted that his daughter had a low chance of recovering from a procedure to address a serious complication.

He was asked if he would prefer a "peaceful" death and not proceed with the surgery. Jessica recovered and affirmed Carl's belief in her will to live. In the words of a parent of a child with a rare disease, "We recognize the fatalness of the rare disease, but choose to focus on what is possible versus what cannot be done."

- **Pediatric ACP conversations can be emotional for facilitators.**
  Of course, I had experienced emotionally-laden conversations with
  adults, but pACP conversations felt different, and at times I wore
  my emotions on my sleeve. Facilitators who become self-aware of
  personal emotions and experiences can prepare to manage them
  appropriately. Facilitators have often asked the question, "Is it
  acceptable to show emotion during pACP conversations?"

  While the answer to this question is personal, I think that the display
  of sincere emotion can communicate empathy if it does not distract
  from the parent's needs. For example, Kate and I had a connection
  that only mothers who are faced with making life-sustaining treatment decisions for a child can have.

  I have told my personal story (in Part Four) of being asked to decide
  whether to remove the ventilator from my son who was suspected
  to have permanent brain damage. I was intimately reminded of the
  angst of that decision during my conversation with Kate and her
  strength. I was aware that I was an ACP facilitator with personal
  experiences that flooded into my memories — an important lesson to
  learn in preparing other facilitators for pACP conversations.

A recurring personal theme for me throughout all the adult and pediatric
ACP conversations I have facilitated has been the uncertainty of the impact
of the conversation. I have been the "lady doing the research" who desires
to learn more and use this information to provide recommendations and
programmatic implementation strategies. But these experiences have created
internal tension for me at times, stimulating questions as "Was I effective as
a facilitator?" Was I helpful?" "Did any of my communication skills cause
undue stress or anxiety?" and "What happened after the conversation?"

A few days after my conversation with Kate, I received the following note
— additional information Kate wanted included in her ongoing plans for
Nolan's care and treatment:

- I do not want Nolan to waste any of his precious time with us doing anything which does not add value to his life. Examples may include things like attending public school when he could learn in a home school setting with more focus on him and less on working the system.

- I am concerned about over-medicating his care and life. Let's keep it simple and beneficial. We could spend hours a week traveling to and receiving care from therapists and others.

- I am concerned that in the case Nolan's health deteriorates to a critical point that his providers' internal biases may prevent us from making the best choices for Nolan.

I am convinced in the enduring power of these conversations as another recurring theme; conversations that continue to promote critical thinking, enhance relationships, support caregivers, and evaluate dynamic goals of care over time. I am convinced of the imperative to seamlessly integrate pACP conversations into the care management of children with complex medical conditions.

Chapter 44: Honoring a Child's Decision Revisited and Future Directions in Pediatric ACP

In a culture of person-centered decision-making, my nephew's story would look different:

A 17-year-old male had battled cystic fibrosis since birth, managing an arduous medical treatment regime, multiple hospitalizations, and disruption of daily activities. As his illness progressed and life-sustaining treatments became the norm, a palliative care team provided ongoing support to manage his increased symptoms and assistance in planning for future complications.

Through ongoing family conversations, the patient decided the burdens of treatment outweighed the benefits and wanted to stop efforts to fight his disease — a decision supported by his parents and healthcare providers. In arranging for home hospice care, the palliative care team facilitated a conversation with the patient and his family about management of the symptoms of the dying process, preparing them for the options of providing medications to treat anxiety and breathing difficulties, and allowing the patient to express his preferences. In addition, the team offered bereavement strategies that included how to say good-bye, how to manage the grief of losing a child, and after-death support.

Summary: The Value of Pediatric Advance Care Planning

Pediatric ACP programs are effective and essential to be implemented as a routine standard of care for parents of children with life-threatening illness, including AYAs with serious illness, from initial diagnosis throughout the twisted course of the illness trajectories. My understanding and perspectives of the ACP needs of the pediatric population have been impacted by clinical experiences, quality improvement and research studies, and by facilitating person-centered decision-making conversations. I am forever grateful for those that have shared their expertise, personal struggles, and suggestions in the pursuit of creating an ACP standard of care for all patients and their families.

Pediatric ACP helps families engage in emotional and challenging conversations, opens the door for ongoing communication, does not create undue stress or anxiety, gives AYAs a voice in their treatment and care and, in this pediatric subgroup, increases congruence between AYAs and their parent/guardian in making treatment decisions.

There are multiple aspects of the pACP strategies described in this Part that tackle the long-standing barriers to pACP outlined in Chapter 40:

1) Early and proactive ACP conversations serve to normalize the conversation, gradually increasing the ability to open channels of communication and strengthen relationships between the patient, family, and healthcare team. The first conversation is typically the most difficult. If this first conversation occurs in a time of stressful decision-making, at a time when a parent or child is facing the reality of a dismal outcome, it will be confronted with suspicion and ineffectiveness. As Greg (We have to be prepared: Heather and Greg's Story) stated, "This is about education. It can open channels of communication and build relationships between parents and the healthcare team."

Ongoing conversations matter. In the words of Kate Detwiller:

> These conversations are individual building blocks that when put together, create something beautiful and strong; the peace

of knowing that I cared for my child throughout his life and those cumulative moments will bring me peace at the end.

The FACE interventions include strategies to help normalize the conversation. For example, the Lyons ACP survey in Session 1 functions as an "ice-breaker" to expose the AYA and their parents to sensitive topics that may have never been raised and prepare the dyad for more specific, follow up conversations. In addition, the FACE Rare intervention begins with the Carer Support Needs Assessment (CSNAT) to identify the kind and level of support parents feel is needed to care for their child. Once these priority needs are uncovered, the parent can more readily focus on ACP planning conversations.[1]

2) The RC Next Steps pACP Conversation for AYAs and parents of children with life-threatening illnesses explores the dyad's understanding of the AYAs illness trajectory and potential complications, thereby helping to close the gap in understanding of prognosis and identifying questions for the physician and healthcare team.

3) The pACP intervention includes the use of skilled facilitators who adhere to standardized and consistent communication guidelines and skills; skills that open communication channels, improve the quality of decision-making, and potentially ease the guilt, fear, or incompetence in making and honoring life-sustaining treatment decisions for a child.

4) The pACP intervention offers an adjunct service to the treating physicians and other members of the healthcare team, providing a communication bridge for more specific conversations, questions, and support for creating and understanding a plan for future care and treatment.

In an editorial following the publication of the FACE-TC study, Chris Feudtner offers additional insights into why the FACE ACP intervention works:[2] 1) such conversations are valued by patients and parents; 2) the conversation was not triggered by an acute event or end of life situation; it was presented during a period of non-crisis; 3) the hypothetical situations presented likely provided "crucial emotional distance from the fears and anxieties that patients and families would normally confront in a crisis situation"; 4) the hypothetical situations did not require prognostication, allowing the focus to be on the identification and articulation of the adolescents goals and values; 5) the "facilitator" was not a member of the patient's clinical healthcare team and may have felt safer for open conversations; and 6) the conversation was scheduled at a non-clinical time, allowing all parties to be focused on goals and values.

Despite ample evidence, I will always regret the inability to garner support for widespread dissemination of pACP as a standard of care for all parents and children living with life-threatening illness.

Personal Exercises

1) Describe an experience with a parent(s) who was struggling to make treatment decisions for his/her child with a life-threatening condition.

2) What gaps do you see in providing decision-making assistance for parents of children with life-threatening conditions?

3) How can healthcare professionals gain insight into the emotional and personal struggles of parents who care for children with life-threatening illness?

Notes

All websites were last accessed on March 14, 2020.
Page details may have changed.

Foreword

1. Institute of Medicine. Crossing the Quality Chasm: A New Health System for the 21st Century. Vol. 6. Washington, DC: National Academy Press; 2001

Introduction: Who Am I and Why Do I Have Something to Say?

1. *About Us*. Respecting Choices. (2018, May 3). https://respectingc-hoices.org/about-us/.
2. Institute of Medicine. Crossing the Quality Chasm: A New Health System for the 21st Century. Vol. 6. Washington, DC: National Academy Press; 2001
3. Feudtner, C. (2005). Hope and the Prospects of Healing at the End of Life. *The Journal of Alternative and Complementary Medicine*, *11*(supplement 1). https://doi.org/10.1089/acm.2005.11.s-23

Chapter 1: Preparation for an Undefined Future

1. Canterbury v. Spence (464 F.2d. 772, 782 D.C. Cir. 1972)
2. Besch, L. Informed Consent: A Patient's Right. Nursing Outlook 27(1): 32-35, Jan 1979.
3. In Re Quinlan, 355 A.2d 647 (N.J. 1976)

4.	Colby, W. H. (2002). *Long goodbye: the deaths of Nancy Cruzan.* Hay House

5.	Colby, W. H. (2002). *Long goodbye: the deaths of Nancy Cruzan.* Hay House. P.37

6.	Colby, W. H. (2002). *Long goodbye: the deaths of Nancy Cruzan.* Hay House. p. 391

7.	Home. Leading the Way to Zero | The Joint Commission. (n.d.). http://www.jointcommission.org/.

Chapter 2: A Clinician's Moral Distress

1.	Savel, R. H., & Munro, C. L. (2015). Moral Distress, Moral Courage. *American Journal of Critical Care, 24*(4), 276–278. https://doi.org/10.4037/ajcc2015738

2.	Levine-Ariff, J., & Groh, D. (1990). *Creating an ethical environment* (Vol. 2, No. 1). Williams & Wilkins. p. 8

3.	*Home.* RWHC. (n.d.). http://www.rwhc.com/.

4.	Hammes, B. J., & Rooney, B. L. (1998). Death and End-of-Life Planning in One Midwestern Community. *Archives of Internal Medicine, 158*(4), 383–390. https://doi.org/10.1001/archinte.158.4.383

Chapter 4: The Promise of Leadership in Building a Culture of Person-Centered Decision-Making

1.	Institute of Medicine. Crossing the Quality Chasm: A New Health System for the 21st Century. Vol. 6. Washington, DC: National Academy Press; 2001

2.	Frampton S, Guastello S, Brady C, Hale M, Horowitz S, Bennett Smith S, Stone S. *Patient-Centered Care Improvement Guide.* Derby, Connecticut: Planetree; October 2008.

3.	*Conversation with Planetree Founder Angelica Thieriot.* Planetree International Conversation with Planetree Founder Angelica Thieriot Comments. (n.d.).

https://www.planetree.org/certification-resources/
conversation-with-planetree-founder-angelica-thieriot.

4. *Certification for Excellence in Person-Centered Care.* Planetree Certification for Excellence in Person-Centered Care. (n.d.). https://www.planetree.org/certification.

5. *History & Impact of Picker in Europe & the USA.* Picker. (2020, March 9). https://www.picker.org/about-us/ our-history-impact/.

6. Frampton S, Guastello S, Brady C, Hale M, Horowitz S, Bennett Smith S, Stone S. *Patient-Centered Care Improvement Guide.* Derby, Connecticut: Planetree; October 2008.

7. Frampton, S. B., Guastello, S., Hoy, L., Naylor, M., Sheridan, S., & Johnston-Fleece, M. (2017). Harnessing Evidence and Experience to Change Culture: A Guiding Framework for Patient and Family Engaged Care. *NAM Perspectives,* 7(1). https://doi. org/10.31478/201701f

8. Dapspro. (2009, July 4). *Don Berwick - What Patient Centred Care Really Means.* YouTube. https://www.youtube.com/ watch?v=SSauhroFTpk.

9. *Improving Health and Health Care Worldwide: IHI.* Institute for Healthcare Improvement. (n.d.). http://www.ihi.org/.

10. Berwick, D. M., Nolan, T. W., & Whittington, J. (2008). The Triple Aim: Care, Health, And Cost. *Health Affairs,* 27(3), 759–769. https://doi.org/10.1377/hlthaff.27.3.759.

11. *The Triple Aim or the Quadruple Aim? Four Points to Help Set Your Strategy.* Institute for Healthcare Improvement. (n.d.). http://www.ihi.org/communities/blogs/the-triple-aim-or-the-quadruple-aim-four-points-to-help-set-your-strategy.

12. 10 IHI Innovations to Improve Health and Health Care. Cambridge, Massachusetts: Institute for Healthcare Improvement; 2017. (Available at www.ihi.org)

13. *Person Centered Care: Advance Care Planning: Shared Decision Making.* Respecting Choices. (2021, June 10). https://respectingc-hoices.org/.

14. Hauser, K., Koerfer, A., Kuhr, K., Albus, C., Herzig, S., & Matthes, J. (2015). Outcome-Relevant Effects of Shared Decision Making. *Deutsches Aerzteblatt Online*. https://doi.org/10.3238/arztebl.2015.0665

15. Hauser, K., Koerfer, A., Kuhr, K., Albus, C., Herzig, S., & Matthes, J. (2015). Outcome-Relevant Effects of Shared Decision Making. *Deutsches Aerzteblatt Online*, p. 669. https://doi.org/10.3238/arztebl.2015.0665

Chapter 5: Initial Leadership Recommendations in Building a Culture of Person-Centered Decision-Making

1. Zennouche, M., & Zhang, J. (2014). Evolution of Leadership and Organizational Culture Research on Innovation Field: 12 Years of Analysis. *Open Journal of Social Sciences*, 02(04), 388–392. https://doi.org/10.4236/jss.2014.24044

2. foundry4. (n.d.). *foundry4*. Home Page | foundry4. https://disruptionhub.com/transformational-change-in-your-organisations-culture/.

3. Schein, E. H. (1999). *The corporate culture survival guide sense and nonsense about culture change.* Jossey-Bass. p. 126

4. Schein, E. H. (1999). *The corporate culture survival guide sense and nonsense about culture change.* Jossey-Bass. p. 126

5. Jerome Parisse-Brassens Jerome is the Regional Director for Walking the Talk Asia Pa. (n.d.). *The 3 levels of change required to shift culture.* Human Synergistics. https://www.humansynergistics.com/blog/culture-university/details/culture-university/2018/08/07/the-3-levels-of-change-required-to-shift-culture.

6. *Culture Change in the Workplace for Sustained Results.* Deloitte United States. (2019, August 6). https://www2.deloitte.com/us/en/pages/human-capital/articles/culture-change-in-the-workplace-for-sustained-results.html?id=us%3A2ps%3A3bi%3Aconfidence%3Aeng%3Acons%3A41819%3Anonem%3Ana%3AOT-

jN56Nz%3A1149431367%3A77378218282586%3Abe%3AR
LSA_Future_of_Work%3AHCT_Intro_A_Exact%3Anb.

7. Herrin, J., Harris, K. G., Kenward, K., Hines, S., Joshi, M. S., &
    Frosch, D. L. (2015). Patient and family engagement: a survey
    of US hospital practices. *BMJ Quality & Safety, 25*(3), 182–189.
    https://doi.org/10.1136/bmjqs-2015-004006

8. Merriam-Webster. (n.d.). *Engage*. Merriam-Webster. https://
    www.merriam-webster.com/dictionary/engage#synonyms.

9. Maclean, N. (1993). *Young Men & Fire*. University of
    Chicago Press.

10. IHIOpenSchool. (2009, March 13). *Escape Fire: 1999 IHI
    National Forum address by Former IHI National Forum ,
    IHI President and CEO*. YouTube. https://www.youtube.com/
    watch?v=00aa6xcOXf4.

Chapter 6: Leadership Recommendations for Program Dissemination and Sustainability

1. Merriam-Webster. (n.d.). *Courage*. Merriam-Webster. https://
    www.merriam-webster.com/dictionary/courage.

2. Hinchey, K. Zahn, D., Lustbader, N., Thomas, S., Ramjohn, D.,
    Chin, M. (2008). *Factors contributing to sustaining and spread-
    ing learning collaborative improvements: Results of a Qualitative
    Research Study*. Primary Care Development Corporation.

3. Scheirer, M. A. (2005). Is Sustainability Possible? A Review and
    Commentary on Empirical Studies of Program Sustainability.
    American Journal of Evaluation, 26(3), 320–347. https://doi.
    org/10.1177/1098214005278752

4. Hinchey, K. Zahn, D., Lustbader, N., Thomas, S., Ramjohn, D.,
    Chin, M. (2008). *Factors contributing to sustaining and spread-
    ing learning collaborative improvements: Results of a Qualitative
    Research Study*. Primary Care Development Corporation.

5. Hinchey, K. Zahn, D., Lustbader, N., Thomas, S., Ramjohn, D.,
    Chin, M. (2008). *Factors contributing to sustaining and spreading*

learning collaborative improvements: Results of a Qualitative Research Study. Primary Care Development Corporation.

6.   *#5 - The Importance of Vision.* John Graham. (n.d.). https://www.johngraham.org/coach/5-the-importance-of-vision.

7.   *Drive: Daniel H. Pink.* Daniel H. Pink | The official site of author Daniel Pink. (2017, October 19). https://www.danpink.com/books/drive/. /

8.   *Strategy: Patient engagement & quality improvement in care.* Picker. (2019, September 2). https://www.picker.org/working-with-us/strategy-setting.

9.   Almutairi, A. F., Salam, M., Adlan, A., & Alturki, A. (2019). Prevalence of severe moral distress among healthcare providers in Saudi Arabia. *Psychology Research and Behavior Management, Volume 12,* 107–115. https://doi.org/10.2147/prbm.s191037. p. 112

10. Almutairi, A. F., Salam, M., Adlan, A., & Alturki, A. (2019). Prevalence of severe moral distress among healthcare providers in Saudi Arabia. *Psychology Research and Behavior Management, Volume 12,* 107–115. https://doi.org/10.2147/prbm.s191037. p. 110

Chapter 8: The History and Evolution of the Respecting Choices Program: A Personal and Professional Journey

1.   Hammes, B. J., & Rooney, B. L. (1998). Death and End-of-Life Planning in One Midwestern Community. *Archives of Internal Medicine, 158*(4), 383. https://doi.org/10.1001/archinte.158.4.383

2.   Hunsaker and Mann, 2013

3.   A controlled trial to improve care for seriously ill hospitalized patients. The study to understand prognoses and preferences for outcomes and risks of treatments (SUPPORT). The SUPPORT Principal Investigators. JAMA. 1995 Nov 22-29;274(20):1591-8. Erratum in: JAMA 1996 Apr 24;275(16):1232. PMID: 7474243.

4. Last Acts (Organization) (2002). Means to a better end: a report on dying in America today. Retrieved January 3, 2007, from the Robert Wood Johnson Foundation website: http://www.rwjf.org/files/publications/other/meansbetterend.pdf

5. *Last Acts Program Assessment.* RWJF. (2018, May 23). https://www.rwjf.org/en/library/research/2002/10/assessment-of-last-acts-r--program-provides-recommendations-for-.html.

6. ABC News Network. (n.d.). ABC News. https://abcnews.go.com/GMA/story?id=8250195&page=1.

7. *About Us.* C-TAC. (2021, February 9). https://www.thectac.org/about/.

8. WiserCare, I. (2020, January 14). WiserCare and Respecting Choices Partner to Expand Reach of Advance Care Planning. https://www.prnewswire.com/news-releases/wisercare-and-re-specting-choices-partner-to-expand-reach-of-advance-care-planning-300986290.html.

9. *Physician Skills: Advance Care Planning.* Physician Skills | Advance Care Planning | Center to Advance Palliative Care. (n.d.). https://www.capc.org/training/building-physician-skills-basic-advance-care-planning/.

10. *Building Public Engagement and Access to Palliative & End-of-Life Care.* The John A. Hartford Foundation. (n.d.). http://www.johnahartford.org/grants-strategy/building-public-engagement-and-access-to-palliative-end-of-life-care.

Chapter 9: The Promise of System Redesign in Building a Culture of Person-Centered Decision-Making

1. Holt, G. E., Sarmento, B., Kett, D., & Goodman, K. W. (2017). An Unconscious Patient with a DNR Tattoo. New England Journal of Medicine, 377(22), 2192–2193. https://doi.org/10.1056/nejmc1713344

2.   Cooper, L., & Aronowitz, P. (2012). DNR tattoos: a cautionary tale. *Journal of general internal medicine*, *27*(10), 1383. https://doi.org/10.1007/s11606-012-2059-8

3.   Hammes B, Briggs L, Silvester W, Wilson K, Shettle S, Maycroft J, Sandoval J, Orders A, Stern M. *Implementing a care planning system: How to fix the most pervasive errors in health care.* Health Affairs Blog. 2015; January 2. DOI: 10.1377/hblog20150102.043563

4.   nationalacademies.org. (n.d.). https://www.nationalacademies.org/event/10-26-2020/advance-care-planning-challenges-and-opportunities-a-workshop
     nationalacademies.org. (n.d.). https://www.nationalacademies.org/event/11-02-2020/advance-care-planning-challenges-and-opportunities-second-webinar.

5.   *Mildred Z. Solomon.* The Hastings Center. (2021, May 28). https://www.thehastingscenter.org/team/mildred-z-solomon-ed-d/.

6.   Deming, W. E. (1989). *Out of the Crisis.* M I T Press.
     Harris, S. G. (1990). The fifth discipline: The art and practice of the learning organization, by Peter Senge, New York: Doubleday/Currency, 1990. *Human Resource Management, 29*(3), 343–348. https://doi.org/10.1002/hrm.3930290308
     Wheatley, M. J. (1992). *Leadership and the new science: Learning about organization from an orderly universe.* Berrett-Koehler Publishers.

7.   Nelson, E. C., Batalden, P. B., Huber, T. P., Mohr, J. J., Godfrey, M. M., Headrick, L. A., & Wasson, J. H. (2002). Microsystems in Health Care: Part 1. Learning from High-Performing Front-Line Clinical Units. *The Joint Commission Journal on Quality Improvement, 28*(9), 472–493. https://doi.org/10.1016/s1070-3241(02)28051-7. p 473.

8.   Nelson, E. C., Batalden, P. B., Huber, T. P., Mohr, J. J., Godfrey, M. M., Headrick, L. A., & Wasson, J. H. (2002). Microsystems in Health Care: Part 1. Learning from High-Performing Front-Line Clinical Units. *The Joint Commission Journal on*

Quality Improvement, 28(9), 472–493. https://doi.org/10.1016/s1070-3241(02)28051-7

9.   *What Is Design Thinking? A Comprehensive Beginner's Guide.* What Exactly Is Design Thinking? (Updated Guide for 2021). (n.d.). https://careerfoundry.com/en/blog/ux-design/what-is-design-thinking-everything-you-need-to-know-to-get-started/.

10.   *History.* IDEO. (n.d.). https://designthinking.ideo.com/history.

Chapter 10: Microsystem #1: Leadership Expectations to "Grow" Microsystems That Promote Person-Centered Decision-Making

1.   Nelson, E. C., Batalden, P. B., Huber, T. P., Mohr, J. J., Godfrey, M. M., Headrick, L. A., & Wasson, J. H. (2002). Microsystems in Health Care: Part 1. Learning from High-Performing Front-Line Clinical Units. *The Joint Commission Journal on Quality Improvement, 28*(9), 472–493. https://doi.org/10.1016/s1070-3241(02)28051-7. p. 490.

2.   Palmer, J. A., Parker, V. A., Mor, V., Volandes, A. E., Barre, L. R., Belanger, E., Carter, P., Loomer, L., McCreedy, E., & Mitchell, S. L. (2019). Barriers and facilitators to implementing a pragmatic trial to improve advance care planning in the nursing home setting. *BMC Health Services Research, 19*(1). https://doi.org/10.1186/s12913-019-4309-5

3.   Palmer, J. A., Parker, V. A., Mor, V., Volandes, A. E., Barre, L. R., Belanger, E., Carter, P., Loomer, L., McCreedy, E., & Mitchell, S. L. (2019). Barriers and facilitators to implementing a pragmatic trial to improve advance care planning in the nursing home setting. *BMC Health Services Research, 19*(1). https://doi.org/10.1186/s12913-019-4309-5

4.   Hickman, S. E., Torke, A. M., Sachs, G. A., Sudore, R. L., Tang, Q., Bakoyannis, G., Smith, N. H., Myers, A. L., & Hammes, B. J. (2020). Do Life-sustaining Treatment Orders Match Patient and Surrogate Preferences? The Role of POLST. *Journal of General*

Internal Medicine, 36(2), 413–421. https://doi.org/10.1007/
s11606-020-06292-1

5.   NQF: National Quality Partners Shared Decision Making Action
     Team. (n.d.). http://www.qualityforum.org/National_Quality_
     Partners_Shared_Decision_Making_Action_Team_.aspx.

6.   nationalacademies.org. (n.d.). https://www.nationalacade-
     mies.org/event/11-02-2020/advance-care-planning-challeng-
     es-and-opportunities-second-webinar.

Chapter 11: Microsystem #2: The Design or Redesign of Planning Documents

1.   Gostin L. O. (1997). Deciding life and death in the courtroom.
     From Quinlan to Cruzan, Glucksberg, and Vacco--a brief
     history and analysis of constitutional protection of the 'right
     to die'. *JAMA, 278*(18), 1523–1528. https://doi.org/10.1001/
     jama.278.18.1523

2.   Castillo, L. S., Williams, B. A., Hooper, S. M., Sabatino, C. P.,
     Weithorn, L. A., & Sudore, R. L. (2011). Lost in Translation: The
     Unintended Consequences of Advance Directive Law on Clinical
     Care. *Annals of Internal Medicine, 154*(2), 121. https://doi.
     org/10.7326/0003-4819-154-2-201101180-00012

3.   *Forms Information - Advance Directives.* Wisconsin Department
     of Health Services. (2018, March 27). https://www.dhs.wisconsin.
     gov/forms/advdirectives/f00085.pdf.

4.   Wisconsin Legislature: Chapter 154. (n.d.). https://docs.legis.
     wisconsin.gov/statutes/statutes/154.

5.   South Carolina Bar. (n.d.). *Free Forms and Publications.* South
     Carolina Bar. https://www.scbar.org/public/get-legal-help/
     free-forms-and-publications/.

6.   *Health-Care Decisions Act.* Health-Care Decisions Act - Uniform
     Law Commission. (n.d.). https://www.uniformlaws.org/commit-
     tees/community-home?CommunityKey=63ac0471-5975-49b0-8a
     36-6a4d790a4edf.

7. Sabatino, C. P. (2018). Overcoming the Balkanization of State Advance Directive Laws. *Journal of Law, Medicine & Ethics*, *46*(4), 978–987. https://doi.org/10.1177/1073110518821999

8. Kalanithi, P. (2019). *When Breath Becomes Air*. Random House.

9. Hammes, B. J., Rooney, B. L., & Gundrum, J. D. (2010). A comparative, retrospective, observational study of the prevalence, availability, and specificity of advance care plans in a county that implemented an advance care planning microsystem. *Journal of the American Geriatrics Society, 58*(7), 1249–1255. https://doi.org/10.1111/j.1532-5415.2010.02956.x

10. Health Care Directives. (n.d.). https://www.honoringchoices.org/health-care-directives.

11. *Advance Health Care Directive.* Advance Health Care Directive | Life Care Plan | Kaiser Permanente. (n.d.). https://healthy.kaiserpermanente.org/health-wellness/life-care-plan/advance-health-care-directive#.

12. Advanced Solutions International, I. (n.d.). Honoring Choices. https://www.wismed.org/wisconsin/wismed/about-us/honoring-choices/wismed/about-us/honoring-choices.aspx.

13. *University of Wisconsin Hospitals and Clinics.* University of Wisconsin Hospitals and Clinics | UW Health. (n.d.). https://www.uwhealth.org/files/uwhealth/docs/patient_guide/power_of_attorney_HA-74449-17.pdf.

14. *Forms Information - Advance Directives.* Wisconsin Department of Health Services. (2018, March 27). https://www.dhs.wisconsin.gov/forms/advdirectives/index.htm.

15. *Portable medical orders for seriously ill or frail individuals.* POLST. (2021, March 16). http://www.polst.org/.

16. *Programs in Your State.* POLST. (2021, June 19). https://polst.org/programs-in-your-state/?pro=1.

17. *National POLST Form: Portable Medical Order.* POLST. (2021, March 17). https://polst.org/national-form/.

18. *Portable medical orders for seriously ill or frail individuals.* POLST. (2021, March 16). https://polst.org/wp-content/

uploads/2020/10/2020.10.19-National-POLST-Form-Adoption. pdf.

19. Hammes, B. J., Rooney, B. L., Gundrum, J. D., Hickman, S. E., & Hager, N. (2012). The POLST Program: A Retrospective Review of the Demographics of Use and Outcomes in One Community Where Advance Directives Are Prevalent. *Journal of Palliative Medicine, 15*(1), 77–85. https://doi.org/10.1089/jpm.2011.0178..

20. *Programs in Your State.* POLST. (2021, June 19). https://polst.org/ programs-in-your-state/?pro=1.

21. *Advance Care Planning Resources for Clinicians.* Gundersen Health System. (n.d.). https://www.gundersenhealth.org/ for-clinicians-professionals/advance-care-planning/.

Chapter 12: Microsystem #3: Medical Record Storage and Retrieval

1.   Anderson J. G. (2007). Social, ethical and legal barriers to e-health. *International journal of medical informatics, 76*(5-6), 480–483. https://doi.org/10.1016/j.ijmedinf.2006.09.016

2.   HealthManagement.org. (2021, June 22). *Health IT Stimulus: Obama's Dream or Nightmare.* HealthManagement. https://healthmanagement.org/c/it/issuearticle/ health-it-stimulus-obama-s-dream-or-nightmare.

3.   *ONC: Office of the National Coordinator for Health Information Technology.* HealthIT.gov. (n.d.). https://www.healthit.gov/sites/ default/files/pdf/health-information-technology-fact-sheet.pdf.

4.   *ONC: Office of the National Coordinator for Health Information Technology.* HealthIT.gov. (n.d.). https://www.healthit.gov/sites/ default/files/pdf/privacy/privacy-and-security-guide.pdf.

5.   *ACP Facilitator Manual,* 2007

6.   Hammes, B. J., & Briggs, L. A. (2011). *Building a systems approach to advance care planning* (1st ed.). Chapter 2. La Crosse, WI: Gundersen Lutheran Medical Foundation.

7.   *About Us.* Epic. (n.d.). https://www.epic.com/about.

8. Lakin, J. R., Isaacs, E., Sullivan, E., Harris, H. A., McMahan, R. D., & Sudore, R. L. (2016). Emergency Physicians' Experience with Advance Care Planning Documentation in the Electronic Medical Record: Useful, Needed, and Elusive. *Journal of Palliative Medicine, 19*(6), 632–638. https://doi.org/10.1089/jpm.2015.0486

9. Hammes, B. J., & Briggs, L. A. (2011). *Building a systems approach to advance care planning* (1st ed.). Chapter 2. La Crosse, WI: Gundersen Lutheran Medical Foundation.

10. Hammes, B. J., & Briggs, L. A. (2011). *Building a systems approach to advance care planning* (1st ed.). Chapter 2. La Crosse, WI: Gundersen Lutheran Medical Foundation.

11. Discussion of Advance Directives/Advance Care Planning. (n.d.). https://manual.jointcommission.org/releases/TJC2018A/DataElem0613.html.

12. Meisel, A., Snyder, L., Quill, T., & American College of Physicians--American Society of Internal Medicine End-of-Life Care Consensus Panel (2000). Seven legal barriers to end-of-life care: myths, realities, and grains of truth. *JAMA, 284*(19), 2495–2501. https://doi.org/10.1001/jama.284.19.2495

13. Chen, H., Butler, E., Guo, Y., George, T., Jr, Modave, F., Gurka, M., & Bian, J. (2019). Facilitation or Hindrance: Physicians' Perception on Best Practice Alerts (BPA) Usage in an Electronic Health Record System. *Health communication, 34*(9), 942–948. https://doi.org/10.1080/10410236.2018.1443263

Chapter 13: Microsystem #4: A Person-Centered Decision-Making Interprofessional Team

1. Naylor MD, Coburn KD, Kurtzman ET, et al. (March 24-25, 2011) *Inter-professional team-based primary care for chronically ill adults: State of the science.* Unpublished white paper presented at the ABIM Foundation meeting to Advance

Team-Based Care for the Chronically Ill in Ambulatory Settings. Philadelphia, PA

2. Sean Morrison, R. (2020). Advance Directives/Care Planning: Clear, Simple, and Wrong. *Journal of Palliative Medicine, 23*(7), 878–879. https://doi.org/10.1089/jpm.2020.0272

3. *ANA Enterprise: American Nurses Association.* ANA. (n.d.). https://www.nursingworld.org/~4af159/globalassets/docs/ana/ethics/issue-brief_patient-centered-team-based-health-care_2016.pdf.

4. Mitchell, P., M. Wynia, R. Golden, B. McNellis, S. Okun, C.E. Webb, V. Rohrbach, and I. Von Kohorn. 2012. Core principles & values of effective team-based health care. *NAM Perspectives.* Discussion Paper, National Academy of Medicine, Washington, DC. https://doi.org/10.31478/201210c

5. Sudore, R. L., Stewart, A. L., Knight, S. J., McMahan, R. D., Feuz, M., Miao, Y., & Barnes, D. E. (2013). Development and Validation of a Questionnaire to Detect Behavior Change in Multiple Advance Care Planning Behaviors. *PLoS ONE, 8*(9). https://doi.org/10.1371/journal.pone.0072465

Chapter 14: Honoring an Individual's Request for DNR Revisited

1. Montgomery C, Hickman SE, Wilkins C, Fromme EK, Anderson S. Response to Morrison, Advance Directives/Care Planning: Clear, Simple, and Wrong (DOI: 10.1089/jpm.2020.0272). J Palliat Med. 2020 Sep 1. doi: 10.1089/jpm.2020.0523. Epub ahead of print. PMID: 32881594

Chapter 15: The Promise of Education and Certification in Building a Culture of Person-Centered Decision-Making

1. Weiner, J. S., & Cole, S. A. (2004). Three Principles to Improve Clinician Communication for Advance Care Planning: Overcoming Emotional, Cognitive, and Skill Barriers. *Journal*

of Palliative Medicine, 7(6), 817–829. https://doi.org/10.1089/
jpm.2004.7.817

2. Back, A. L., Fromme, E. K., & Meier, D. E. (2019). Training
Clinicians with Communication Skills Needed to Match Medical
Treatments to Patient Values. *Journal of the American Geriatrics
Society, 67*(S2). https://doi.org/10.1111/jgs.15709

Chapter 16: Setting Standards for Person-Centered Communication Education and Certification: It is Time

1. aacn.org. (n.d.). https://www.aacn.org/education.

2. Schwarz, J. (2020, February 20). *How on-the-
job training became the new graduate degree.* Fast
Company. https://www.fastcompany.com/90465141/
how-on-the-job-training-became-the-new-graduate-degree.

3. *ACLS Certification Online: ACLS.com by CareerCert.* ACLS.com.
(2021, May 20). https://acls.com/acls-certification.

4. *What is Accreditation.* The Joint Commission. (n.d.). https://
www.jointcommission.org/accreditation-and-certification/
become-accredited/what-is-accreditation/.

5. *Comprehensive Cardiac Center Certification.* The Joint
Commission. (n.d.). https://www.jointcommission.org/certifica-
tion/comprehensive_cardiac_center_certification.aspx.

6. *Facts About Patient-Centered Communications.* The Joint
Commission. (n.d.). https://www.jointcommission.org/
facts_about_patient-centered_communications/.

7. Back, A. L., Fromme, E. K., & Meier, D. E. (2019). Training
Clinicians with Communication Skills Needed to Match Medical
Treatments to Patient Values. *Journal of the American Geriatrics
Society, 67*(S2). https://doi.org/10.1111/jgs.15709.

8. National Academies Press. (2015). *Dying in America: improving quality and honoring individual preferences at the end of
life: Committee on Approaching Death: addressing key end-of-
life issues.*

9. Gilligan, T., Coyle, N., Frankel, R. M., Berry, D. L., Bohlke, K., Epstein, R. M., Finlay, E., Jackson, V. A., Lathan, C. S., Loprinzi, C. L., Nguyen, L. H., Seigel, C., & Baile, W. F. (2017). Patient-Clinician Communication: American Society of Clinical Oncology Consensus Guideline. *Journal of Clinical Oncology*, 35(31), 3618–3632. https://doi.org/10.1200/jco.2017.75.2311

Chapter 17: The Development, Evolution, and Dissemination of Competency-Based Person-Centered Decision-Making Communication Programs: The Respecting Choices Experience

1. If I Only Knew: A Patient Education Program on Advance Directives. Copyright 1989, *Lutheran Hospital-La Crosse*.
2. Kak, Neeraj & Burkhalter, Bart & Cooper, Merri-Ann. (2001). *Measuring the Competence of Healthcare Providers*. Operations Research Issue Paper. 2.
3. Albanese, M. A., Mejicano, G., Mullan, P., Kokotailo, P., & Gruppen, L. (2008). Defining characteristics of educational competencies. *Medical Education*, 42(3), 248–255. https://doi.org/10.1111/j.1365-2923.2007.02996.x
4. Gruppen, L. D., Mangrulkar, R. S., & Kolars, J. C. (2012). The promise of competency-based education in the health professions for improving global health. *Human Resources for Health*, 10(1). https://doi.org/10.1186/1478-4491-10-43
5. Gundersen Lutheran Medical Foundation, Inc., 2007-2015; All rights reserved. RC 1100_FSFcltrPPt_v6.15
6. Hammes, B. J., & Briggs, L. A. (2011). *Building a systems approach to advance care planning* (1st ed.). Chapter 2. La Crosse, WI: Gundersen Lutheran Medical Foundation.
7. Donovan, H. S., Ward, S. E., Song, M. K., Heidrich, S. M., Gunnarsdottir, S., & Phillips, C. M. (2007). An update on the representational approach to patient education. *Journal of nursing scholarship : an official publication of Sigma Theta Tau*

International Honor Society of Nursing, 39(3), 259–265. https://doi.org/10.1111/j.1547-5069.2007.00178.x

Chapter 18: Program Delivery Adaptations: From the Classroom to Virtual Learning Platforms: The Respecting Choices Experience

1. Pierce 01/11/17, D. (n.d.). *What Effective Blended Learning Looks Like*. THE Journal. https://thejournal.com/articles/2017/01/11/what-effective-blended-learning-looks-like.aspx.

2. Gasevic, Dragan & Siemens, George & Dawson, Shane. (2015). *Preparing for the digital university: a review of the history and current state of distance, blended, and online learning.* 10.13140/RG.2.1.3515.8483.

3. Defining Critical Thinking. (n.d.). http://www.criticalthinking.org/pages/defining-critical-thinking/766.

4. *Turning New Nurses Into Critical Thinkers*. Turning New Nurses Into Critical Thinkers | Wolters Kluwer. (n.d.). http://lippincottsolutions.lww.com/blog.entry.html/2018/06/05/turning_new_nursesi-UnqI.html.

5. *Current Research Involving Respecting Choices*®. Respecting Choices. (2018, April 19). https://respectingchoices.org/research-and-reports/current-research-involving-respecting-choices/.

Chapter 19: Certification of Instructors as Teachers, Role Models, Mentors and Organizational Resources: The Respecting Choices Experience

1. Gilligan, T., Coyle, N., Frankel, R. M., Berry, D. L., Bohlke, K., Epstein, R. M., Finlay, E., Jackson, V. A., Lathan, C. S., Loprinzi, C. L., Nguyen, L. H., Seigel, C., & Baile, W. F. (2017). Patient-Clinician Communication: American Society of Clinical Oncology Consensus Guideline. *Journal of Clinical Oncology, 35*(31), 3618–3632. https://doi.org/10.1200/jco.2017.75.2311

2.   *AHA Instructors.* cpr.heart.org. (n.d.). https://cpr.heart.org/en/
      resources/aha-instructors.

3.   *Instructor Certification.* Respecting Choices.
      (2021, June 10). https://respectingchoices.org/
      types-of-curriculum-and-certification/instructor-certification/.

4.   Morrison, C. D. (2014). From 'Sage on the Stage' to 'Guide on
      the Side': A Good Start. *International Journal for the Scholarship
      of Teaching and Learning, 8*(1). https://doi.org/10.20429/
      ijsotl.2014.080104

Chapter 20: Organizational Commitment to Competency in Person-Centered Decision-Making Communication

1.   Gruppen, L. D., Mangrulkar, R. S., & Kolars, J. C. (2012). The
      promise of competency-based education in the health profes-
      sions for improving global health. *Human Resources for Health,
      10*(1). https://doi.org/10.1186/1478-4491-10-43. p. 2

Chapter 21: The Power of Person-Centered Decision-Making Communication: Lessons From the Field

1.   *Hospitality.* Henri Nouwen Society. (n.d.). https://henrinouwen.
      org/meditation/hospitality/.

2.   Colby, W. H. (2002). *Long goodbye: the deaths of Nancy Cruzan.*
      Hay House

3.   Briggs, L. (2004). Shifting the Focus of Advance Care Planning:
      Using an In-depth Interview to Build and Strengthen
      Relationships. *Journal of Palliative Medicine, 7*(2), 341–349.
      https://doi.org/10.1089/109662104773709503

4.   Greg Loomis in "One of the most important conversations we
      had." Hammes, B. J. (2012). *Having your own say: getting the
      right care when it matters most.* CHT Press.

5. Greg Loomis in "One of the most important conversations we had." Hammes, B. J. (2012). *Having your own say: getting the right care when it matters most.* CHT Press.

Chapter 23: The Promise of Community Engagement and Education in Building a Culture of Person-Centered Decision-Making

1. Adam. (2010, October 20). *It Takes A Village To Raise A Child.* NGO Pulse. http://www.ngopulse.org/article/ it-takes-village-raise-child.
2. MacQueen, K. M., McLellan, E., Metzger, D. S., Kegeles, S., Strauss, R. P., Scotti, R., Blanchard, L., & Trotter, R. T. (2001). What Is Community? An Evidence-Based Definition for Participatory Public Health. *American Journal of Public Health, 91*(12), 1929–1938. https://doi.org/10.2105/ajph.91.12.1929
3. Bartle, P. (n.d.). *HOME PAGE.* Home Page; Methods to Strengthen Communities; Community Self Management, Empowerment and Development. http://cec.vcn.bc.ca/cmp/index. htm.

Chapter 24: Community Education is Different Than Community Engagement

1. Wikimedia Foundation. (2021, June 21). *Education.* Wikipedia. https://en.wikipedia.org/wiki/Education.
2. Schroeder, E. B., Rosamond, W. D., Morris, D. L., Evenson, K. R., & Hinn, A. R. (2000). Determinants of use of emergency medical services in a population with stroke symptoms: the Second Delay in Accessing Stroke Healthcare (DASH II) Study. *Stroke, 31*(11), 2591–2596. https://doi.org/10.1161/01.str.31.11.2591
3. Vecchio, G. D. (2014, May 12). *Got Milk? Got Fired: 5 Valuable Lessons That All Executives Must Heed.* HuffPost. https://www. huffpost.com/entry/got-milk-got-fired-5-valu_b_4938176.

4. Rao, J. K., Anderson, L. A., Lin, F.-C., & Laux, J. P. (2014, January). *Completion of advance directives among U.S. consumers.* American journal of preventive medicine. https://www.ncbi. nlm.nih.gov/pmc/articles/PMC4540332/pdf/nihms714216.pdf.

5. Respecting Choices. (n.d.). https://respectingchoices.dcopy.net/ product/rc302-e-decision-aid-help-with-breathing.

6. Kreuter, M. W., & Skinner, C. S. (2000). Tailoring: what's in a name?. *Health education research*, *15*(1), 1–4. https://doi. org/10.1093/her/15.1.1

7. Respecting Choices. (n.d.). https://respectingchoices.dcopy.net/ product/cardio-pulmonary-resuscitation-facts.

8. Hibbard, J. H., Stockard, J., Mahoney, E. R., & Tusler, M. (2004). Development of the Patient Activation Measure (PAM): conceptualizing and measuring activation in patients and consumers. *Health services research*, *39*(4 Pt 1), 1005–1026. https://doi. org/10.1111/j.1475-6773.2004.00269.x

9. Phil Bartle, P. D. (n.d.). *CULTURE AND SOCIAL ANIMATION.* Culture And Social Animation. http://cec.vcn.bc.ca/cmp/ modules/emp-cul.htm.

10. Frampton, S. B., Guastello, S., Hoy, L., Naylor, M., Sheridan, S., & Johnston-Fleece, M. (2017). Harnessing Evidence and Experience to Change Culture: A Guiding Framework for Patient and Family Engaged Care. *NAM Perspectives*, *7*(1). https://doi. org/10.31478/201701f. p. 12

11. Carman, K. L., Dardess, P., Maurer, M., Sofaer, S., Adams, K., Bechtel, C., & Sweeney, J. (2013). Patient And Family Engagement: A Framework For Understanding The Elements And Developing Interventions And Policies. *Health Affairs*, *32*(2), 223–231. https://doi.org/10.1377/hlthaff.2012.1133

12. Berwick, Donald. (2002). *A user's manual for the IOM's 'Quality Chasm' report. Health affairs* (Project Hope). 21. 80-90. 10.1377/ hlthaff.21.3.80.

13. (US), I. of M. (1970, January 1). *Engaging Patients to Improve Science and Value in a Learning Health System.* Patients Charting

the Course: Citizen Engagement and the Learning Health System: Workshop Summary. https://www.ncbi.nlm.nih.gov/books/NBK92074/#_ch4_rl1_.

14. U.S. Dept. of Health and Human Services, Public Health Service, National Institutes of Health, National Cancer Institute. (2005). *Theory at a glance: a guide for health promotion practice.* p. 27

Chapter 25: #1 The Intrapersonal Level of Influence on Behavior Change

1. U.S. Dept. of Health and Human Services, Public Health Service, National Institutes of Health, National Cancer Institute. (2005). *Theory at a glance: a guide for health promotion practice.*

2. Carman, K. L., Dardess, P., Maurer, M., Sofaer, S., Adams, K., Bechtel, C., & Sweeney, J. (2013). Patient And Family Engagement: A Framework For Understanding The Elements And Developing Interventions And Policies. *Health Affairs, 32*(2), 223–231. https://doi.org/10.1377/hlthaff.2012.1133. p. 227

3. Mcleod, S. (2020, December 29). *Maslow's Hierarchy of Needs.* Simply Psychology. https://www.simplypsychology.org/maslow.html.

4. U.S. Dept. of Health and Human Services, Public Health Service, National Institutes of Health, National Cancer Institute. (2005). *Theory at a glance: a guide for health promotion practice.*

5. healthstandards.com. (n.d.). http://healthstandards.com/wp-content/uploads/2014/11/HL7Standards-Patient-Engagement-ebook.pdf.

6. *Motivational Interviewing.* Stephen Rollnick. (2020, March 30). https://www.stephenrollnick.com/about-motivational-interviewing/.

7. US Legal, I. (n.d.). *Find a legal form in minutes.* Healthcare. https://healthcare.uslegal.com/informed-consent/from-common-law-to-statute/.

Chapter 26: #2 The Interpersonal Level of Influence on Behavior Change

1. *How more caring, while boys are taught - Best free essay*. Great Essays. (2018, August 28). https://great-home-decorations.com/ethics-of-care-theory-carol-gilligan-nel-noddings/.
2. Respecting Choices. (n.d.). https://respectingchoices.dcopy.net/product/mc520-e-agent-information-card.

Chapter 27: #3 The Organizational Level of Influence on Behavior Change

1. Sharma, U. M., Schroeder, J. E., Al-Hamadani, M., Mathiason, M. A., Meyer, C. M., Frisby, K. A., Meyer, L. A., Sieber, D. L., & Go, R. S. (1970, January 1). *An exploratory study of the use of advance directives by US oncologists*. Mayo Clinic. https://mayoclinic.pure.elsevier.com/en/publications/an-exploratory-study-of-the-use-of-advance-directives-by-us-oncol.
2. Corace, K., & Garber, G. (2014). When knowledge is not enough: Changing behavior to change vaccination results. *Human Vaccines & Immunotherapeutics, 10*(9), 2623–2624. https://doi.org/10.4161/21645515.2014.970076

Chapter 28: #4 The Community Level of Influence on Behavior Change

1. *Fogg Method*. Foggmethod. (n.d.). https://www.foggmethod.com/.
2. Respecting Choices. (n.d.). https://respectingchoices.dcopy.net/category/Patient-Education-Materials-English.
3. NPR. (2016, October 5). *Episode 521: The Town That Loves Death*. NPR. https://www.npr.org/sections/money/2016/10/05/496751771/episode-521-the-town-that-loves-death.

4. *Home.* JCI USA. (n.d.). https://www.jciusa.org/.

5. *Research Resources and Tools.* Research Resources and Tools | Division of Cancer Control and Population Sciences (DCCPS). (n.d.). https://cancercontrol.cancer.gov/brp/research/theories_project/theory.pdf.

6. Caplan, A. (2015, June 11). *Ten Years After Terri Schiavo, Death Debates Still Divide Us: Bioethicist.* NBCNews.com. https://www.nbcnews.com/health/health-news/bioethicist-tk-n333536.

7. *COVID-19 Resources.* Respecting Choices. (2020, December 23). https://respectingchoices.org/covid-19-resources/.

8. *Health Care.* State Bar of Wisconsin. (n.d.). https://www.wisbar.org/forPublic/INeedInformation/Pages/Health-Care.aspx.

9. *Engagement Behavior Framework.* Prepared Patient. (2016, November 17). http://preparedpatient.org/engagement-behavior-framework/.

10. *Guide to Patient and Family Engagement in Hospital Quality and Safety.* AHRQ. (n.d.). https://www.ahrq.gov/professionals/systems/hospital/engagingfamilies/guide.html.

11. *Passport to Planetree.* Planetree. (n.d.). http://planetree.org/wp-content/uploads/2015/08/Passport-to-PlanetreeRev2.pdf.

12. PatientsLikeMe. (n.d.). https://www.patientslikeme.com/.

13. healthstandards.com. (n.d.). http://healthstandards.com/wp-content/uploads/2014/11/HL7Standards-Patient-Engagement-ebook.pdf. p. 2.

14. *Engagement Behavior Framework.* Prepared Patient. (2016, November 17). http://preparedpatient.org/engagement-behavior-framework/.

15. *Engagement Behavior Framework.* Prepared Patient. (2016, November 17). http://preparedpatient.org/engagement-behavior-framework/.

16. *About.* Coda Alliance. (n.d.). https://codaalliance.org/about/.

17. *Go Wish.* Coda Alliance. (n.d.). https://codaalliance.org/go-wish/#faqs.

18. Naveon. (n.d.). https://www.naveonguides.com/our-solution.

Chapter 29: # 5 The Policy Level of Influence on Behavior Change

1. Kelly, M. P., & Barker, M. (2016). Why is changing health-related behaviour so difficult? *Public Health, 136*, 109–116. https://doi.org/10.1016/j.puhe.2016.03.030. p. 1

2. Castillo, L. S., Williams, B. A., Hooper, S. M., Sabatino, C. P., Weithorn, L. A., & Sudore, R. L. (2011). Lost in translation: the unintended consequences of advance directive law on clinical care. *Annals of internal medicine, 154*(2), 121–128. https://doi.org/10.7326/0003-4819-154-2-201101180-00012

3. *Medicare Program; Revisions to Payment Policies Under the Physician Fee Schedule and Other Revisions to Part B for CY 2016.* Federal Register. (2015, November 16). https://www.federalregister.gov/documents/2015/11/16/2015-28005/medicare-program-revisions-to-payment-policies-under-the-physician-fee-schedule-and-other-revisions.

4. ASAPAC Day of Contributing (DoC) Challenge. American Society of Anesthesiologists (ASA). (n.d.). http://www.asahq.org/publicationsAndServices/standards/09.html.

5. Aleccia, J. N. (2020, January 21). Diagnosed With Dementia, She Documented Her Wishes. They Said No. Kaiser Health News. https://khn.org/news/advance-directive-dementia-vsed-assisted-feeding/.

Chapter 30: Global Experiences Engaging Diverse Communities in Person-Centered Decision-Making Activities

1. Frampton, S. B., Guastello, S., Hoy, L., Naylor, M., Sheridan, S., & Johnston-Fleece, M. (2017). Harnessing Evidence and Experience to Change Culture: A Guiding Framework for Patient and Family Engaged Care. *NAM Perspectives, 7*(1). https://doi.org/10.31478/201701f. p. 8

2. Hammes, B. J., & Briggs, L. A. (2011). *Building a systems approach to advance care planning* (1st ed.). Chapter 2. La Crosse, WI: Gundersen Lutheran Medical Foundation.

3. *What Doctors Say About the Care of the Dying.* Lien Foundation. (n.d.). http://www.lienfoundation.org/sites/default/files/What_Doctors_Say_About_Care_of_the_Dying_0.pdf.

4. *Topics.* USCCB. (n.d.). http://www.usccb.org/about/doctrine/ethical-and-religious-directives/upload/ethical-religious-directives-catholic-health-service-sixth-edition-2016-06.pdf.

5. *Topics.* USCCB. (n.d.). http://www.usccb.org/about/doctrine/ethical-and-religious-directives/upload/ethical-religious-directives-catholic-health-service-sixth-edition-2016-06.pdf.

6. *What Matters.* What Matters | Marlene Meyerson JCC Manhattan. (n.d.). https://jccmanhattan.org/what-matters.

7. 2016 NSTE presentation, Minneapolis.

Chapter 32: The Promise of Quality Improvement, Research, and Evidence-Based Practice in Building a Culture of Person-Centered Decision-Making

1. Diaconis P. (2016). I Wish Someone Had Told Us the Risks and Benefits of Replacing My Father's Defibrillator. *JAMA internal medicine, 176*(7), 885. https://doi.org/10.1001/jamainternmed.2016.1926

2. *What Is An Evidence-Based Program?* Project Enhance. (n.d.). https://projectenhance.org/what-is-an-evidence-based-program/.

3. Institute of Medicine (US) Committee on Standards for Developing Trustworthy Clinical Practice Guidelines. (1970, January 1). *Clinical Practice Guidelines We Can Trust.* National Center for Biotechnology Information. https://www.ncbi.nlm.nih.gov/books/NBK209539/.

4. Institute of Medicine (US) Committee on Standards for Developing Trustworthy Clinical Practice Guidelines. (1970,

January 1). *Clinical Practice Guidelines We Can Trust*. National Center for Biotechnology Information. https://www.ncbi.nlm. nih.gov/books/NBK209539/.

5. *Practice guidelines, standards, consensus statements, position papers: What they are, how they differ*. American Nurse. (2017, October 6). https://www.myamericannurse.com/practice-guide-lines-standards-consensus-statements-position-papers-what-they-are-how-they-differ/.

6. Florida, U. of S. (n.d.). *Child & Family Studies: University of South Florida*. Child & Family Studies | University of South Florida. http://cfs.cbcs.usf.edu/_docs/publications/ OutcomesRoundtableBrief.pdf.

7. Batalden, P. B., & Davidoff, F. (2007). What is "quality improvement" and how can it transform healthcare? *Quality and Safety in Health Care, 16*(1), 2–3. https://doi.org/10.1136/ qshc.2006.022046. p. 1

8. Going Lean in Health Care: IHI. Institute for Healthcare Improvement. (n.d.). http://www.ihi.org/resources/Pages/ IHIWhitePapers/GoingLeaninHealthCare.aspx.

9. *The CAHPS Ambulatory Care Improvement Guide: Practical Strategies for Improving Patient Experience*. AHRQ. (n.d.). https:// www.ahrq.gov/cahps/quality-improvement/improvement-guide/ improvement-guide.html.

10. Balas, E. A., & Boren, S. A. (2000). Managing Clinical Knowledge for Health Care Improvement. *Yearbook of medical informatics*, (1), 65–70.

11. Eccles, M. P., & Mittman, B. S. (2006). Welcome to Implementation Science. *Implementation Science, 1*(1). https:// doi.org/10.1186/1748-5908-1-1

12. Bauer, M. S., Damschroder, L., Hagedorn, H., Smith, J., & Kilbourne, A. M. (2015). An introduction to implementation science for the non-specialist. *BMC Psychology, 3*(1). https://doi. org/10.1186/s40359-015-0089-9

National Adult and Influenza Immunization Summit.

National Adult and Influenza Immunization Summit |. (2021, April 16). https://www.izsummitpartners.org/content/ uploads/2015/02/Implementation-science-health-care-chapter-Mittman-10-02-2014.pdf.

Feldstein, A. C., & Glasgow, R. E. (2008). A practical, robust implementation and sustainability model (PRISM) for integrating research findings into practice. *Joint Commission journal on quality and patient safety, 34*(4), 228–243. https://doi.org/10.1016/ s1553-7250(08)34030-6

13. Bauer, M. S., Damschroder, L., Hagedorn, H., Smith, J., & Kilbourne, A. M. (2015). An introduction to implementation science for the non-specialist. *BMC psychology, 3*(1), 32. https:// doi.org/10.1186/s40359-015-0089-9. p. 4

14. Bauer, M. S., Damschroder, L., Hagedorn, H., Smith, J., & Kilbourne, A. M. (2015, September 16). *An introduction to implementation science for the non-specialist.* BMC Psychology. http://bmcpsychology.biomedcentral.com/articles/10.1186/ s40359-015-0089-9.

Chapter 33: The Respecting Choices Principles for Quality Improvement, Evidence-Based Practice, and Research

1. *Advance Directives and Advance Care Planning: Report to Congress.* ASPE. (2017, February 21). https://aspe.hhs.gov/ basic-report/advance-directives-and-advance-care-planning-report-congress.

Institute of Medicine; Committee on Approaching Death: Addressing Key End-of-Life Issues. (2014, September 17). Dying in America: Improving Quality and Honoring Individual Preferences Near the End of Life. Improving Quality and Honoring Individual Preferences Near the End of Life | The National Academies Press. http://www.nap.edu/catalog. php?record_id=18748.

2. Research and Reports. Respecting Choices. (2018, May 3). https://respectingchoices.org/research-and-reports/.

3. *Evidence-Based Program Review Process: Assessing if Applicants Meet the Administration for Community Living's (ACL) Health Promotion Program Criteria.* Thurston Arthritis Research Center. (2021, January 4). https://www.med.unc.edu/tarc/research/clinical-and-epidemiological-science-1/acl-health-promotion-evidence-based-program-review/.

4. Kirchhoff, K. T., Hammes, B. J., Kehl, K. A., Briggs, L. A., & Brown, R. L. (2012). Effect of a Disease-Specific Advance Care Planning Intervention on End-of-Life Care. *Journal of the American Geriatrics Society, 60*(5), 946–950. https://doi.org/10.1111/j.1532-5415.2012.03917.x

    Hammes, B. J., Rooney, B. L., & Gundrum, J. D. (2010, July 2). *A Comparative, Retrospective, Observational Study of the Prevalence, Availability, and Specificity of Advance Care Plans in a County that Implemented an Advance Care Planning Microsystem.* American Geriatrics Society. http://onlinelibrary.wiley.com/doi/10.1111/j.1532-5415.2010.02956.x/abstract.

    Detering, K. M., Hancock, A. D., Reade, M. C., & Silvester, W. (2010, March 24). *The impact of advance care planning on end of life care in elderly patients: randomised controlled trial.* The BMJ. http://www.bmj.com/content/340/bmj.c1345.

    Lyon, M. E., Squires, L., Scott, R. K., Benator, D., Briggs, L., Greenberg, I., D'Angelo, L. J., Cheng, Y. I., & Wang, J. (2020). Effect of FAmily CEntered (FACE®) Advance Care Planning on Longitudinal Congruence in End-of-Life Treatment Preferences: A Randomized Clinical Trial. *AIDS and Behavior, 24*(12), 3359–3375. https://doi.org/10.1007/s10461-020-02909-y

5. Pecanac, K. E., Repenshek, M. F., Tennenbaum, D., & Hammes, B. J. (2014). Respecting Choices® and Advance Directives in a Diverse Community. *Journal of Palliative Medicine, 17*(3), 282–287. https://doi.org/10.1089/jpm.2013.0047

in der Schmitten, J., Lex, K., Mellert, C., Rothärmel, S., Wegscheider, K., & Marckmann, G. (2014). Implementing an Advance Care Planning Program in German Nursing Homes. *Deutsches Aerzteblatt Online*. https://doi.org/10.3238/arztebl.2014.0050

Huang, C.-H. S., Crowther, M., Allen, R. S., DeCoster, J., Kim, G., Azuero, C., Ang, X., & Kvale, E. (2016). A Pilot Feasibility Intervention to Increase Advance Care Planning among African Americans in the Deep South. *Journal of Palliative Medicine*, *19*(2), 164–173. https://doi.org/10.1089/jpm.2015.0334

Teo, W.-S. K., Raj, A. G., Tan, W. S., Ng, C. W., Heng, B. H., & Leong, I. Y.-O. (2014). Economic impact analysis of an end-of-life programme for nursing home residents. *Palliative Medicine*, *28*(5), 430–437. https://doi.org/10.1177/0269216314526270

Lyon, M. E., Jacobs, S., Briggs, L., Cheng, Y. I., & Wang, J. (2013). Family-Centered Advance Care Planning for Teens With Cancer. *JAMA Pediatrics*, *167*(5), 460. https://doi.org/10.1001/jamapediatrics.2013.943

Lyon, M. E., D'Angelo, L. J., Dallas, R. H., Hinds, P. S., Garvie, P. A., Wilkins, M. L., Garcia, A., Briggs, L., Flynn, P. M., Rana, S. R., Cheng, Y. I., & Wang, J. (2017). A randomized clinical trial of adolescents with HIV/AIDS: pediatric advance care planning. AIDS Care, 29(10), 1287–1296. https://doi.org/10.1080/09540121.2017.1308463.

6.   Hickman, S. E., Unroe, K. T., Ersek, M. T., Buente, B., Nazir, A., & Sachs, G. A. (2016). An Interim Analysis of an Advance Care Planning Intervention in the Nursing Home Setting. *Journal of the American Geriatrics Society*, *64*(11), 2385–2392. https://doi.org/10.1111/jgs.14463

Rocque, G. B., Dionne-Odom, J. N., Sylvia Huang, C.-H., Niranjan, S. J., Williams, C. P., Jackson, B. E., Halilova, K. I., Kenzik, K. M., Bevis, K. S., Wallace, A. S., Lisovicz, N., Taylor, R. A., Pisu, M., Partridge, E. E., Butler, T. W., Briggs, L. A., Kvale, E. A., Jackson, L., Scott, Z., … Partridge, E. E. (2017).

Implementation and Impact of Patient Lay Navigator-Led Advance Care Planning Conversations. *Journal of Pain and Symptom Management, 53*(4), 682–692. https://doi.org/10.1016/j.jpainsymman.2016.11.012

7. Person Centered Care: Advance Care Planning: Shared Decision Making. Respecting Choices. (2021, June 10). https://respectingchoices.org/.

8. Wikimedia Foundation. (2021, June 21). A Prairie Home Companion. Wikipedia. https://en.wikipedia.org/wiki/A_Prairie_Home_Companion.

9. Heyland, D. K. (2013). Failure to engage hospitalized elderly patients and their families in advance care planning. JAMA Internal Medicine, 173(9), 778. https://doi.org/10.1001/jamainternmed.2013.180

10. Hickman, S. E., Torke, A. M., Heim Smith, N., Myers, A. L., Sudore, R. L., Hammes, B. J., & Sachs, G. A. (2021). Reasons for discordance and concordance between polst orders and current treatment preferences. Journal of the American Geriatrics Society, 69(7), 1933–1940. https://doi.org/10.1111/jgs.17097

11. Heyland, D. K. (2013). Failure to engage hospitalized elderly patients and their families in advance care planning. JAMA Internal Medicine, 173(9), 758. https://doi.org/10.1001/jamainternmed.2013.180

12. Richardson, D. K., Fromme, E., Zive, D., Fu, R., & Newgard, C. D. (2014). Concordance of out-of-hospital and emergency department cardiac arrest resuscitation with documented end-of-life choices in Oregon. *Annals of emergency medicine, 63*(4), 375–383. https://doi.org/10.1016/j.annemergmed.2013.09.004
Pedraza, S. L., Culp, S., Falkenstine, E. C., & Moss, A. H. (2016). POST Forms More Than Advance Directives Associated With Out-of-Hospital Death: Insights From a State Registry. *Journal of pain and symptom management, 51*(2), 240–246. https://doi.org/10.1016/j.jpainsymman.2015.10.003

Hickman, S. E., Nelson, C. A., Moss, A. H., Tolle, S. W., Perrin, N. A., & Hammes, B. J. (2011). The consistency between treatments provided to nursing facility residents and orders on the physician orders for life-sustaining treatment form. *Journal of the American Geriatrics Society, 59*(11), 2091–2099. https://doi.org/10.1111/j.1532-5415.2011.03656.x

13. Hickman, S. E., Hammes, B. J., Torke, A. M., Sudore, R. L., & Sachs, G. A. (2017). The Quality of Physician Orders for Life-Sustaining Treatment Decisions: A Pilot Study. *Journal of Palliative Medicine, 20*(2), 155–162. https://doi.org/10.1089/jpm.2016.0059

14. Hickman, S. E., Torke, A. M., Sachs, G. A., Sudore, R. L., Tang, Q., Bakoyannis, G., Smith, N. H., Myers, A. L., & Hammes, B. J. (2020). Do Life-sustaining Treatment Orders Match Patient and Surrogate Preferences? The Role of POLST. *Journal of General Internal Medicine, 36*(2), 413–421. https://doi.org/10.1007/s11606-020-06292-1

15. Lyon, M. E., Squires, L., Scott, R. K., Benator, D., Briggs, L., Greenberg, I., D'Angelo, L. J., Cheng, Y. I., & Wang, J. (2020). Effect of FAMILY CEntered (face®) Advance CARE planning On Longitudinal CONGRUENCE in End-of-Life Treatment Preferences: A randomized clinical trial. *AIDS and Behavior, 24*(12), 3359–3375. https://doi.org/10.1007/s10461-020-02909-y

16. Nelson, E. C., Batalden, P. B., Huber, T. P., Mohr, J. J., Godfrey, M. M., Headrick, L. A., & Wasson, J. H. (2002). Microsystems in Health Care: Part 1. Learning from High-Performing Front-Line Clinical Units. *The Joint Commission Journal on Quality Improvement, 28*(9), 472–493. https://doi.org/10.1016/s1070-3241(02)28051-7. p. 473.

17. *The CAHPS Ambulatory Care Improvement Guide: Practical Strategies for Improving Patient Experience.* AHRQ. (n.d.). https://www.ahrq.gov/cahps/quality-improvement/improvement-guide/improvement-guide.html.

Chapter 34: Quality Improvement Experiences in Person-Centered Decision-Making

1. Fried, T. R., & Bradley, E. H. (2003). What Matters to Seriously Ill Older Persons Making End-of-Life Treatment Decisions?: A Qualitative Study. *Journal of Palliative Medicine, 6*(2), 237–244. https://doi.org/10.1089/109662103764978489

2. Donovan, H. S., & Ward, S. (2001). A representational approach to patient education. Journal of nursing scholarship : an official publication of Sigma Theta Tau International Honor Society of Nursing, 33(3), 211–216. https://doi.org/10.1111/j.1547-5069.2001.00211.x

3. Leventhal, Howard & Steele, Ds. (1984). *Illness Representations and Coping with Health Threats.* Handbook of psychology and health volume IV social psychology aspects of health. 4. Lau, R. R., Bernard, T. M., & Hartman, K. A. (1989). Further explorations of common-sense representations of common illnesses. *Health psychology : official journal of the Division of Health Psychology, American Psychological Association, 8*(2), 195–219. https://doi.org/10.1037//0278-6133.8.2.195

4. Briggs, L. A., Kirchhoff, K. T., Hammes, B. J., Song, M.-K., & Colvin, E. R. (2004). Patient-centered advance care planning in special patient populations: a pilot study. *Journal of Professional Nursing, 20*(1), 47–58. https://doi.org/10.1016/j.profnurs.2003.12.001

5. *Shifting the focus of advance care planning: Using an in-depth interview to build and strengthen relationships. Innovations in End-of-Life Care.* EDC. (2021, June 22). www.edc.org/lastacts.

6. Kirchhoff, K. T., Hammes, B. J., Kehl, K. A., Briggs, L. A., & Brown, R. L. (2010). Effect of a Disease-Specific Planning Intervention on Surrogate Understanding of Patient Goals for Future Medical Treatment. *Journal of the American Geriatrics Society, 58*(7), 1233–1240. https://doi.org/10.1111/j.1532-5415.2010.02760.x

7. Song, M.-K., Kirchhoff, K. T., Douglas, J., Ward, S., & Hammes, B. (2005). A Randomized, Controlled Trial to Improve Advance Care Planning Among Patients Undergoing Cardiac Surgery. *Medical Care*, *43*(10), 1049–1053. https://doi.org/10.1097/01. mlr.0000178192.10283.b4

8. Song, M.-K., Ward, S. E., Happ, M. B., Piraino, B., Donovan, H. S., Shields, A.-M., & Connolly, M. C. (2009). Randomized controlled trial of SPIRIT: An effective approach to preparing African-American dialysis patients and families for end of life. *Research in Nursing & Health*, *32*(3), 260–273. https://doi. org/10.1002/nur.20320

9. *The Results and Impact of a Death Chart Audit in an Academic Health Care System*. Respecting Choices. (2021, June 10). https:// respectingchoices.org/wp-content/uploads/2018/10/2018-10-25-14.30-C4-3b-The-Results-and-Impact-of-a-Death-Chart-Audit-in-an-Academic-Health-Care-System-Sanders-Burstein.pdf.

10. Boettcher, I., Turner, R., & Briggs, L. (2014). Telephonic advance care planning facilitated by health plan case managers. *Palliative and Supportive Care*, *13*(3), 795–800. https://doi.org/10.1017/ s1478951514000698

    Abstracts from Center to Advance Palliative Care National Seminar Palliative Care Everywhere: Bridging the Gaps November 12–14, 2015 San Antonio, TX. (2016). *Journal of Palliative Medicine*, *19*(5). https://doi.org/10.1089/ jpm.2016.0088

11. Respecting Choices. (n.d.). https://respectingchoices.dcopy.net/ product/Building-Physician-Skills-in-Basic-ACP-Cert-Adv-Practitioners.

12. Personal communication with Carole Montgomery

Chapter 35: Adaptations of the Respecting Choices Evidence-Based ACP Program

1. *Welcome To ACF.* Administration for Children & Families. (n.d.). https://www.acf.hhs.gov/sites/default/files/fysb/prep-making-adaptations-ts.pdf.
2. Home. (n.d.). https://honoringchoices.org/.
3. Wilson, K. S., Kottke, T. E., & Schettle, S. (2014). Honoring Choices Minnesota: Preliminary Data from a Community-Wide Advance Care Planning Model. *Journal of the American Geriatrics Society, 62*(12), 2420–2425. https://doi.org/10.1111/jgs.13136. p. 2421
4. Home. (n.d.). https://honoringchoices.org/.
5. Implementing A Care Planning System: How To Fix The Most Pervasive Errors In Health Care, Health Affairs Blog, January 2, 2015. DOI: 10.1377/hblog20150102.043563
6. *Welcome to Life Care Planning.* Life care planning | Kaiser Permanente. (n.d.). https://healthy.kaiserpermanente.org/health-wellness/life-care-plan.

Chapter 36: Adaptations of the Respecting Choice ACP Program: International Examples

1. Andreasen, P., Finne-Soveri, U. H., Deliens, L., Van den Block, L., Payne, S., Gambassi, G., Onwuteaka-Philipsen, B. D., Smets, T., Lilja, E., Kijowska, V., & Szczerbińska, K. (2019). Advance directives in European long-term care facilities: a cross-sectional survey. BMJ Supportive & Palliative Care. https://doi.org/10.1136/bmjspcare-2018-001743
2. Hammes, B. J., & Silvester, W. (2012). Respecting Patient Choices: Scaling Care Planning to a Whole Country. In *Having your own say: getting the right care when it matters most* (pp. 57–66). essay, CHT Press.

3. Hammes, B. J., & Silvester, W. (2012). Respecting Patient
    Choices: Scaling Care Planning to a Whole Country. In *Having
    your own say: getting the right care when it matters most* (pp.
    58–59). essay, CHT Press.

4. Detering, K. M., Hancock, A. D., Reade, M. C., & Silvester,
    W. (2010). The impact of advance care planning on end of life
    care in elderly patients: randomised controlled trial. BMJ,
    340(mar23 1), c1345–c1345. https://doi.org/10.1136/bmj.c1345

5. *A National Framework for Advance Care Directives*. Advance
    Care Planning Australia. (n.d.). https://www.advancecare-
    planning.org.au/docs/default-source/acpa-resource-library/
    acpa-publications/a-national-framework-for-advance-care-direc-
    tives_september-2011.pdf?sfvrsn=2.

6. Royal Commission into Aged Care Quality and Safety.
    (n.d.). https://agedcare.royalcommission.gov.au/publications/
    Documents/background-paper-5.pdf.

7. ACP Framework. ACP in Canada | PPS au Canada. (2020,
    November 17). https://www.advancecareplanning.ca/
    acp-framework/.

8. *Home - ACP in Canada: PPS au Canada*. ACP in
    Canada | PPS au Canada. (2020, November 17).
    https://www.advancecareplanning.ca/across-canada/
    episode-three-history-advance-care-planning-canada/.

9. *About Fraser Health*. Fraser Health. (n.d.). https://www.fraser-
    health.ca/about-us/about-fraser-health.

10. Talking About Advance Care Planning. Fraser Health. (n.d.).
    https://www.fraserhealth.ca/health-topics-a-to-z/advance-care-
    planning/advance-care-planning-talking-about-the-future#.
    XrAG1ahKg2w.

11. Advance Care Planning Greensleeve. MyHealth.Alberta.ca
    Government of Alberta Personal Health Portal. (n.d.). https://
    myhealth.alberta.ca/Alberta/Pages/advance-care-planning-
    green-sleeve.aspx.

12. Grant, S., Barwich, D., Rush, J. L., & Tayler, C. (2007). Advance Care Planning: What's All the Talk About? *Canadian Journal of Medical Radiation Technology, 38*(4), 5–10. https://doi.org/10.1016/s0820-5930(09)60254-1

13. Canada, H. (2009, September 30). Government of Canada. Canada.ca. https://www.canada.ca/en/health-canada/services/health-care-system/reports-publications/palliative-care/implementation-guide-advance-care-planning-canada-case-study-two-health-authorities-2008.html.

14. Resources and Tools - ACP in Canada: PPS au Canada. ACP in Canada | PPS au Canada. (2020, July 20). https://www.advance-careplanning.ca/resource/researchers/.

15. *Caregiving at Home.* Caregiving. (n.d.). https://www.aic.sg/caregiving/caregiving-at-home/Plan%20Ahead.

16. Tan, W. S., Bajpai, R., Ho, A. H., Low, C. K., & Car, J. (2019). Retrospective cohort analysis of real-life decisions about end-of-life care preferences in a Southeast Asian country. *BMJ Open, 9*(2). https://doi.org/10.1136/bmjopen-2018-024662

17. Tan, W. S., Bajpai, R., Ho, A. H., Low, C. K., & Car, J. (2019). Retrospective cohort analysis of real-life decisions about end-of-life care preferences in a Southeast Asian country. *BMJ Open, 9*(2). https://doi.org/10.1136/bmjopen-2018-024662

18. in der Schmitten, J., Lex, K., Mellert, C., Rothärmel, S., Wegscheider, K., & Marckmann, G. (2014). Implementing an Advance Care Planning Program in German Nursing Homes. Deutsches Aerzteblatt Online. https://doi.org/10.3238/arztebl.2014.0050

19. Rietjens, J. A., Korfage, I. J., Dunleavy, L., Preston, N. J., Jabbarian, L. J., Christensen, C. A., de Brito, M., Bulli, F., Caswell, G., Červ, B., van Delden, J., Deliens, L., Gorini, G., Groenvold, M., Houttekier, D., Ingravallo, F., Kars, M. C., Lunder, U., Miccinesi, G., Mimić, A., … van der Heide Pl, A. (2016). Advance care planning--a multi-centre cluster randomised clinical trial: the research protocol of the

ACTION study. *BMC cancer, 16,* 264. https://doi.org/10.1186/
s12885-016-2298-x

20.   Korfage, I. J., Carreras, G., Arnfeldt Christensen, C. M.,
      Billekens, P., Bramley, L., Briggs, L., Bulli, F., Caswell, G., Červ,
      B., van Delden, J. J., Deliens, L., Dunleavy, L., Eecloo, K., Gorini,
      G., Groenvold, M., Hammes, B., Ingravallo, F., Jabbarian, L. J.,
      Kars, M. C., ... Rietjens, J. A. (2020). Advance care planning in
      patients with advanced cancer: A 6-country, cluster-randomised
      clinical trial. *PLOS Medicine, 17*(11). https://doi.org/10.1371/jour-
      nal.pmed.1003422

21.   Zwakman, M., Pollock, K., Bulli, F., Caswell, G., Červ, B., van
      Delden, J. J., Deliens, L., van der Heide, A., Jabbarian, L. J., Koba-
      Čeh, H., Lunder, U., Miccinesi, G., Arnfeldt, C. A., Seymour, J.,
      Toccafondi, A., Verkissen, M. N., & Kars, M. C. (2019). Trained
      facilitators' experiences with structured advance care plan-
      ning conversations in oncology: an international focus group
      study within the ACTION trial. *BMC Cancer, 19*(1). https://doi.
      org/10.1186/s12885-019-6170-7

22.   *Verken uw wensen voor zorg en behandeling.* Verken
      uw wensen voor zorg en behandeling | Thuisarts.
      nl. (n.d.). https://www.thuisarts.nl/keuzehulp/
      verken-uw-wensen-voor-zorg-en-behandeling.

23.   Personal communication with Ida Korfage

24.   Judez, J., Vivancos, L., Antunez, C., Quesada, M., Novoa, A.,
      Feito, L., & Ogando, B. (2011, June 1). Advance care plan-
      ning in life limiting illness. BMJ Supportive & Palliative
      Care. https://spcare.bmj.com/content/1/1/68.3.

Chapter 37: ACP Research: Measurement Conundrums and Future Directions

1.   Jimenez, G., Tan, W. S., Virk, A. K., Low, C. K., Car, J., & Ho,
      A. (2018). Overview of Systematic Reviews of Advance Care
      Planning: Summary of Evidence and Global Lessons. Journal of

pain and symptom management, 56(3), 436–459.e25. https://doi.org/10.1016/j.jpainsymman.2018.05.016

2. Weathers, E., O'Caoimh, R., Cornally, N., Fitzgerald, C., Kearns, T., Coffey, A., Daly, E., O'Sullivan, R., McGlade, C., & Molloy, D. W. (2016). Advance care planning: A systematic review of randomised controlled trials conducted with older adults. *Maturitas, 91*, 101–109. https://doi.org/10.1016/j.maturitas.2016.06.016

McMahan, R. D., Tellez, I., & Sudore, R. L. (2020). Deconstructing the Complexities of Advance Care Planning Outcomes: What Do We Know and Where Do We Go? A Scoping Review. *Journal of the American Geriatrics Society, 69*(1), 234–244. https://doi.org/10.1111/jgs.16801

3. Weathers, E., O'Caoimh, R., Cornally, N., Fitzgerald, C., Kearns, T., Coffey, A., Daly, E., O'Sullivan, R., McGlade, C., & Molloy, D. W. (2016). Advance care planning: A systematic review of randomised controlled trials conducted with older adults. *Maturitas, 91*, 101–109. https://doi.org/10.1016/j.maturitas.2016.06.016

4. McMahan, R. D., Tellez, I., & Sudore, R. L. (2020). Deconstructing the Complexities of Advance Care Planning Outcomes: What Do We Know and Where Do We Go? A Scoping Review. *Journal of the American Geriatrics Society, 69*(1), 234–244. https://doi.org/10.1111/jgs.16801

5. Brinkman-Stoppelenburg, A., Rietjens, J. A. C., & van der Heide, A. (2014). The effects of advance care planning on end-of-life care: A systematic review. *Palliative Medicine, 28*(8), 1000–1025. https://doi.org/10.1177/0269216314526272

6. Sudore, R. L., Stewart, A. L., Knight, S. J., McMahan, R. D., Feuz, M., Miao, Y., & Barnes, D. E. (2013). Development and Validation of a Questionnaire to Detect Behavior Change in Multiple Advance Care Planning Behaviors. *PLoS ONE, 8*(9). https://doi.org/10.1371/journal.pone.0072465

7. Sudore, R. L., Stewart, A. L., Knight, S. J., McMahan, R. D., Feuz, M., Miao, Y., & Barnes, D. E. (2013). Development and Validation of a Questionnaire to Detect Behavior Change in Multiple Advance Care Planning Behaviors. *PLoS ONE, 8*(9). https://doi.org/10.1371/journal.pone.0072465. p. 72465

8. Sudore, R. L., Heyland, D. K., Lum, H. D., Rietjens, J. A. C., Korfage, I. J., Ritchie, C. S., Hanson, L. C., Meier, D. E., Pantilat, S. Z., Lorenz, K., Howard, M., Green, M. J., Simon, J. E., Feuz, M. A., & You, J. J. (2018). Outcomes That Define Successful Advance Care Planning: A Delphi Panel Consensus. *Journal of Pain and Symptom Management, 55*(2). https://doi.org/10.1016/j.jpainsymman.2017.08.025

9. McMahan, R. D., Tellez, I., & Sudore, R. L. (2020). Deconstructing the Complexities of Advance Care Planning Outcomes: What Do We Know and Where Do We Go? A Scoping Review. *Journal of the American Geriatrics Society, 69*(1), 234–244. https://doi.org/10.1111/jgs.16801

10. McMahan, R. D., Tellez, I., & Sudore, R. L. (2020). Deconstructing the Complexities of Advance Care Planning Outcomes: What Do We Know and Where Do We Go? A Scoping Review. *Journal of the American Geriatrics Society, 69*(1), 234–244. https://doi.org/10.1111/jgs.16801

11. Jimenez, G., Tan, W. S., Virk, A. K., Low, C. K., Car, J., & Ho, A. (2018). Overview of Systematic Reviews of Advance Care Planning: Summary of Evidence and Global Lessons. Journal of pain and symptom management, 56(3), 436–459.e25. https://doi.org/10.1016/j.jpainsymman.2018.05.016

12. McMahan, R. D., Tellez, I., & Sudore, R. L. (2020). Deconstructing the Complexities of Advance Care Planning Outcomes: What Do We Know and Where Do We Go? A Scoping Review. *Journal of the American Geriatrics Society, 69*(1), 234–244. https://doi.org/10.1111/jgs.16801

13. Heyland, D. K. (2020). Advance Care Planning (ACP) vs. Advance Serious Illness Preparations and Planning (ASIPP).

Healthcare, 8(3), 218. https://doi.org/10.3390/healthcare8030218. p.4

14. Commissioner, O. of the. (n.d.). U.S. Food and Drug Administration. http://www.fda.gov/downloads/Drugs/Guidances/UCM193282.pdf.

15. Our Story. (2021, April 12). https://www.pcori.org/about-us/our-story.

16. Chen, J., Ou, L., & Hollis, S. J. (2013). A systematic review of the impact of routine collection of patient reported outcome measures on patients, providers and health organisations in an oncologic setting. BMC Health Services Research, 13(1). https://doi.org/10.1186/1472-6963-13-211

Chapter 38: Respecting Choices Research Partnerships: What Lessons Have Been Learned?

1. Sudore, R. L., Lum, H. D., You, J. J., Hanson, L. C., Meier, D. E., Pantilat, S. Z., Matlock, D. D., Rietjens, J., Korfage, I. J., Ritchie, C. S., Kutner, J. S., Teno, J. M., Thomas, J., McMahan, R. D., & Heyland, D. K. (2017). Defining Advance Care Planning for Adults: A Consensus Definition From a Multidisciplinary Delphi Panel. Journal of pain and symptom management, 53(5), 821–832.e1. https://doi.org/10.1016/j.jpainsymman.2016.12.331

2. Sean Morrison, R. (2020). Advance Directives/Care Planning: Clear, Simple, and Wrong. Journal of Palliative Medicine, 23(7), 878–879. https://doi.org/10.1089/jpm.2020.0272

3. Heyland, D. K. (2020). Advance Care Planning (ACP) vs. Advance Serious Illness Preparations and Planning (ASIPP). *Healthcare, 8*(3), 218. https://doi.org/10.3390/healthcare8030218. p. 3

4. Sean Morrison, R. (2020). Advance Directives/Care Planning: Clear, Simple, and Wrong. Journal of Palliative Medicine, 23(7), 878–879. https://doi.org/10.1089/jpm.2020.0272. p. 879

5. Personal communication with Kate Detwiller

6. MacKenzie, M. A., Smith-Howell, E., Bomba, P. A., & Meghani, S. H. (2017). Respecting Choices and Related Models of Advance Care Planning: A Systematic Review of Published Evidence. American Journal of Hospice and Palliative Medicine®, 35(6), 897–907. https://doi.org/10.1177/1049909117745789

7. Korfage, I. J., Carreras, G., Arnfeldt Christensen, C. M., Billekens, P., Bramley, L., Briggs, L., Bulli, F., Caswell, G., Červ, B., van Delden, J. J., Deliens, L., Dunleavy, L., Eecloo, K., Gorini, G., Groenvold, M., Hammes, B., Ingravallo, F., Jabbarian, L. J., Kars, M. C., ... Rietjens, J. A. (2020). Advance care planning in patients with advanced cancer: A 6-country, cluster-randomised clinical trial. PLOS Medicine, 17(11). https://doi.org/10.1371/journal.pmed.1003422. p. 4

8. Korfage, I. J., Carreras, G., Arnfeldt Christensen, C. M., Billekens, P., Bramley, L., Briggs, L., Bulli, F., Caswell, G., Červ, B., van Delden, J. J., Deliens, L., Dunleavy, L., Eecloo, K., Gorini, G., Groenvold, M., Hammes, B., Ingravallo, F., Jabbarian, L. J., Kars, M. C., ... Rietjens, J. A. (2020). Advance care planning in patients with advanced cancer: A 6-country, cluster-randomised clinical trial. *PLOS Medicine*, *17*(11). https://doi.org/10.1371/journal.pmed.1003422. p. 12

9. Slaughter, S. E., Hill, J. N., & Snelgrove-Clarke, E. (2015). What is the extent and quality of documentation and reporting of fidelity to implementation strategies: a scoping review. *Implementation Science*, *10*(1). https://doi.org/10.1186/s13012-015-0320-3. p. 19

10. *Implementation Science Health Care Chapter*. National Adult and Influenza Immunization Summit |. (2021, April 16). https://www.izsummitpartners.org/content/uploads/2015/02/Implementation-science-health-care-chapter-Mittman-10-02-2014.pdf.

11. Kars, M. C., van Thiel, G. J. M. W., van der Graaf, R., Moors, M., de Graeff, A., & van Delden, J. J. M. (2015). A systematic review of reasons for gatekeeping in palliative care research. *Palliative Medicine*, *30*(6), 533–548. https://doi.org/10.1177/0269216315616759

Chapter 39: If I Only Knew Revisited

1. If I Only Knew: A Patient Education Program on Advance Directives. Copyright 1989, *Lutheran Hospital-La Crosse*.
2. Hammes, B. J., & Rooney, B. L. (1998). Death and End-of-Life Planning in One Midwestern Community. *Archives of Internal Medicine, 158*(4), 383. https://doi.org/10.1001/archinte.158.4.383

Chapter 40: The Promise of Pediatric Advance Care Planning

1. Halfon, N., & Newacheck, P. W. (2010). Evolving notions of childhood chronic illness. *JAMA, 303*(7), 665–666. https://doi.org/10.1001/jama.2010.130
2. Feudtner, C. (2007). Collaborative Communication in Pediatric Palliative Care: A Foundation for Problem-Solving and Decision-Making. *Pediatric Clinics of North America, 54*(5), 583–607. https://doi.org/10.1016/j.pcl.2007.07.008
3. Feudtner, C. (2007). Collaborative Communication in Pediatric Palliative Care: A Foundation for Problem-Solving and Decision-Making. *Pediatric Clinics of North America, 54*(5), 583–607. https://doi.org/10.1016/j.pcl.2007.07.008
4. Cohen, E., Kuo, D. Z., Agrawal, R., Berry, J. G., Bhagat, S. K., Simon, T. D., & Srivastava, R. (2011). Children With Medical Complexity: An Emerging Population for Clinical and Research Initiatives. *PEDIATRICS, 127*(3), 529–538. https://doi.org/10.1542/peds.2010-0910
5. American Academy of Pediatrics, Committee on Bioethics and Committee on Hospital Care. (2000). *Palliative Care for Children*. Pediatrics 106, 351-357
    Institute of Medicine (US) Committee on Palliative and End-of-Life Care for Children and Their Families, Field, M. J., & Behrman, R. E. (Eds.). (2003). *When Children Die: Improving Palliative and End-of-Life Care for Children and Their Families*. National Academies Press (US).

6. Society, C. P. (n.d.). *Advance care planning for paediatric patients: Canadian Paediatric Society*. Advance care planning for paediatric patients | Canadian Paediatric Society. https://www.cps.ca/en/documents/position/advance-care-planning.

7. Durall, A., Zurakowski, D., & Wolfe, J. (2012). Barriers to Conducting Advance Care Discussions for Children With Life-Threatening Conditions. *Pediatrics, 129*(4). https://doi.org/10.1542/peds.2011-2695

8. Hilden, J. M., Emanuel, E. J., Fairclough, D. L., Link, M. P., Foley, K. M., Clarridge, B. C., Schnipper, L. E., & Mayer, R. J. (2001). Attitudes and practices among pediatric oncologists regarding end-of-life care: results of the 1998 American Society of Clinical Oncology survey. *Journal of clinical oncology : official journal of the American Society of Clinical Oncology, 19*(1), 205–212. https://doi.org/10.1200/JCO.2001.19.1.205

9. Kimberly, M. B., Forte, A. L., Carroll, J. M., & Feudtner, C. (2005). Pediatric do-not-attempt-resuscitation orders and public schools: a national assessment of policies and laws. *The American journal of bioethics : AJOB, 5*(1), 59–65. https://doi.org/10.1080/15265160590900605

10. Child Abuse Prevention and Treatment Act, 42 USC 5106g (1996)

11. American Medical Association Journal of Ethics, Volume 12, Number 7 (July 2010): 564-568
    Legal Restrictions on Decision Making for Children with Life-Threatening Illnesses—CAPTA and the Ashley Treatment. (2010). *AMA Journal of Ethics, 12*(7), 564–568. https://doi.org/10.1001/virtualmentor.2010.12.7.hlaw1-1007

12. Badzek, L., & Kanosky, S. (2002). Mature minors and end-of-life decision making: a new development in their legal right to participation. *Journal of nursing law, 8*(3), 23–29.
    Rosato JL. *The ultimate test of autonomy: Should minors have a right to make decisions regarding life-threatening treatment.* Rutgers Law Rev 1996;49:1-103

13.   Hinds, P. S., Drew, D., Oakes, L. L., Fouladi, M., Spunt, S.
       L., Church, C., & Furman, W. L. (2005). End-of-Life Care
       Preferences of Pediatric Patients With Cancer. *Journal of
       Clinical Oncology, 23*(36), 9146–9154. https://doi.org/10.1200/
       jco.2005.10.538
       Wiener, L., Zadeh, S., Battles, H., Baird, K., Ballard, E., Osherow,
       J., & Pao, M. (2012). Allowing Adolescents and Young Adults
       to Plan Their End-of-Life Care. *PEDIATRICS, 130*(5), 897–905.
       https://doi.org/10.1542/peds.2012-0663

14.   Caplan, A. L. (2007, January 1). *Challenging Teenagers' Right
       to Refuse Treatment.* Journal of Ethics | American Medical
       Association. https://journalofethics.ama-assn.org/article/
       challenging-teenagers-right-refuse-treatment/2007-01.

15.   Legislative Information System. (n.d.). HB 2319 Abraham's Law.;
       parents' right to make medical decisions. https://lis.virginia.gov/
       cgi-bin/legp604.exe?071%2Bsum%2BHB2319.

16.   Marron, J. M., Meyer, E. C., & Kennedy, K. O. (2021). The
       Complicated Legacy of Cassandra Callender. *JAMA Pediatrics,
       175*(4), 343. https://doi.org/10.1001/jamapediatrics.2020.4812

17.   Wharton, R. H., Levine, K. R., Buka, S., & Emanuel, L. (1996).
       Advance care planning for children with special health care
       needs: a survey of parental attitudes. *Pediatrics, 97*(5), 682–687.

18.   Hammes, B. J., Klevan, J., Kempf, M., & Williams, M. S. (2005).
       Pediatric advance care planning. *Journal of palliative medicine,
       8*(4), 766–773. https://doi.org/10.1089/jpm.2005.8.766

19.   DeCourcey, D. D., Silverman, M., Oladunjoye, A., & Wolfe, J.
       (2019). Advance Care Planning and Parent-Reported End-of-Life
       Outcomes in Children, Adolescents, and Young Adults With
       Complex Chronic Conditions*. *Critical Care Medicine, 47*(1),
       101–108. https://doi.org/10.1097/ccm.0000000000003472

20.   Orkin, J., Beaune, L., Moore, C., Weiser, N., Arje, D., Rapoport,
       A., Netten, K., Adams, S., Cohen, E., & Amin, R. (2020). Toward
       an Understanding of Advance Care Planning in Children With

Medical Complexity. *Pediatrics, 145*(3). https://doi.org/10.1542/peds.2019-2241

21. Lyon, M. E., Jacobs, S., Briggs, L., Cheng, Y. I., & Wang, J. (2013). Family-Centered Advance Care Planning for Teens With Cancer. *JAMA Pediatrics, 167*(5), 460. https://doi.org/10.1001/jamapediatrics.2013.943

Lyon, M. E., D'Angelo, L. J., Dallas, R. H., Hinds, P. S., Garvie, P. A., Wilkins, M. L., Garcia, A., Briggs, L., Flynn, P. M., Rana, S. R., Cheng, Y. I., & Wang, J. (2017). A randomized clinical trial of adolescents with HIV/AIDS: pediatric advance care planning. *AIDS Care, 29*(10), 1287–1296. https://doi.org/10.1080/09540121.2017.1308463

Lyon, M. E., Garvie, P. A., D'Angelo, L. J., Dallas, R. H., Briggs, L., Flynn, P. M., Garcia, A., Cheng, Y. I., & Wang, J. (2018). Advance Care Planning and HIV Symptoms in Adolescence. *Pediatrics, 142*(5). https://doi.org/10.1542/peds.2017-3869

22. Friebert, S., Grossoehme, D. H., Baker, J. N., Needle, J., Thompkins, J. D., Cheng, Y. I., Wang, J., & Lyon, M. E. (2020). Congruence Gaps Between Adolescents With Cancer and Their Families Regarding Values, Goals, and Beliefs About End-of-Life Care. *JAMA Network Open, 3*(5). https://doi.org/10.1001/jamanetworkopen.2020.5424

23. Knapp, C., Quinn, G. P., Murphy, D., Brown, R., & Madden, V. (2010). Adolescents With Life-Threatening Illnesses. *American Journal of Hospice and Palliative Medicine®, 27*(2), 139–144. https://doi.org/10.1177/1049909109358310

24. Wiener, L., Zadeh, S., Battles, H., Baird, K., Ballard, E., Osherow, J., & Pao, M. (2012). Allowing Adolescents and Young Adults to Plan Their End-of-Life Care. *PEDIATRICS, 130*(5), 897–905. https://doi.org/10.1542/peds.2012-0663

25. Handy, C. M., Sulmasy, D. P., Merkel, C. K., & Ury, W. A. (2008). The surrogate's experience in authorizing a do not resuscitate order. *Palliative and Supportive Care, 6*(1), 13–19. https://doi.org/10.1017/s1478951508000035

Chapter 41: Pediatric Advance Care Planning: The Early Evidence and Respecting Choices Experience

1. Lotz, J. D., Jox, R. J., Borasio, G. D., & Fuhrer, M. (2013). Pediatric Advance Care Planning: A Systematic Review. PEDIATRICS, 131(3). https://doi.org/10.1542/peds.2012-2394
2. Hammes, B. J., Klevan, J., Kempf, M., & Williams, M. S. (2005). Pediatric Advance Care Planning. *Journal of Palliative Medicine*, 8(4), 766–773. https://doi.org/10.1089/jpm.2005.8.766
3. Personal communication with Dr. Bud Hammes

Chapter 43: The Respecting Choices Research Partnerships in Pediatric Advance Care Planning

1. Lyon ME, Thompkins JD, Fratantoni K, *et al*Family caregivers of children and adolescents with rare diseases: a novel palliative care intervention*BMJ Supportive & Palliative Care* Published Online First: 25 July 2019. doi: 10.1136/bmjspcare-2019-001766
2. csnat.org. (n.d.). http://csnat.org/.
3. Personal communication with Kate Detwiller
4. Rule, A. R. (2018). I Am That Parent. *JAMA, 319*(5), 445. https://doi.org/10.1001/jama.2017.21048
5. Halfon, N., & Newacheck, P. W. (2010). Evolving notions of childhood chronic illness. *JAMA, 303*(7), 665–666. https://doi.org/10.1001/jama.2010.130
6. Lyon, M. E., McCabe, M. A., Patel, K. M., & D'Angelo, L. J. (2004). What do adolescents want? An exploratory study regarding end-of-life decision-making. *The Journal of adolescent health : official publication of the Society for Adolescent Medicine, 35*(6), 529.e1–529.e5296. https://doi.org/10.1016/j.jadohealth.2004.02.009
7. Lyon, M. E., Garvie, P. A., McCarter, R., Briggs, L., He, J., & D'Angelo, L. J. (2009). Who Will Speak for Me? Improving End-of-Life Decision-Making for Adolescents With HIV and

Their Families. *PEDIATRICS, 123*(2). https://doi.org/10.1542/peds.2008-2379

8. Dallas RH, Kimmel A, Wilkins ML, Rana S, Garcia A, Cheng YI, Wang J, Lyon ME, for the Adolescent Palliative Care Consortium. *A Randomized Controlled Trial of FAmily-CEntered (FACE) Advanced Care Planning for Adolescents with HIV/AIDS: Emotions, Acceptability, Feasibility.* Pediatrics 2016 138(6):December:e 20161854

9. Lyon, M. E., Garvie, P. A., McCarter, R., Briggs, L., He, J., & D'Angelo, L. J. (2009). Who Will Speak for Me? Improving End-of-Life Decision-Making for Adolescents With HIV and Their Families. *PEDIATRICS, 123*(2). https://doi.org/10.1542/peds.2008-2379

10. Lyon, M. E., Jacobs, S., Briggs, L., Cheng, Y. I., & Wang, J. (2013). Family-centered advance care planning for teens with cancer. *JAMA pediatrics, 167*(5), 460–467. https://doi.org/10.1001/jamapediatrics.2013.943

11. Thompkins, J. D., Needle, J., Baker, J. N., Briggs, L., Cheng, Y. I., Wang, J., Friebert, S., & Lyon, M. E. (2021). Pediatric advance care planning and families' positive caregiving appraisals: An rct. Pediatrics, 147(6). https://doi.org/10.1542/peds.2020-029330

12. Lyon, M. E., Squires, L., Scott, R. K., Benator, D., Briggs, L., Greenberg, I., D'Angelo, L. J., Cheng, Y. I., & Wang, J. (2020). Effect of FAmily CEntered (FACE®) Advance Care Planning on Longitudinal Congruence in End-of-Life Treatment Preferences: A Randomized Clinical Trial. *AIDS and behavior, 24*(12), 3359–3375. https://doi.org/10.1007/s10461-020-02909-y

13. *Family-Centered Advance Care Planning for Teens with Cancer (FACE-TC).* Family-Centered Advance Care Planning for Teens with Cancer (FACE-TC) | Evidence-Based Cancer Control Programs (EBCCP). (n.d.). https://rtips.cancer.gov/rtips/programDetails.do?programId=17054015.

14. *About This Site.* About This Site | Evidence-Based Cancer Control Programs (EBCCP). (n.d.). https://rtips.cancer.gov/rtips/about. do.

Chapter 44: Honoring a Child's Decision Revisited and Future Directions in Pediatric ACP

1. csnat.org. (n.d.). http://csnat.org/.
2. Walter, J. K., Rosenberg, A. R., & Feudtner, C. (2013). Tackling Taboo Topics. *JAMA Pediatrics, 167*(5), 489. https://doi. org/10.1001/jamapediatrics.2013.1323